# INSTRUCTOR'S RESOURCE MANUAL & TEST BANK *to accompany*

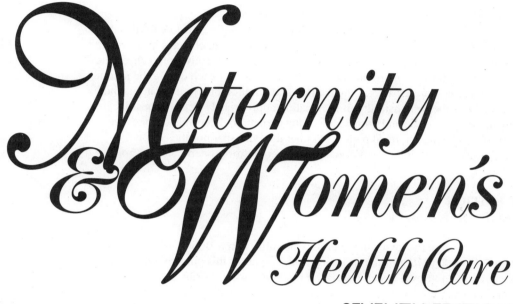

# *Maternity & Women's Health Care*

## SEVENTH EDITION

**DEITRA LEONARD LOWDERMILK,** RNC, PHD, FAAN

**SHANNON E. PERRY,** RN, CNS, PHD, FAAN

**IRENE M. BOBAK,** RN, PHD, FAAN

*Prepared by*
**KAREN A. PIOTROWSKI,** RNC, MSN
Assistant Professor of Nursing
D'Youville College
Buffalo, New York

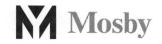
Mosby

*A Harcourt Health Sciences Company*

St. Louis   London   Philadelphia   Sydney   Toronto

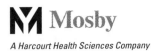

A Harcourt Health Sciences Company

*Vice President, Nursing Editorial Director:* Sally Schrefer
*Senior Editor:* Michael S. Ledbetter
*Senior Developmental Editor:* Laurie K. Muench
*Project Manager:* Gayle May Morris
*Designer:* Amy Buxton

**NOTICE:**

Pharmacology is an ever-changing field. Standard safety precautions must be followed, but as new research and clinical experience broaden our knowledge, changes in treatment and drug therapy may become necessary or appropriate. Readers are advised to check the most current product information provided by the manufacturer of each drug to be administered to verify the recommended dose, the method and duration of administration, and contraindications. It is the responsibility of the treating appropriately licensed health care provider, relying on experience and knowledge of the patient, to determine dosages and the best treatment for each individual patient. Neither the Publisher nor the editor assumes any liability for any injury and/or damage to persons or property arising from this publication.

**SEVENTH EDITION**
**Copyright © 2000 by Mosby, Inc.**

Printed in the United States of America

Mosby, Inc.
*A Harcourt Health Sciences Company*
11830 Westline Industrial Drive
St. Louis, Missouri 63146
www.mosby.com

**International Standard Book Number**
0-323-00962-X

00 01 02 03 04 BD/ EB 9 8 7 6 5 4 3 2 1

# INTRODUCTION

This instructor's manual is designed to accompany the seventh edition of *Maternity & Women's Health Care*. The three separate sections included in this manual are the chapters section, the case studies, and the test bank. A study guide and CD-ROM are available for students and can be used by faculty to facilitate student learning.

I. The **CHAPTERS SECTION** consists of 42 chapters that are keyed to the text. Each chapter includes the following sections:

- **Summary of the Key Concepts** highlights the essential content presented in each chapter in the text.
- **Learning Objectives** lists the objectives as they appear at the beginning of each chapter in the text.
- **Outline of Chapter Content with Course Guidelines** lists the content headings in the chapter. This outline may be used as the basis for constructing a lecture outline. Since some maternity and women's health care courses will be unable to cover the entire text in the time allotted, the outline may also be used to select the topics most appropriate for individual nursing curriculums. Each of the content headings is classified according to the following system:
  - **A:** denotes content absolutely essential to a basic understanding of maternity and women's health care
  - **B:** denotes content that must be mastered to achieve a strong knowledge base
  - **C:** denotes content that should be included to ensure a thorough understanding of all aspects of maternity and women's health care
- **Teaching Strategies** identify a variety of approaches that can be used to present essential content in interesting and creative ways. Suggestions for class discussions, student presentations, demonstrations, out-of-class activities for students, and guest speakers are included.
- **Suggested Student Learning Activities** include a variety of activities that can be the focus for individual or group projects by students. These activities can be used as required course assignments, as a way of earning extra credit, or as a means of providing service to the community. Many of the activities require investigation of community resources and services; contact with health care professionals, clients, and families; observation of health care activities in the agencies where student clinical experiences take place; creation of class outlines; and the design of written materials to inform clients and provide resources for registered nurses. Activities that require students to choose a nursing article or research study and prepare a bibliography card help them to appreciate that nursing ideas and research findings can be used to enhance and improve the quality health care.
- **Topics for Discussion** raise timely issues reflected in the content of the chapter. These topics could be discussed during class, seminars, and post-conferences, or the topics could be the basis for written assignments or essay questions. The chosen topics are designed to facilitate the development of student critical thinking skills as they consider, debate, and discuss the ramifications of important issues facing the health care system, health care professionals, and the public. In addition, students should be encouraged to examine and define their views regarding these issues and to listen to and respect the views of others.

Hopefully, a discussion of these issues will help students appreciate the critical role of the nurse as caregiver, teacher, and advocate for women and their families. When discussing the topics, students should support their positions or answer with concepts and research findings from professional literature, information from the mass media, including magazines, newspapers, and television or radio presentations, and knowledge gained from personal and professional experiences (as a student nurse) with the health care system and health care providers.

- **MERLIN Projects** are activities designed to help students develop skill in the use of the Internet and expand their knowledge in relation to the chapter content, developing an appreciation for the Internet as a valuable resource for client information and support.

II. **CASE STUDIES** reflect selected content areas from the text. Answer guidelines are included for each case study. Additional case studies are found in the Critical Thinking Exercises section of each chapter in the study guide and in the CD-ROM that accompanies the textbook. Case studies can be used to present content in the classroom and as a focus for discussions in class, seminars, and clinical conferences. This teaching strategy encourages students to think critically, apply nursing knowledge, and share ideas and creative solutions with other students. The client care situations that students encounter during their clinical experiences can be additional sources for case studies.

III. **The TEST BANK** contains multiple-choice questions. As on the NCLEX-RN examination, the questions are situation based and independent of each other. Answers for each question are included in the Test Bank Answer Key.

## STUDY GUIDE

A separate study guide is available to accompany the seventh edition of *Maternity & Women's Health Care*. The Study Guide includes activities that are designed to facilitate student learning by identifying critical information and terms presented in each chapter and by testing student knowledge and ability to apply critical content. Three types of learning and study activities are provided for each chapter:

I. **Chapter Review Activities** focus on recall and application of critical concepts and essential terminology. These activities are specifically designed to help students identify the important content of the chapter and test their level of knowledge and understanding after reading the chapter. Completion of each of the activities will provide students with an excellent resource to use when reviewing important content before course examinations. The knowledge that is attained by completing the activities will help develop the theoretic foundation that students will need to answer the critical thinking exercises, to successfully pass course examinations and the NCLEX-RN examination and to manage the client care in the clinical setting. Answers or answer guidelines for the activities are provided in the Answer Key located at the end of this study guide.

II. **Critical Thinking Exercises** focus primarily on the application of critical chapter content. Typical client care situations are presented, and students are required to apply the concepts found in the chapter to solve problems, make decisions concerning care management, and provide responses to clients' questions and concerns. These exercises may be completed individually or within study groups. Completing the critical thinking exercises will help prepare students for clinical experiences, course examinations, and the NCLEX-RN examination, all of which focus on problem solving and application of nursing knowledge. Guidelines for completing the exercises and specific chapter sections, boxes, or tables where the content for the answers are found are provided in the Answer Key located at the end of this study guide.

III. **MERLIN Projects** that are different from those in the instructor's manual are found in each chapter of the study guide. They are designed with the same purposes in mind.

## CD-ROM

A CD-ROM accompanies the textbook. It is composed of interactive case studies, multiple-choice questions in NCLEX format with answers and rationales, and a variety of fill-in-the-blank and matching exercises.

## SUGGESTED STUDENT READING ASSIGNMENTS

Student reading assignments are often adjusted, based on the time frame allotted to cover maternal, women's health, and newborn content within the nursing curriculum. Suggested student reading assignments for two typical maternal, women's health, and newborn course time frames are outlined below.

I. **Suggested reading assignment for a 6- to 7-week course**—suggestions are based on 4 to 6 hours per week for lecture or small group discussion.
  A. The following reading assignments will be covered in lecture and most are essential for clinical preparation:
   **Week 1:** Chapter 1 (contemporary issues in maternity and women's health care); Chapter 6 (assessment of women); Chapter 14 (conception, fetal development, and genetics)
   **Week 2:** Chapters 15, 16, and 17 (pregnancy); Chapter 9 (abortion)
   **Week 3:** Chapters 18, 19, 20, 21, and 22 (childbirth)
   **Week 4:** Chapters 23, 24, and 25 (postpartum); Chapter 9 (contraception)
   **Week 5:** Chapters 26, 27, and 28 (newborn)
   **Weeks 6 and 7:** Selected complications from Chapters 30 through 38
   **Option:** Chapters 7, 8, 10, 12, and 13 (women's health issues); Chapters 39, 40, and 41 (newborn complications) should be covered in the child health content of the curriculum
  B. The following chapters are recommended for small group discussions:
   **Week 2:** Chapter 2 (the family and culture); Chapter 11 (violence against women)
   **Week 5:** Chapter 5 (health promotion and prevention); Chapter 4 (alternative and complimentary therapies)
   **Weeks 6 and 7:** Chapter 29 (assessment for risk factors); Chapter 3 (community and home care); Chapter 42 (loss and grief)

II. **Suggested reading assignment for a 14- to 16-week course**—suggestions are based on 3 hours per week for lecture or small group discussion.

    A. The following reading assignments will be covered in lecture and most are essential for clinical preparation:

      **Week 1:** Chapter 1 (contemporary issues in maternity and women's health care); Chapter 5 (health promotion and prevention)

      **Week 2:** Chapter 6 (assessment of women); Chapter 14 (conception, fetal development, and genetics)

      **Week 3:** Chapter 15 (anatomy and physiology of pregnancy)

      **Week 4:** Chapter 17 (nursing care during pregnancy); Chapter 16 (maternal/fetal nutrition); Chapter 18 (childbirth education)

      **Week 5:** Chapters 19 and 22 (process of labor and nursing care)

      **Week 6:** Chapters 20 and 21 (discomfort, fetal assessment)

      **Week 7:** Chapters 23, 24, and 25 (postpartum)

      **Week 8:** Chapter 26, 27, and 28 (newborn characteristics and care)

      **Week 9:** Chapters 29 (assessment for risk factors)

      **Week 10:** Chapter 30 and 31 (selected pregnancy complications)

      **Week 11:** Chapters 32, 33, 34, and 35 (selected pregnancy complications)

      **Week 12:** Chapter 36, 37, and 38 (preterm labor and birth, labor and birth complications, postpartum complications)

      **Week 13:** Chapter 39, 40, and 41 (selected newborn complications); ideally the content related to the high risk newborn should be covered in the child health section of the curriculum—this will increase time available to cover women's health issues

      **Week 14:** Chapters 7, 8, 10, 12, and 13 (women's health concepts including infertility)

    B. The following chapters are recommended for small group discussions:

      **Week 4:** Chapter 2 (the family and culture); Chapter 42 (loss and grief)

      **Week 9:** Chapter 9 (contraception)

      **Week 10:** Chapter 9 (abortion)

      **Week 11:** Chapter 4 (alternative and complementary therapies)

      **Week 12:** Chapter 11 (violence against women)

      **Week 13:** Chapter 3 (community and home care)

## MERLIN: *MATERNITY & WOMEN'S HEALTH CARE,*
## SEVENTH EDITION WEB SITE

Throughout the textbook are references to the web address for the Lowdermilk: *Maternity & Women's Health Care,* seventh edition home page. This site provides information about the text, biosketches about the authors, links to related Mosby titles and WebLinks, and related sections for students, clinicians, and faculty.

Specially designed to accompany the textbook are the Student Station, the Faculty Forum, and the Clinician's Corner. These are locations where special information is posted and where users of the text may communicate with Mosby and the authors. The Student Station and the Faculty Forum contain sections on "Teaching Tips," "Content Updates," and "New WebLinks" that have been located and posted. Additionally, faculty using the text have the opportunity at these sites to ask questions and post teaching tips that they have found useful. These tips are then reviewed by the authors and posted for all users to access. The Faculty Forum contains links to Mosby author guidelines, reviewer and contributor inquiry forums, and a location where faculty may bring their ideas for publication.

## WEBLINKS

A new feature to accompany *Maternity & Women's Health Care,* seventh edition is WebLinks, which brings the textbook alive by permitting students to access new information located on the Internet and participate in multimedia learning. Each identified web site has been selected to reinforce and/or supplement materials in the text. An off-site developer has created and posted each site. Although each site has been screened for appropriateness to the content of the textbook, Mosby is not responsible for the content of the web sites. The sites are continuously scanned for updates and changes in URL addresses.

## GETTING TO THE WEBLINKS

WebLinks are mentioned throughout the textbook. Inside the front cover of the textbook, opposite the title page, is a pull-off tab with a passcode number. Instructors and students will need to register at the designated web site before accessing WebLinks pages. To directly access WebLinks, the user must have an Internet account.

## WHAT IS AVAILABLE AT THE WEBLINKS SITE?

Once registered at the textbook home page, the user is able to access WebLinks. The links have been organized to parallel the table of contents of the textbook. When the user double-clicks on the table-of-content headings (chapter titles), a second screen appears with the WebLinks addresses. Double-clicking on any of the annotated WebLinks addresses will take the user directly to the web sites. The contents of the WebLinks sites are the property of the individual developers or organizations. Mosby has made no attempt to modify or screen the materials except for their relevance to the subject matter in the textbook.

Hopefully, users will share addresses of additional appropriate sites located while "cruising" the Internet so that the sites can be posted for other users. These can be e-mailed to Mosby at the designated area on the textbook home page.

## MOSBY'S ELECTRONIC IMAGE COLLECTION
## TO ACCOMPANY *MATERNITY & WOMEN'S HEALTH CARE,* SEVENTH EDITION

Now available to accompany the textbook is Mosby's Electronic Image Collection, containing electronic versions of over 200 photographs and illustrations from the text to assist in lecture and classroom presentations. Each image may be selected from the CD-ROM and imported into a Power Point presentation or printed to a paper hard copy or transparency acetate. Complete instructions for the use of the electronic image collection and a list of the figure numbers and legends are provided in the pamphlet packaged with the CD-ROM.

# CONTENTS

## Chapter

# 1

# Contemporary Issues in Maternity and Women's Health Care

## SUMMARY OF KEY CONCEPTS

The primary focus of Chapter 1 is the importance of the professional nurse as a provider of holistically based health care to women, infants, and their families. The responsibilities of the nurse are described along with the changing roles of the nurse within today's health care system.

Biostatistical data, including birth rates and fertility rates, maternal and infant mortality rates, and trends regarding health and health care, are presented as a way of illustrating the current state of health and health care for women and infants. The shortcomings of the nation's health care system and the areas in which interventions are directed toward change and improvement are identified. Chapter 1 describes the trends and issues facing today's health care system and health care providers, including greater client involvement, the increase in home care and the use of high technology for care, escalation of high risk pregnancies, higher costs, limitations on the ability to pay and access to health care, and expansion of managed care approaches. A discussion of trends in nursing practice focuses on the classification of nursing interventions, evidence-based practice, outcomes orientation, clinical benchmarking, and telemedicine. Overviews of standards of practice, legal and ethical issues, and research into practice conclude the chapter. Students are introduced to the vital need to establish a research base to guide maternity, women's health care, and infants' health care. The importance of promoting research funding, conducting research, and using research to improve practice is emphasized.

## LEARNING OBJECTIVES

Define the key terms.
Describe the scope of maternity and women's health nursing.
Evaluate contemporary issues and trends in maternity and women's health nursing.
Describe sociopolitical issues affecting the care of women and infants.
Compare selected biostatistical data among races.
Examine social concerns in maternity and women's health care.
Explain quality management and standards of practice in the delivery of nursing care.
Debate ethical issues in perinatal nursing.
Identify topics for nursing research related to maternity and women's health nursing.

# OUTLINE OF CHAPTER CONTENT WITH COURSE GUIDELINES

| CONTENT | GUIDELINE |
|---|:---:|
| Contemporary issues and trends | |
|   – Changing health care delivery structure | B |
|   – Integrative health care | B |
|   – Changing childbirth practices | B |
|   – Changing women's health practices | B |
|   – Trends in fertility, birthrate, and infant and maternal mortality | B |
|   – Trends of consumer involvement, self-care, and focus on health care | B |
|   – Trend toward earlier prenatal care | B |
|   – Trend toward high-technology care | C |
|   – Home health care flourishes | B |
|   – High risk pregnancies escalate | B |
|   – Managed care expands | B |
|   – Trends and issues of high costs | B |
|   – Access to care problems | B |
| Trends in nursing practice | |
|   – Nursing interventions classification | C |
|   – Evidence-based practice | B |
|   – Outcomes orientation | C |
|   – Best practices as goal of care | C |
|   – Clinical benchmarking | C |
|   – Telemedicine | C |
|   – A global perspective | C |
| Standards of practice and legal issues in delivery of care | A |
| Ethical issues in perinatal nursing | A |
| Research in maternity and women's health | A |
| Research into practice | A |
| Bias in health research | B |

# TEACHING STRATEGIES

1. Describe how health care patterns have changed locally. Give examples of new and changing roles, responsibilities, and work settings for nurses.

2. Invite a nurse-midwife to discuss how her or his approach to care of pregnant women and their families differs from that of a physician. Request the nurse-midwife to give a description of the care management process used to provide health care to pregnant women and their families.

3. Compare local biostatistical rates with state and national rates and trends. Compare national bio-statistical rates and trends with several other countries. Include both industrialized countries and third-world countries in the comparison. Identify factors that could be responsible for differences in rates and trends.

4. Discuss how consumer involvement has influenced changes in perinatal and women's health care.

5. Provide specific examples of high-tech care in the hospital and in the home. Arrange for students to observe nurses involved in high-tech care in a variety of settings.

6. Give examples of how nurses provide perinatal care in the home.

7. Contrast the cost of a low risk pregnancy and birth with that of a high risk pregnancy and birth. Use client care situations that students have encountered in the clinical setting as examples. Discuss how costs could have been reduced while still maintaining quality of health care for the women, their infants, and families.

8. Distribute examples of standards of care from a variety of nursing organizations. Discuss how and why nurses should be using standards to ensure and improve the quality of care.

9. Identify several ethical issues affecting perinatal health care. Use examples from student clinical experiences and the media to illustrate each ethical issue identified. Discuss how nurses confronting these issues should respond.

10. Use several nursing research studies to illustrate how nursing research improves and influences the health care of women, infants, and childbearing families. Indicate how research findings facilitate evidence-based practice.

## SUGGESTED STUDENT LEARNING ACTIVITIES

1. *INTERVIEW* a nurse practicing in the area of maternity, women's health care, and/or infants' health care (e.g., neonatal clinical nurse specialist, women's health nurse-practitioner, nurse-midwife, lactation consultant, maternal-newborn staff nurse, labor and delivery nurse, etc.). Through the interview process, determine this nurse's:
   - Educational background and certification status
   - Philosophy (beliefs) regarding nursing in general and in the area of specialty and/or expanded practice
   - Reason for choosing this area of health care for practice
   - Day-to-day activities that fulfill the nursing role elements of caregiver, teacher/educator, advocate, manager of care, researcher, political activist for health care reform, and change agent
   - Views regarding the priorities for change related to maternity and women and infant's health care
   - Views regarding promoting and conducting research and using research findings to enhance and improve practice
   - Methods used to maintain expertise in this area of health care
   - Ethical issues encountered in practice and how he or she dealt with the issue

2. GATHER your city, county, and state's biostatistics related to maternal, infant, and women's health. With the statistical data that you obtain, do the following:
   - COMPARE the statistical data with national trends.
   - CREATE a table or graph that illustrates your findings.
   - DISCUSS the actions taken by your community or that should be taken to address any inadequacies in health care reflected by the statistical data you gathered.
   - IDENTIFY improvements in health care that you would recommend based on your analysis of the data.

3. INVESTIGATE the types of childbirth options available in your community.
   - COMPARE your findings with the trends and changes described in this chapter.
   - IDENTIFY options that you feel should be made available in your community. GIVE the rationale for your suggestions.

4. SEARCH the nursing literature for articles related to maternity, women's health care, and infants' health care, such as the following: benefits of care, barriers, improving access, services offered, and models of care. Choose one article, and complete a bibliography card that includes the following:
   - Summary of the article's key points
   - Personal reaction to the ideas presented in the article
   - How the professional nurse could use the information presented to enhance and improve health care

5. SEARCH the literature for articles related to ethical issues encountered in women's health care and perinatal health care. Choose one article, and complete a bibliography card that includes the following:
   - Summary of the issue
   - Approaches used by health care providers to deal with the issue
   - Personal reaction to the issue and the approaches taken
   - Action you would have taken if faced with the same issue

## TOPICS FOR DISCUSSION

1. *Support this statement:* Nurses play a critical role in shaping the health care system to ensure its responsiveness to the needs of contemporary women and their infants. Use current nursing literature as well as examples of the activities and contributions of professional nurses and nursing organizations in formulating your response.

2. *Discuss this question:* Have changing childbirth practices had a positive impact on women's perceptions of their childbirth experiences? Gather information for your answer by interviewing women who recently gave birth (e.g., your clients, family members, and friends) and interviewing women who gave birth many years ago. Compare their experiences and the impressions they have of their births.

3. *Discuss this question:* Have changing childbirth practices had a positive impact on men's perceptions of their partners' childbirth experiences? Use the format suggested in the previous question to formulate your answer.

4. *Support this statement:* Research can validate that nursing care measures are effective. Use examples from current nursing research and their findings in formulating your response. Describe how nursing can use its body of research to improve the effectiveness and quality of care administered.

## MERLIN PROJECT

1. Use MERLIN to connect to the web site of a health care organization dedicated to improving the quality of health care provided to women and infants. Describe this organization's:
   • Purpose and mission
   • Accomplishments and current activities
   • Services provided to health care professionals and lay persons
   • Web site with regard to its usefulness in providing information and services related to the health care of women and infants
2. Explore an ethical issue currently facing health care professionals involved in women's health care and perinatal health care. Use the Internet to obtain information about the issue and how health care providers around the country are dealing with this issue in their practice.
3. Write a three- to four-page paper related to the Women's Health Equity Act (WHEA) using the Internet to gather your information. The paper should include each of the following:
   • Summary of the legislation, including when it was proposed and the benefits that it proposes to provide to enhance the health of women and infants
   • Major sponsors of the legislation in both the House of Representatives and the Senate
   • Current status of the legislation (contact one of the sponsors of the legislation)

# Chapter

## 2

# The Family and Culture

## SUMMARY OF KEY CONCEPTS

The focus of Chapter 2 is the family as a unit of care for perinatal health nurses. Definitions of the concept of family are presented along with a description of a variety of family forms including nuclear, extended, single-parent, binuclear, reconstituted, and homosexual. Family functions are identified and extend over the following five areas: affective, socialization, reproductive, economic, and health care. These functions operate within a structure of beliefs, values, and sentiments that are developed by the family and serve as a guide for their actions. Stages of the family life cycle, according to Carter and McGoldrick, are presented in a concise table format. Students are also introduced to the concept of family dynamics, in terms of delegation of roles, boundaries and channels with external systems, nurturing and socialization of children, communication patterns, and problem-solving protocols that incorporate values, attitudes, power allocation, and hierarchies. A short form of the Friedman Family Assessment Model is included, illustrating the process of determining a family's developmental stage, environment, structure, functions, stress, and coping.

The family systems theory, family developmental theory, and family stress theory and their implications for maternity nursing are discussed. A description of how families function within a cultural context includes cultural beliefs and practices related to childbearing and parenting for Hispanic, African-American, Asian, Caucasian/European-American, and Native American families.

## LEARNING OBJECTIVES

Define the key terms.

Identify key factors in determining the quality of family health.

Identify and describe the key characteristics of various family forms.

Explain the functions carried out by a family for the well-being of its members and society.

Explain components of family dynamics and how these contribute to accomplishing family functions.

Explain three theoretic approaches (family systems theory, family developmental theory, and family stress theory) for working with childbearing families. Describe the nursing implications of each theory.

Relate the role and impact of culture on childbearing families.

Identify topics for nursing research related to the family and culture.

# OUTLINE OF CHAPTER CONTENT WITH COURSE GUIDELINES

| CONTENT | GUIDELINE |
|---|---|
| Defining the family | B |
| – Nuclear family | B |
| – Extended family | B |
| – Alternative family forms | B |
| Family functions | B |
| Family dynamics | B |
| Family theories | |
| – Family systems theory | C |
| – Family developmental theory | C |
| – Family stress theory | C |
| Key factors in family health | B |
| – Cultural factors | B |
| – Cultural context of the family | B |
| – Childbearing beliefs and practices | B |

# TEACHING STRATEGIES

1. Assign students to write their definitions of family, including a list of persons they consider to be family members. During the class discussion of family, have students present their definitions. Compare similarities and differences among the definitions.

2. Create several genograms using family case studies. Assign each student to create a genogram representing his or her family history.

3. Discuss how each family form can influence parents and their ability to care for and nurture their children. Identify areas of potential conflict and/or problems of each family form. Describe measures that families can use to prevent or effectively deal with these conflicts and problems.

4. Discuss how a family's form could influence the health care provider and the quality of care that the family receives.

5. Divide students into groups, and assign to each group a specific family theory. In addition, provide each group with a family case study. Each group should then assess the family using the assigned theory. Have each student group report their findings during the class discussion of family theories.

6. Illustrate factors affecting family health by having students identify the factors that they feel enhanced or hindered the health of the families they cared for in the clinical setting.

7. Invite a nurse working in a transcultural setting to discuss how the culture of women and their families influences their health and the attitudes of caregivers who provide the health care that they receive.

8. Arrange for a panel discussion of women representing several cultures to discuss how their culture affects family structure and function, childbearing beliefs and practices, and approaches to parenting.

## SUGGESTED STUDENT LEARNING ACTIVITIES

1. Your family serves as a critical influencing factor on your development as a person and on the formation of your value and belief system. *DESCRIBE* your family using the following factors:
   - Classification of family form
   - Family functions
   - Environment
   - Stage within the family life cycle (include the manner in which developmental tasks have been and are being met)
   - Family dynamics: roles and role function, boundaries and channels, nurturing and socialization of children, communication patterns, protocols for problem solving

   Create a genogram of your family.

2. *ASSESS* the pregnancy, childbearing, and parenting values, beliefs, and practices of a specific cultural group.
   - *SUMMARIZE* this group's values, beliefs, and practices; include the references and sources used to obtain your information.
   - *DISCUSS* how you would use this information when planning culturally sensitive care for the women of this culture and their families.

3. *VIEW* the film *Birth in the Squatting Position* (Polymorph Films).
   - *DESCRIBE* the cultural characteristics related to birthing exhibited by the women depicted in this film.
   - *CONTRAST* this type of birthing with the typical American manner of giving birth as it was in the past and how it has changed.

4. *DESCRIBE* the family of one of your postpartum clients using the family systems theory and the family stress theory. *SPECIFY* how this family has changed with the baby as a new family member.

5. *ASSESS* a family using the Freidman Family Assessment Model. Based on an analysis of the assessment findings, identify one nursing diagnosis. Using the nursing diagnosis identified, develop a care management plan that includes expected outcomes and proposed interventions.

6. *SEARCH* the nursing literature for articles related to the importance of the family as a source of support for the pregnant woman and the family's need for care. CHOOSE one article, and complete a bibliography card that includes the following:
   - Summary of the article's key points
   - Your personal reaction to the ideas presented in the article
   - How the professional nurse can use the information in the article to enhance and improve health care

7. *SEARCH* the literature for nursing research related to the influence of family form on the health and well being of its members, the socialization of its children, and its relationship with the society in which it lives. Choose one research study, and complete a bibliography card that includes the following:
   - Hypothesis; research question
   - Summary of the methodology used and key findings
   - Reliability of the study and its findings
   - Recommendations for further research
   - How the professional nurse can use the study's findings to enhance and improve health care for families

## TOPICS FOR DISCUSSION

1. *Discuss this question:* How can the application of family theories help nurses to appropriately manage the care of families after childbirth? Use one specific family theory to illustrate the value of family theory in managing the care of a postpartum woman, her newborn, and her family.

2. *Consider this statement:* Definitions of family vary among family theorists and among people in general. Contrast your definition of family with the variety of definitions held by family theorists, your nursing program, and people in general, including family members, friends, fellow students, and clients. Discuss the importance of identifying and respecting each client's personal definition of family.

3. *Consider this statement:* Providing culturally sensitive care is an important goal for nurses as health care providers. Discuss how you used the care management approach (assessment, identification of nursing diagnoses and expected outcomes, interventions, and evaluation) to develop a family-focused, culturally sensitive plan of care for one of your antepartal, intrapartal, or postpartal clients. (A group discussion where each student presents a client representing a different subcultural group would be an effective approach.)

## MERLIN PROJECT

Using the Chapter 2 section of MERLIN as a starting point, search the Internet for web sites designed to provide families with parenting information and support.

1. Prepare a report that includes the following:
   - A list of web sites that you found and their addresses
   - Sponsor of each of the sites—person(s), agency, or organization
   - Clarity, accuracy, accessibility (ease of use), relevance, depth, and value of the information provided by the site
   - Currency of the site—frequency of site updates
   - Variety of links to other relevant sites
   - Ability of persons visiting the site to obtain additional information and individualized support through services such as e-mail and chat rooms
2. Discuss how you would use this information when teaching parenting classes.

# 3 Community and Home Care

## SUMMARY OF KEY CONCEPTS

Health and wellness of the community and perinatal home care are the primary topics for discussion in Chapter 3. The concept of community is defined, emphasizing the three characteristics of people, place, and interaction or function. Students are informed that community assessment can be accomplished using the "windshield" (or walking) survey. The survey facilitates the gathering of data regarding the community's sociocultural characteristics and the environment, housing, transportation, and local community agencies. A table outlining the windshield survey components can be used by the student to assess a community. Health status indicators focusing on biostatistical data related to common health problems (e.g., the infant mortality rate and the mortality rates for specific health problems and the incidence of certain infections) and risk factors are suggested as a way of determining the health and wellness of a community. Analysis of a community's health status indicators can assist health care providers in targeting vulnerable populations or high risk aggregates for intervention and care. Such populations or aggregates include the homeless, migrants, and refugees and immigrants.

The second half of Chapter 3 discusses perinatal home care. An overview regarding current trends and historic perspectives, methods of communication, guidelines for nursing practice, and perinatal services is included in the discussion. Care management of a home visit is described in terms of the process of admission to home care, preparing for the home visit, conducting the visit itself, and finally postvisit interventions and documentation. One box provides the student with a concise outline for conducting a perinatal home visit while another box outlines a psychosocial assessment that can be used during the visit. The student is also alerted to the safety and infection control issues that the home care nurse must consider.

## LEARNING OBJECTIVES

Define the key terms.
Compare community-based health care and community health (population or aggregate focused) care.
Select appropriate methods of community assessment for specific situations.
List health indicators of community health status and their relevance to perinatal health care.
Explain how age, gender, socioeconomic status, health status, and life experiences can predispose people to vulnerability.

Discuss perinatal concerns and related nursing interventions for selected vulnerable populations: homeless, migrant laborers, and refugees.

Define *service learning* and describe opportunities across the perinatal health continuum.

List the potential advantages and disadvantages of home visits.

Explore telephonic nursing care options in perinatal nursing.

Describe the way home care fits into the maternity continuum of care.

Discuss types of agencies providing home care.

Identify and define common perinatal conditions amenable to home care.

Discuss safety and infection control principles as they apply to the care of clients in their homes.

Describe the nurse's role in perinatal home care.

Identify topics of nursing research related to perinatal home care.

## OUTLINE OF CHAPTER CONTENT WITH COURSE GUIDELINES

| CONTENT | GUIDELINE |
|---|---|
| Assessing levels of community wellness | |
| – Definitions of community | C |
| – Methods of community assessment | C |
| Health and wellness in the community | |
| – Community health status indicators | C |
| – Population-focused or aggregate-focused care | C |
| – High risk aggregates or vulnerable populations | C |
| Home care across the perinatal continuum of care | |
| – Current trends and historic perspectives | C |
| – Communication to bridge the continuum | B |
| – Guidelines for nursing practice | A |
| – Perinatal services | A |
| Care management | |
| – First home care visit | A |
| – Assessment and nursing diagnoses | A |
| – Expected outcomes of care | A |
| – Plan of care and interventions | A |
| – Nursing considerations | A |
| – Evaluation | A |

## TEACHING STRATEGIES

1. Divide students into groups. Assign each group to assess the health and well-being of a variety of communities including the community in which the college is located, an urban community, and a rural community by using the windshield survey and community health status indicators and risk factors.
   - Arrange for students to present their findings to the class

- Assist students in doing the following:
  - Comparing the community that they assessed with national health status indicators
  - Identifying the high risk aggregates or vulnerable populations in the community assessed and the types of services available to meet the needs of these groups for health care
  - Using the care management approach to identify one community-related nursing diagnosis, along with expected outcomes for care, planned interventions, and evaluation strategies

2. Invite a nurse involved in perinatal home care to discuss the protocol that he or she follows when making a home visit to a high risk pregnant woman and to a postpartum woman, her newborn, and family. The nurse should include in the discussion the impact of changes in the health care system on his or her ability to provide care services to clients.

## SUGGESTED STUDENT LEARNING ACTIVITIES

1. *SURVEY* your community for home care agencies that are available for women during and after pregnancy and for the compromised newborn. *GATHER* information related to each service identified. *DESIGN* a table that includes the following information for each agency:
   - Type of home care agency
   - Method of referral
   - Clients cared for by the agency and the criteria used for admission
   - Services provided
   - Method of payment
   - Health care providers used to deliver care and their qualifications

2. *ACCOMPANY* a nurse on a high-tech home care visit to a high risk pregnant woman or a compromised newborn. *PREPARE* a report that includes the following:
   - Description of this nurse's qualifications and typical caseload
   - Summary of the client's health problem and care requirements
   - Description of how the nurse prepared for the visit
   - Specific actions of the nurse in the home that represented the roles of caregiver, teacher, and advocate
   - Method of documentation used by the nurse
   - Reaction of the client and family to the nurse and to the home visit
   - Manner in which the nurse met infection control precautions and addressed safety issues

3. *SEARCH* the nursing literature for articles related to perinatal home care issues including early discharge and use of technology in the home. *CHOOSE* one article, and complete a bibliography card that includes the following:
   - Summary of the article's key points
   - Personal reaction to the ideas presented in the article
   - How the professional nurse could use the information presented to enhance and improve health care

4. *SURVEY* your community in terms of the extent to which hospitals have implemented early discharge and home care programs.
   - *DESCRIBE* the types of services that have been established to support families participating in early discharge programs.
   - *SUMMARIZE* your findings.
   - *COMPARE* your community with national trends.

5. *INTERVIEW* a nurse involved in home care of postpartum women. *DESCRIBE* this nurse's views regarding the following:
   - Criteria that should be met by the woman and her newborn before being discharged from the hospital or birthing center and then from home care
   - Advantages and disadvantages of early discharge and home care
   - Perceived client satisfaction or dissatisfaction with this method of health care delivery
   - Care management techniques used to facilitate the safety of the mother and her newborn
   - Community resources used to enhance home care after early discharge

6. *ACCOMPANY* a nurse on a home visit. *DESCRIBE* the home visit in terms of the following:
   - When after birth the visit took place
   - Who was present during the visit and how they participated
   - How the nursing process was used to manage the health care of the mother, her newborn, and her family
   - The value that the home visit had for the woman, her newborn, and her family
   - Changes that you would propose to enhance the effectiveness of the visit

7. *CONDUCT* a postdischarge telephone follow-up with one of your postpartum clients.
   - *USE* the information presented in the chapter to organize the assessment and intervention format that will guide your telephone follow-up.
   - *SUMMARIZE* the outcome of your call, including the client's reaction as well as your own.
   - *DISCUSS* the value of your follow-up call and what you would do the next time to improve its effectiveness.

## LEARNING OBJECTIVES

1. *Address this question:* How should the determination be made that a client is ready for discharge from the hospital and is a candidate for home care? How should the determination be made that the client no longer requires home care services?

2. *Consider this question:* What are the ethical and legal responsibilities of the nurse who believes that a home care client needs to be cared for in a hospital or who believes that a home care client needs to continue to receive care and not be discharged from the service?

3. *Consider this question:* What can the home care nurse do to reduce the stressors encountered by the home caregiver and family?

4. *Debate these issues:*
   - Early discharge and home care—an advantage or disadvantage for the postpartum woman, her newborn, and family?
   - Home care versus hospital care for the high risk pregnant woman

5. *Address this question:* What community services should be available before implementing an early discharge program for postpartum women, their newborns, and their families? Give the rationale for the services that you propose.

## MERLIN PROJECT

Use MERLIN to assist you in searching MEDLINE for research studies related to the effectiveness of home care for the high risk pregnant woman.
- Create an annotated bibliography of at least five research studies.
- Choose one of the research studies, and complete a bibliography card that includes the following:
  - Hypothesis; research question
  - Summary of the methodology used and key findings
  - Reliability of the study and its findings
  - Recommendations for further research
  - How the professional nurse can use the study's findings to enhance and improve health care

# 4 Alternative and Complementary Therapies

## SUMMARY OF KEY CONCEPTS

Chapter 4 provides the student with a concise overview of the most common alternative and complementary therapies available in health care today. Dissatisfaction with the impersonal, high-technology approach of traditional health care and a growing appreciation of the value of health and the connection of mind-body-spirit are cited as major factors in a growing demand by consumers for alternative and complementary therapies to promote, maintain, and restore their health. A table presents definitions of terms essential to the understanding of alternative therapies. The concepts shared by many alternative health care options are cited, and the basis for the effectiveness of these options is explained. The need for research data to prove effectiveness is emphasized. A box identifies several Internet resources for alternative therapies such as therapeutic touch, interactive imagery, and holistic nursing. The chapter concludes with a discussion of holistic nursing and the most common holistic therapies and modalities used by nurses. Touch and energetic therapies and mind-body healing approaches found to be beneficial in women's health care are described.

## LEARNING OBJECTIVES

Define the key terms.
Describe the differences between standard (allopathic or Western) and holistic health care.
Define the biopsychosocial and spiritual implications of holistic health care.
Outline the advantages of a holistic philosophy.
Compare and contrast touch and energetic, mind-body, and alternative pharmacologic healing modalities.
Discuss the limitations of research in holistic healing.
Identify the appropriate modalities for integrative women's health care.
Propose appropriate topics for holistic nursing research.

# OUTLINE OF CHAPTER CONTENT WITH COURSE GUIDELINES

| CONTENT | GUIDELINE |
|---|:---:|
| Overview of alternative and complementary modalities | C |
| – Integrative health care | C |
| – Research efforts | C |
| – The nurse's role: holistic nursing | B |
| Alternative and complementary therapies in women's health care | |
| – Overview | B |
| – Touch and energetic healing | B |
| – Mind-body healing | B |
| – Alternative pharmacologic modalities | B |
| – Applications in women's health care | A |
| – Implications for nursing practice | A |

# TEACHING STRATEGIES

1. Identify services in your community that offer consumers the option of alternative and complementary therapy. Invite a practitioner from two of these services and two consumers of these services to participate in a panel discussion regarding approaches used and their effectiveness. Encourage students to share their experiences with this type of health care.

2. Invite a nurse involved in holistic nursing to discuss how he or she approaches health care, including the following:
   - Characteristics of the clients served and the health problems that they are experiencing
   - Types of holistic care measures used and their effectiveness
   - Use of and need for research to validate the effectiveness of holistic nursing approaches

3. Discuss the manner in which traditional and alternative health care approaches can be combined to provide clients with high quality health care. Cite several examples that illustrate how health care is enhanced by an integrative approach that combines alternative and traditional health care modalities.

4. Cite research studies that validate the effectiveness of alternative and complementary therapies. Identify the role OAM and NCCAM play in fostering and disseminating this research.

# SUGGESTED STUDENT ACTIVITIES

1. *VISIT* an alternative or complementary health care service in your community.
   A. *INTERVIEW* a provider of this service to determine the following:
      - Education and background of the provider including preparation for the service that he or she offers
      - Clients served and health care problems that they are experiencing

- Perceived effectiveness of the service provided in managing the health problem that the patients are experiencing
- Cost and accessibility of the service
- Use of research findings in providing services and participation in research studies to validate effectiveness of the services

B. *PREPARE* a report that summarizes the information gathered in your interview and includes your assessment of the effectiveness of the service offered.

2. *EVALUATE* the health care agencies where you have your clinical rotations. *IDENTIFY* the alternative and complementary therapies used in combination with traditional or standard health care. *PREPARE* a report that includes the following:
- Types of therapies used, including a description of each therapy, the agency where it was used, the client that used the therapy, and the perceived effectiveness of the therapy in modifying the health problem for which it was used
- Types of therapies that you would suggest including a description of the therapy and the client and health problem for which you would recommend it; state the rationale for each of your suggestions and/or recommendations

3. *SEARCH* the nursing literature for articles related to the use of alterative and complementary therapies in the health care of women. *CHOOSE* one article, and complete a bibliography card that includes the following:
- Summary of the article's key points
- Personal reaction to the ideas presented in the article
- How the professional nurse can use the article's ideas to enhance and improve the quality of health care

## TOPICS FOR DISCUSSION

1. *Debate the issue:* Complementary and alternative therapies—a help or hindrance to traditional health care?

2. *Support this statement:* Nurses are more likely to incorporate holistic approaches when providing health care than are physicians.

## MERLIN PROJECT

1. Use MERLIN to assist you in searching the literature for research studies that validate the effectiveness of alternative and complementary therapies.
- Create an annotated bibliography of at least five research studies.
- Choose one research study, and complete a bibliography card that includes the following:
  - Hypothesis; research question
  - Summary of the methodology used and key findings
  - Reliability of the study and its findings
  - Recommendations for further research
  - How the professional nurse can use the study's findings to enhance and improve health care

2. Using the Chapter 4 section of MERLIN, search the Internet for web sites related to alternative and complementary therapies. Prepare a report that includes the following:
   - List of web sites with addresses and sponsor
   - Summary of the information provided at each site
   - Value and accessibility of the information provided for both consumers of health care and for health care providers
   - Ability of persons visiting each site to obtain additional information through services such as links to other relevant sites, e-mail, and chat rooms

## Chapter

# 5 Health Promotion and Prevention

## SUMMARY OF KEY CONCEPTS

Chapter 5 introduces students to the concept of well-woman health care. The reasons why women enter the health care system are explained along with the financial, cultural, and gender issues that can interfere with women seeking and obtaining needed health care. The demographics of women's health care are described in terms of age, social and cultural factors, health behaviors, sexual practices, medical and gynecologic conditions, environmental and workplace hazards, and violence. A discussion of anticipatory guidance emphasizes the importance of women becoming active participants in their own health promotion and illness prevention and the essential role of nurses in helping women to accomplish these tasks by educating women and motivating them to take control of their health management. Students are provided with a description of specific health promotion and illness prevention activities that includes the rationale for the effectiveness of each activity.

## LEARNING OBJECTIVES

Define the key terms.

Describe factors influencing a woman's contact with the health care system.

Identify reasons for women to enter the health care delivery system.

Discuss financial, cultural, and gender barriers to seeking health care.

Explain conditions and characteristics that increase health risks for women during their childbearing years.

Analyze programs of anticipatory guidance that promote health and prevention.

Outline health screening schedules for women in the childbearing years.

Identify topics for nursing research related to health promotion in women.

# OUTLINE OF CHAPTER CONTENT WITH COURSE GUIDELINES

| CONTENT | GUIDELINE |
|---|:---:|
| Reasons for entering the health care system | |
|   – Preconception counseling | A |
|   – Pregnancy | A |
|   – Well-woman care | B |
|   – Fertility control and infertility | A |
|   – Menstrual problems | B |
|   – Perimenopause | B |
| Barriers to seeking health care | |
|   – Financial issues | B |
|   – Cultural issues | B |
|   – Gender issues | B |
| Conditions and characteristics that increase health risks | |
|   in the childbearing years | |
|   – Demographics | A |
|   – Age | A |
|   – Social/cultural | A |
|   – Health behaviors | A |
|     – Smoking | A |
|     – Substance use and abuse | A |
|     – Nutrition | A |
|     – Stress | A |
|   – Sexual practices | A |
|   – Medical conditions | A |
|   – Gynecologic conditions affecting pregnancy | A |
|   – Environmental and workplace hazards | A |
|   – Violence against women | A |
| Anticipatory guidance for health promotion and prevention | |
|   – Nutrition | A |
|   – Exercise | A |
|   – Stress management | A |
|   – Substance use cessation | A |
|   – Safer sex practices | A |
|   – Health screening schedule | B |
|   – Health risk prevention | A |
|   – Health promotion | A |

# TEACHING STRATEGIES

1. Identify the types of agencies in your community that provide health care for women. Describe the specific services offered by each of these agencies.

2. Invite a women's health nurse-practitioner to discuss her or his approach to the care management of women, including measures used to empower women to participate as full partners in their care.

3. Use case studies to illustrate barriers faced by women that interfere with their seeking and obtaining the health care that they require. Discuss how nurses caring for women can help them to overcome these barriers.

4. Encourage students to participate in a discussion of the health promotion and illness prevention activities that they engage in—why they engage in these activities, how they learned about them, and barriers that they experience when trying to fully implement these activities in their daily lives. Discuss the strategies that students can use to counsel women to participate in these types of activities to promote their own health and prevent illness.

5. Involve students in identifying changes that they would need to make in their own health and lifestyle habits to prepare themselves for conception and pregnancy. Discuss the process that the students could follow in making these changes, including the use of a professional health care provider.

## SUGGESTED STUDENT LEARNING ACTIVITIES

1. *VISIT* a woman's health clinic. Shadow a nurse who is working in an expanded role as a provider of women's health services. *PREPARE* a report that describes each of the following:
   - Health assessment and screening methods routinely used by the nurse
   - Typical women's health problems managed by the nurse
   - Manner in which the nurse approaches the assessment and care of women in his or her caseload, including the use of therapeutic communication techniques, health teaching, the nursing process, and research findings
   - Types of health promotion and illness prevention activities offered by the clinic
   - Types of alternative and complementary therapies integrated into the standard health care offered by the clinic
   - Atmosphere and environment of the facility: how does it facilitate the holistic care of women's health and health problems, provide for the woman's comfort and privacy, and enhance a woman's ability to learn about her health?
   - Degree to which women are encouraged to (and expected to) actively participate in their own health care
   - Changes that you would propose to enhance the agency's role as a provider of women's health care services; state the rationale for each change you propose

2. *DESIGN* a pamphlet for women regarding health promotion and illness prevention activities. The pamphlet should explain each activity, noting how it influences health status, what it entails, and what measures can be used to incorporate the activity into the woman's lifestyle.

3. *VISIT* a local bookstore or library to assess the literature available related to women and their health. *CREATE* a list of the books that you found to be the most appealing. *CHOOSE* one book and prepare a report that includes the following:
   - Summary of the important concepts covered in the book
   - Readability, currency, accuracy, and comprehensiveness of the content presented
   - Credentials of the author or authors; cost
   - Personal reaction to the information in the book, including the effect that the book could have on empowering women to take responsibility for their own health
   - How the book could be used by nurses who work in women's health care services to plan and administer more effective client care

4. *PREPARE* a class for a group of young adult women that will provide them with the information required to encourage them to be active participants in their own health promotion and illness prevention.
   - *LIST* the expected outcomes of the class.
   - *OUTLINE* in detail the content to be covered in the class.
   - *STATE* the teaching methodologies that you would use, including class format (lecture, group discussion), demonstrations, role playing, audiovisual presentations, and written materials.
   - *CONDUCT* the class, if possible, and evaluate its effectiveness in terms of the expected outcomes that you identified.

5. *SEARCH* the nursing literature for articles related to types of women's health care services available in the United States. *CHOOSE* one article, and complete a bibliography card that includes the following:
   - Summary of the article's key points
   - Your personal reaction to the ideas presented in the article
   - How the professional nurse could use the information to enhance and improve health care

## TOPICS FOR DISCUSSION

1. *Support this statement:* Women should be empowered to become active partners with their health care providers in the promotion and maintenance of their own health.

2. *Consider this question:* What is the benefit of full insurance coverage for regular health assessment and screening of women that includes such assessment methods as clinical breast examination, pelvic examination, mammograms, and Papanicolaou smears?

3. *Discuss this issue:* The nursing profession needs to take a leadership role in removing barriers that limit access of women to needed health care.

## MERLIN PROJECT

Use the Chapter 5 section of MERLIN as a starting point to search the Internet for web sites designed to inform women about health issues as well as health promotion and illness prevention measures. Prepare a report that includes the following:
   - List of at least five sites
   - Evaluation of two sites in terms of the following:
     - Sponsoring person(s), agency, or organization
     - Clarity, accuracy, accessibility (ease of use), value, and depth of information provided
     - Currency of information presented—frequency of site updates
     - Variety of links to relevant web sites
     - Ability of persons visiting the site to obtain additional information through services such as e-mail and chat rooms
   - Discussion of how the professional nurse can use these web sites and the information that they provide to enhance and improve health care for women

# Chapter

# Assessment of Women

## SUMMARY OF KEY CONCEPTS

Chapter 6 introduces the student to anatomy and physiology of the female reproductive system, human sexuality, immunology, and the health assessment of women. A variety of illustrations, tables, and diagrams facilitate student learning.

The female reproductive system is presented in terms of internal and external structures, breasts, and the physiologic changes that occur within the menstrual cycle. The discussion includes function and typical characteristics as well as variations related to developmental stage and parity.

The student is provided with an overview of the four phases of the human sexual response cycle. A table summarizes the female and male reactions during each of the phases. A basic review of immunological principles focuses on body defenses to infection and different types of immunity

The discussion of health assessment of women focuses on the health history interview, physical examination, and laboratory and diagnostic procedures. Students are alerted to the necessity of considering the unique needs of women with emotional and physical disorders, women who are abused, and older women. The influence of a woman's cultural beliefs on her approach to health care and on her manner of communication is described.

## LEARNING OBJECTIVES

Define the key terms.
Identify the structures and functions of the female reproductive system.
Summarize the menstrual cycle in relation to hormonal, ovarian, and endometrial response.
Identify the four phases of the sexual response.
Compare natural and acquired immunity.
Discuss the effects of age, lifestyle, environment, and nutrition on the immune system.
Identify cultural and communication variations that may affect a woman's decision to seek and follow through with health care.
Discuss how history and physical examination can be adapted for women with special needs.
List strategies for teaching safety and injury prevention during routine health examinations.
Identify indications of abuse, appropriate screening, and referral to community agencies.
Define components of taking a woman's history and performing a physical examination.

Identify the correct procedure for assisting with and collecting Papanicolaou smear specimens.

Review client teaching of breast self-examination.

Identify risk factors for osteoporosis.

Identify topics for nursing research related to health assessment of women.

## OUTLINE OF CHAPTER CONTENT WITH COURSE GUIDELINES

| CONTENT | GUIDELINE |
|---|---|
| Female reproductive system | |
| – External structures | A |
| – Internal structures | A |
| Breasts | A |
| Menstruation and menopause | A |
| – Menarche and puberty | A |
| – Menstrual cycle | A |
| – Endometrial cycle | A |
| – Hypothalamic-pituitary cycle | A |
| – Ovarian cycle | A |
| – Prostaglandins | A |
| – Climacteric and menopause | A |
| Sexual response | B |
| Immunology | B |
| – Body defenses | B |
| – Types of immunity | B |
| – Factors associated with immunological disease | B |
| Health assessment | A |
| – Interview | A |
| – Biographic information | A |
| – Cultural considerations and communication variations | A |
| – Women with special needs | A |
| – Age-related considerations | A |
| – History | A |
| – Physical examination | A |
| – Pelvic examination | A |
| – Laboratory and diagnostic procedures | A |

## TEACHING STRATEGIES

1. Use anatomical illustrations (e.g., transparencies, large charts) and models to illustrate the internal and external structures of the breasts and female reproductive system. Use videos that demonstrate assessment of the female breasts, reproductive system, and breast self-examination (BSE). (NOTE: Assessment videos that accompany *Mosby's Guide to Physical Examination* and breast self-examination videos from the American Cancer Society are good sources to use.)

2. Demonstrate breast self-examination, using breast models to detect masses.

3. Use diagrams and charts (transparencies) of the menstrual cycle to illustrate fluctuations in hormonal levels and physiologic changes that occur during the cycle.

4. Use case studies to illustrate variations in menstrual cycle beliefs and changes as described by different women. Encourage students to share their beliefs and experiences with the menstrual cycle. Male students can discuss their beliefs and impressions of the menstrual cycle as experienced by the women in their lives.

5. Invite a sexual counselor to discuss effective counseling methods and measures that he or she uses to put clients at ease and develop rapport and how they reconcile their sexual beliefs and practices with those of the clients when a conflict exists. Encourage students to describe their feelings when they need to discuss topics of a sexual nature with clients.

6. Bring a variety of abuse assessment screening tools to class. Discuss how students should incorporate such screens in their health assessment of women.

7. Invite a women's health nurse-practitioner to discuss measures that she or he uses to facilitate the health assessment of women.

8. Identify measures that nurses can use to assist women to enhance their body's ability to resist or prevent infection.

## SUGGESTED STUDENT LEARNING ACTIVITIES

1. *PREPARE* a class related to sexuality and reproductive development and health for a group of early-adolescent girls who are approaching puberty. The class that you prepare should reflect the following:
   - A detailed outline of content that you consider to be essential for understanding of the topic
   - Developmental considerations
   - A variety of teaching methods, including audiovisual aids, role playing, and group discussions

2. *SEARCH* the nursing literature for articles related to the topic of human sexuality and reproduction. *CHOOSE* one article, and complete a bibliography card that includes the following:
   - Summary of the article's key points
   - Your personal reaction to the ideas presented in the article
   - How the professional nurse can use the article's ideas to enhance and improve the quality of health care

3. *DESIGN* a pamphlet for women regarding health assessment and screening methods. The pamphlet should explain each method, why it is performed, what it entails, and the schedule for its performance. Self-assessment techniques such as BSE and vulvar self-examination (VSE) should be fully explained and illustrated in the pamphlet.

## TOPICS FOR DISCUSSION

1. *Support this statement:* Myths and folklore often influence a woman and her beliefs and practices related to the menstrual cycle and sexuality. These myths and folklore can influence health practices and sexual function.

2. *Explore this question:* What can nurses do to facilitate communication and enhance their own comfort and their clients' comfort during discussions of intimate topics related to reproductive anatomy and physiology and sexuality?

## MERLIN PROJECT

Using the Chapter 6 section of MERLIN as a starting point, search the Internet for web sites designed to educate women regarding self-assessment techniques such as BSE and VSE, and inform them regarding current recommendations for healthy women assessments to be conducted by health care providers. Discuss how you would use this information when providing health care for women that focuses on health promotion and illness prevention activities.

# Chapter

# 7 Common Reproductive Concerns

## SUMMARY OF KEY CONCEPTS

Chapter 7 focuses on the menstrual cycle in terms of changes and common disorders that occur over the life span. The chapter begins with a discussion of common menstrual disorders that focuses on hypogonadotropic amenorrhea, dysmenorrhea, premenstrual syndrome, and endometriosis. Each disorder is explained according to its typical clinical manifestations, pathophysiologic basis, and appropriate care management. Plans of care related to premenstrual syndrome (PMS) and endometriosis illustrate the use of the nursing process for the care management of women experiencing these problems. The plan of care for PMS considers the nursing diagnoses of fluid volume excess, pain (breast discomfort), and situational low self-esteem. The plan of care for endometriosis considers the nursing diagnoses of pain, knowledge deficit, and situational low self-esteem. An overview of alterations in cyclical bleeding concludes the discussion of menstrual disorders. Each cyclical bleeding alteration is described in terms of its characteristics, etiology, and common care management approaches.

Menopause is discussed in detail in the second part of the chapter. Changes experienced by a woman as she progresses through the perimenopausal period to the postmenopausal period are described according to clinical manifestations, physiologic basis, and care management. The benefits and risks of menopausal hormone therapy are identified. An overview of the care management of perimenopausal women uses the nursing process format. Suggested interventions focus on nursing support measures, sexual counseling, midlife support groups, nutrition, exercise, and alternative therapies.

## LEARNING OBJECTIVES

Define the key terms.
Develop a nursing care plan for the woman with primary dysmenorrhea.
Outline client teaching about premenstrual syndrome.
Relate the pathophysiology of endometriosis to associated symptoms.
Develop an assessment guide for perimenopausal women.
Develop a nursing care plan for the postmenopausal woman.
Outline client teaching about menopausal hormone therapy.
Outline client teaching about prevention of osteoporosis.
Evaluate the use of alternative therapies for menstrual disorders and menopausal symptoms.
Identify topics for nursing research related to menstrual disorders and menopause.

# OUTLINE OF CHAPTER CONTENT WITH COURSE GUIDELINES

| CONTENT | GUIDELINE |
|---|:---:|
| Common menstrual disorders | A |
| – Amenorrhea | A |
| – Dysmenorrhea | B |
| – Premenstrual syndrome | A |
|    – Plan of care—PMS | A |
| – Endometriosis | A |
|    – Plan of care—endometriosis | A |
| – Alterations in cyclical bleeding | A |
|    – Care management | A |
| Menopause | A |
| – Physiology | A |
| – Physical changes during the perimenopausal period | A |
| – Mood and behavioral responses | A |
| – Health risks of perimenopausal women | A |
| – Menopausal hormonal therapy (MHT) | A |
| – Alternative therapies | A |
| – Care management | A |
|    – Assessment and nursing diagnoses | A |
|    – Expected outcomes of care | A |
|    – Plan of care and interventions | A |
|       – Sexual counseling | A |
|       – Nutrition | A |
|       – Exercise | A |
|       – Midlife support groups | A |
| – Evaluation | A |

# TEACHING STRATEGIES

1. Identify services and support groups that are available in your community to assist women who have menstrual problems such as PMS, dysmenorrhea, and endometriosis.

2. Use case studies to illustrate the impact that specific menstrual problems can have on a woman's lifestyle, relationships, self-esteem, and emotions. Focus on the essential role of the nurse in assisting women to manage these problems in a healthy manner.

3. Invite a representative from a PMS support group to discuss the impact of PMS on women and their families, typical signs and symptoms, and management approaches that women have found helpful and have even developed themselves.

4. Assign students to collect information about the perimenopausal period that can be found in the media (print, television, and radio). Involve students in a discussion of the impact that these media presentations can have on women approaching or experiencing the perimenopausal period. Identify measures that nurses can use to reinforce positive media images and refute those that are negative.

5. Assemble a panel of perimenopausal women to discuss their experiences with the characteristic changes of this period in their lives. Encourage women to share alternative therapies that they have tried and their degree of effectiveness.

## SUGGESTED STUDENT LEARNING ACTIVITIES

1. *ATTEND* a meeting of a PMS support group, and *INTERVIEW* the group's leader. *PREPARE* a report that includes a description of each of the following points:
   - How the group was founded: who, when, and why?
   - Purpose and mission of the group
   - The manner in which the group provides support for women experiencing PMS
   - The group dynamics operant during the meeting
   - The PMS symptomatology experienced by the women and the coping strategies used
   - The role that a nurse could play in facilitating the support efforts of the group

2. *DESIGN* a pamphlet regarding the perimenopausal and postmenopausal periods that can be used as a teaching aid by nurses who work with women who have reached this period in their lives. The pamphlet should utilize a holistic approach and include each of the following:
   - Typical physical, sexual, and emotional changes that occur; include the physiologic basis for each of the changes identified
   - Current management approaches including MHT, calcium supplementation, nutrition, exercise, and alterative therapies
   - Midlife support groups available in the community
   - Internet sites designed to educate and support perimenopausal women
   - Annotated bibliography of recommended literature

3. *VISIT* a local bookstore or library to assess the type, quality, and quantity of literature available for women seeking information on menstrual disorders, perimenopause, and postmenopause. *CREATE* a list of the books that you found to be the most appealing. *CHOOSE* one book, and prepare a report that includes the following:
   - Summary of the important concepts covered in the book
   - Readability, currency, accuracy, and comprehensiveness of the content presented
   - Credentials of the author(s); cost
   - Personal reaction to the information in the book, including the effect that the book could have on enhancing a woman's self-esteem and self-worth during this period of her life
   - How the book could be used by nurses who work with women to plan and administer more effective health care

4. *READ* the book *The Silent Passage: Menopause* or *Passages* by Gail Sheehy. *PREPARE* a report that summarizes the important points presented by the author, and evaluate the effectiveness of the book in helping women to cope with the changes that accompany this period in their lives.

5. *SEARCH* the nursing literature for articles related to the menstrual concerns discussed in this chapter. *CHOOSE* one article, and complete a bibliography card that includes the following:
   - Summary of the article's key points
   - Personal reaction to the ideas presented in the article
   - How the professional nurse can use the article's ideas to enhance and improve the quality of health care

6. *CREATE* a pamphlet for women about PMS that includes typical signs and symptoms and management approaches that incorporate a variety of pharmacologic, nonpharmacologic, and alternative treatments.

7. *INTERVIEW* a woman who has a diagnosis of and is being treated for endometriosis.
   - *GATHER* information regarding the following:
     - The woman's description of the impact that endometriosis has had on her health and well-being and on her partner and family
     - Coping mechanisms that the woman and her partner or family use to deal with the stressors encountered as a result of the diagnosis and treatment for endometriosis
     - The support measures, people, and services that she and her partner or family found helpful, those that they found to be lacking or not helpful, and those that they wished would have been offered
     - Her impressions of the impact that the health care system and health care providers had on her health and well-being during the diagnosis and treatment for endometriosis
   - *DESCRIBE* how you would use this information to plan care that is effective in dealing not only with the woman's physical needs but also with the woman, her partner, and family's psychosocial and emotional needs. How would you use this information to care for other women with this diagnosis?

## TOPICS FOR DISCUSSION

1. *Address these questions:*
   - What is society's view of women who experience premenstrual syndrome? Consider the impact this view could have on a woman's ability to advance in her career.
   - How are perimenopausal women viewed by society? Discuss how this view can affect a woman's response to her own approaching menopause.

2. *Support this statement:* Nurses are in a key position to advance a more positive image of women as they experience the changes of the perimenopause and postmenopausal periods.

3. *Debate the issue:* Hormone replacement therapy and alternative therapies—safe and effective or unsafe and ineffective for the treatment of perimenopausal changes?

## MERLIN PROJECT

1. Use MERLIN to assist you in searching the literature for research studies related to effective treatment approaches for women experiencing menopause.
   - Create an annotated bibliography of at least five research studies.
   - Choose one of the research studies, and complete a bibliography card that includes the following:
     - Hypothesis; research question
     - Summary of the methodology used and the key findings
     - Reliability of the study and its findings
     - Recommendations for further research
     - How the professional nurse can use the study's findings to enhance and improve health care
2. Imagine that you are conducting a support group for women experiencing the signs and symptoms associated with premenstrual syndrome. How would you use the Internet to extend the education and support needed by these women into their homes?

# Chapter

# 8

# Sexually Transmitted Diseases and Other Infections

## SUMMARY OF KEY CONCEPTS

Chapter 8 focuses on the concept of infection as it affects women, including those who are pregnant. A variety of tables, illustrations, and boxes facilitate student learning and review.

Sexually transmitted diseases (STDs) and vaginal infections are presented in terms of the major causative organisms, namely bacteria, viruses, and fungi. Each infection is described according to incidence, mode(s) of transmission, clinical manifestations and effects for the woman and her fetus or newborn, screening and diagnosis, and management. An overview of group B streptococcus and the TORCH infections is included in the chapter. The nursing process is used as a framework for the care management of women with infections. Risk identification, prevention, and treatment measures are described. A plan of care illustrates the use of the nursing process in managing the care of a woman with a sexually transmitted infection. The nursing diagnoses of altered health maintenance, impaired social interaction, and impaired tissue integrity are considered.

The chapter concludes with an overview of infection control measures with an emphasis on Standard Precautions and precautions for invasive procedures, including specific childbearing precautions.

## LEARNING OBJECTIVES

Define the key terms.
Describe prevention of sexually transmitted infections in women.
Differentiate signs, symptoms, diagnosis, and management of women with sexually transmitted infections.
Identify differences in management for pregnant women with sexually transmitted infections.
Summarize the care of women with selected viral infections (human immunodeficiency virus; hepatitis A, B, C).
Discuss the effect of group B streptococcus (GBS) on pregnancy and management of pregnant clients with GBS.
Compare and contrast signs, symptoms, and management of selected vaginal infections.
Review principles of infection control.
Identify topics for nursing research related to sexually transmitted infections.

# OUTLINE OF CHAPTER CONTENT WITH COURSE GUIDELINES

| CONTENT | GUIDELINE |
|---|:---:|
| Sexually transmitted diseases (STDs) | |
| – Prevention | A |
| – Safer sex practices | A |
| Bacterial sexually transmitted diseases | |
| – Chlamydia | A |
| – Gonorrhea | A |
| – Syphilis | B |
| – Pelvic inflammatory disease | A |
| Viral sexually transmitted infections | |
| – Human papillomavirus | A |
| – Herpes simplex virus | A |
| – Viral hepatitis | A |
| – Human immunodeficiency virus | A |
| Group B streptococcus | A |
| Vaginal infections | |
| – Bacterial vaginosis | B |
| – Candidiasis | A |
| – Trichomoniasis | B |
| Effects of sexually transmitted infections on pregnancy and the fetus | A |
| – TORCH infections | A |
| Care management | |
| – Assessment and nursing diagnoses | A |
| – Expected outcomes of care | A |
| – Plan of care and interventions | A |
| – Evaluation | A |
| Plan of care—sexually transmitted diseases | A |
| Infection control: Standard Precautions | A |

# TEACHING STRATEGIES

1. Use statistical data to describe the incidence of STDs. Compare statistics for geographic area, age, and gender.

2. Create a chart that compares the expected assessment findings, impact, diagnostic tests, and management for STDs and vaginal infections. Review CDC guidelines for treating and preventing reproductive tract infections.

3. Discuss the legal guidelines for HIV testing during pregnancy in your state and community. Discuss the impact that these guidelines have on women and health care providers.

4. Identify HIV health care services in your community and nationally that address the unique needs of the HIV-positive nonpregnant and pregnant woman.

5. Discuss the importance of preventive measures and early detection of reproductive tract infections emphasizing safer sex practices and genital self-examination. Identify strategies that students can use to teach and encourage women and men to practice safer sex and regular genital self-examination.

## SUGGESTED STUDENT LEARNING ACTIVITIES

1. *DEVELOP* a teaching program aimed at young adolescents for the purpose of alerting them to STDs—what they are, signs and symptoms, prevention and treatment measures, and impact on general and reproductive health now and in the future. Your program should reflect not only relevant information but also teaching methodologies appropriate to this age group.

2. *SURVEY* your community with regard to STDs, both bacterial and viral, in terms of their incidence and the prevention and treatment services available.
   - *CREATE* a graph or table that illustrates the statistical data. Data should reflect general incidence as well as incidence among various population groups and areas. *COMPARE* local incidence with state and national incidence.
   - *DESCRIBE* the educational programs and services designed to alert the public about STDs and effective preventive measures. *INDICATE* the availability of these educational programs to various population groups.
   - *DESCRIBE* assessment and treatment services available according to type, location, accessibility, cost, and effectiveness.

3. *VISIT* a health care facility that serves the public's need for STD assessment, treatment, prevention, and education.
   - *DESCRIBE* the manner in which this facility offers its services.
   - *SPECIFY* changes that you would propose to improve and enhance this facility's mission; *INCLUDE* the rationale for each change that you propose.
   - *INTERVIEW* a nurse who provides care at this facility to determine how he or she views his or her role and fulfills it.

4. *EVALUATE* the measures used by you and other health care providers to prevent and control infection at the agency where you have your maternity clinical experience. *PREPARE* a report that includes the following:
   - A description of the infection control practices and infection prevention measures used
   - A comparison of these practices and measures with the concepts and standards discussed in this chapter
   - Identification of changes that need to be made in order to improve these practices and measures and facilitate their effectiveness; indicate the rationale for each change recommended

5. *SEARCH* the nursing literature for articles related to infection as it relates to maternity and newborn, and women's health care. *CHOOSE* one article and complete a bibliography card that includes the following:
   - Summary of the article's key points
   - Personal reaction to the ideas presented in the article
   - How the professional nurse could use the information to enhance and improve health care

# TOPICS FOR DISCUSSION

1. *Consider these questions:*
   - What can nurses do to reduce the incidence of STDs and their impact on the reproductive health of women?
   - How can preconception care be used to reduce the incidence and impact of infection during pregnancy?

2. *Debate these issues:*
   - Only pregnant women who have been clearly identified to be at high risk should be tested for exposure to HIV.
   - Women should be encouraged to self-diagnose and treat simple vaginal infections such as candidiasis in an effort to save money and time.

# MERLIN PROJECT

Explore the Centers for Disease Control and Prevention (CDC) web site.
- Gather information regarding the incidence and recommended management for sexually transmitted infections.
- Based on your findings, identify strategies to reduce the incidence of STDs and ensure prompt diagnosis and treatment. State the rationale for each of the strategies that you propose using statistical data to validate the potential effectiveness of the strategy.

Chapter

9

# Contraception and Abortion

## SUMMARY OF KEY CONCEPTS

Chapter 9 focuses on the concept of fertility control. Contraception, as the voluntary prevention of pregnancy, is viewed in terms of the variety of methods available now with an emphasis on barrier, hormonal, and intrauterine methods. The nursing process is used as the care management approach to assist clients as they choose contraceptive methods that are best for them and to use the method that they choose effectively. Each currently available method is described with regard to mode of action, effectiveness, manner of use for maximum effectiveness, advantages, disadvantages and side effects, nursing considerations, and client teaching. A variety of boxes provide guidelines to follow when using many of the methods presented in the text. This approach makes it easy for the student to learn the method and to present accurate information to clients. A plan of care illustrates the use of the nursing process in the care management of a sexually active couple requiring information regarding contraception and protection from sexually transmitted diseases. Decisional conflict and risk for infection are the nursing diagnoses developed.

The chapter continues with a discussion of sterilization. Methods currently available are described. The care management approach focuses on the use of the nursing process to meet the needs of clients considering sterilization and then undergoing these procedures. Finally, the chapter concludes with a discussion of induced abortion within a nursing process framework. Methods of first and second trimester abortion, possible complications related to induced abortion, and nursing considerations are described.

## LEARNING OBJECTIVES

Define the key terms.
Compare the different methods of contraception.
State the advantages and disadvantages of frequently used methods of contraception.
Explain the common nursing interventions that facilitate contraceptive use.
Recognize the various ethical, legal, cultural, and religious considerations of fertility
    management.
Describe the techniques used for medical and surgical interruption of pregnancy.
Examine the various ethical and legal considerations of elective abortion.
Identify topics in nursing research related to contraception and abortion.

# OUTLINE OF CHAPTER CONTENT WITH COURSE GUIDELINES

| CONTENT | GUIDELINE |
|---|---|
| Contraception | |
| Care management | |
| – Assessment and nursing diagnoses | A |
| – Expected outcomes of care | A |
| – Plan of care and interventions | A |
|   – Coitus interruptus | C |
|   – Periodic abstinence | B |
|   – Barrier methods | A |
|     – Spermicides | A |
|     – Condom | A |
|     – Diaphragm | A |
|     – Cervical cap | A |
|     – Contraceptive sponge | A |
|   – Hormonal methods | A |
|     – Combined estrogen and progesterone contraceptives | A |
|     – Progestin-only contraception | A |
|   – Mifepristone (RU 486) | A |
|   – Intrauterine device (IUD) | A |
|   – Sterilization | A |
|     – Types of sterilization (female and male) | A |
|     – Tubal reconstruction | B |
|   – Laws and regulations | A |
|   – Future trends | B |
| – Evaluation | A |
| Abortion | A |
| – Induced abortion | A |
| – Care management | A |
|   – Assessment and nursing diagnoses | A |
|   – Expected outcomes of care | A |
|   – Plan of care and interventions | A |
|     – First trimester abortion | A |
|     – Second trimester abortion | A |
|     – Complications after abortion | A |
|     – Nursing considerations | A |
|   – Evaluation | A |

# TEACHING STRATEGIES

1. Identify contraceptive services available in your community. Describe each service in terms of population served, services provided, and payment methods.

2. Invite a nurse who practices at Planned Parenthood to discuss how she counsels clients regarding contraceptive choice and how she adjusts her approach according to the developmental status and unique characteristics of her clients.

3. Create a chart related to each type of contraceptive method. Bring samples of a variety of methods to class, including those methods that are available over the counter. Use the chart and samples to describe each method in terms of action, advantages and disadvantages, effectiveness, and guidelines for use to maximize effectiveness.

4. Describe each sterilization method. Discuss the issues that must be considered when guiding an individual or couple through the decision-making process concerning sterilization.

5. Invite a nurse who cares for women who undergo induced abortions to discuss the approach that she uses to help women during the decision-making process regarding their pregnancies and the measures that she uses to provide emotional support for women before, during, and after an induced abortion.

## SUGGESTED STUDENT LEARNING ACTIVITIES

1. *VISIT* a Planned Parenthood clinic in your community.
   - *INTERVIEW* a nurse who is working there to determine his or her role at the clinic.
   - *DESCRIBE* the services offered by this agency and the environment in which they are provided.
   - *WRITE* a report that describes your findings and evaluates the effectiveness of Planned Parenthood in fulfilling its mission. Indicate any changes that you would propose that would enhance or improve the effectiveness of this agency's efforts. State the rationale for each change that you propose.

2. *DETERMINE* one cultural group's beliefs, values, and practices related to fertility and birth control. *DESCRIBE* how you would use this information when planning care for women representing that cultural group.

3. *VISIT* your local pharmacy, and assess the number and types of over-the-counter birth control preparations available.
   - *PREPARE* a report that summarizes your findings, including cost, degree of effectiveness claimed, readability of instructions, how to use effectively, and side effects.
   - *DESCRIBE* how you would use this information when teaching young women and men about birth control and the use of over-the-counter preparations for the purpose of controlling fertility and preventing the transmission of STDs.

4. *SEARCH* the literature for nursing research studies related to the topic of fertility control and nursing measures found to be effective in helping individuals and couples use methods effectively. *CHOOSE* one study, and complete a bibliography card that includes the following:
   - Hypothesis; research question
   - Summary of the methodology used and key findings
   - Reliability of the study and its findings
   - How the professional nurse could use the findings to enhance and improve health care
   - Suggestions for further research

5. *INTERVIEW* a nurse who provides care to women as they make the decision to have an induced abortion. *GATHER* information regarding the following:
   - The techniques used by the nurse to help women make a decision that is appropriate for them
   - Types of abortion procedures performed and the care management approach used before, during, and after each procedure
   - Measures used by the nurse to provide psychosocial and emotional support to women during and after the decision-making process
   - This nurse's reaction to the conflict between the right-to-life and pro-choice movements

6. *SEARCH* the nursing literature for articles related to support measures required by women as they make the decision to have an induced abortion, as they undergo the procedure, and as they recover after the procedure. *CHOOSE* one article, and complete a bibliography card that includes the following:
   - Summary of the article's key points
   - Your personal reaction to the ideas presented in the article
   - How the professional nurse can use the article's ideas to enhance and improve the quality of health care

## TOPICS FOR DISCUSSION

1. *Debate these issues:*
   - Should contraceptive methods be advertised in the print and electronic media?
   - Should contraceptive information, counseling, and products be available in high schools?
   - Should parents give consent before their adolescent children are informed and counseled about the prevention of pregnancy and STDs?
   - Should parents be informed when a pregnant adolescent seeks an induced abortion?

2. *Address this question:* What can nurses who work with women of childbearing age do to help these women achieve pregnancies that are planned rather than a "surprise" associated with improper use of birth control measures?

3. *Support this statement:* Nurses should be aware of their own views of sexuality and control of fertility before counseling others in the use of contraceptive methods.

4. *Consider these questions:* What are the ethical issues involved in the current debate over legislation concerning late pregnancy or partial-birth abortion? Who should be involved in and what criteria should be used when making the decision regarding this type of induced abortion?

# MERLIN PROJECT

Using the Chapter 9 section of MERLIN as a starting point, search the Internet for web sites designed to educate and support women as they make the decision to have or not have an induced abortion. Prepare a report that includes the following:

- List of the relevant sites found during the search
- Description of two of the sites that you found to be the most helpful and supportive regarding the following:
  - Sponsoring person(s), agency, and/or organization
  - Clarity, accuracy, accessibility (ease of use), value, and depth of information
  - Degree to which all available options are presented in an unbiased manner, thereby allowing a woman to make a decision that is best for her
  - Currency—frequency of sites updates
  - Variety of links to other relevant sites
  - Ability of persons visiting the site to obtain additional information and individualized support through such services as e-mail and chat rooms
- Discussion as to how the professional nurse could use these sites as a tool in helping a woman during the decision-making process regarding the course of action that she should take with regard to an unplanned pregnancy

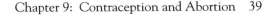

# Chapter

## 10    Infertility

## SUMMARY OF KEY CONCEPTS

Chapter 10 focuses on the concept of infertility, which is defined using contemporary views and incorporating incidence, causation, and psychosocial considerations. The couple is seen as a "biological unit" with the factors contributing to infertility having a male and/or female origin. The process of investigating female and male infertility is discussed in detail. A variety of tables and boxes summarizes this information, facilitating student learning and review. The most common tests and examinations currently in use are fully explained in terms of timing, purpose, method, effects on the client, and the required nursing care and support. Each factor (congenital or developmental, ovarian, tubal/peritoneal, uterine, vaginal-cervical, and seminal) implicated in infertility is described with an emphasis on treatment methods and prognosis for successful resolution of the problem.

The nursing process is used as the organizing framework for the care management of the couple experiencing infertility. The student is informed of the critical role that the nurse plays as a support person, advocate, teacher, and caregiver when working with clients who must cope with impaired ability to conceive and carry a child to term. Table 10-2 in the text suggests therapeutic nursing responses to a couple's grieving behaviors associated with impaired fertility. Nursing considerations to keep in mind when the couple conceives or does not conceive are included in the discussion. The student is introduced to the latest in reproductive alternatives including what they are and their financial, ethical, legal, and emotional impact. A plan of care illustrates the use of the nursing process in the care management of an infertile couple. Knowledge deficit and risk for ineffective individual and family coping are the nursing diagnoses developed.

## LEARNING OBJECTIVES

Define the key terms.
List common causes of infertility.
Discuss the psychologic impact of infertility.
List common diagnoses and treatments for infertility.
Identify reproductive alternatives for couples experiencing infertility.
Recognize the various ethical and legal considerations of infertility.
Identify topics for nursing research related to infertility.

# OUTLINE OF CHAPTER CONTENT WITH COURSE GUIDELINES

| CONTENT | GUIDELINE |
|---|:---:|
| Infertility | |
|   – Incidence | A |
|   – Misconceptions | B |
|   – Factors associated with infertility | |
|     – Female infertility | A |
|     – Male infertility | A |
| Care management | |
|   – Assessment and nursing diagnoses | A |
|     – Diagnostic tests | A |
|     – Assessment of female infertility | A |
|     – Assessment of male infertility | A |
|     – Assessment of the couple | A |
|   – Expected outcomes of care | A |
|   – Plan of care and interventions | A |
|     – Psychosocial | A |
|     – Nonmedical | A |
|     – Medical | A |
|     – Surgical | A |
|     – Reproductive alternatives | A |
|     – Adoption | A |
|   – Evaluation | A |
| Plan of care—infertility | A |

# TEACHING STRATEGIES

1. Use case studies to illustrate the impact of infertility on a couple.

2. Arrange for students to view a variety of infertility diagnostic tests and then report to the class the purpose, protocol, and impact on the client for each of the tests observed. Discuss nursing considerations for each test, including those designed to support the couple before, during, and after the test.

3. Divide students into groups, and assign each group to contact one of the following organizations and prepare a report regarding the purpose of and services provided by the organization chosen. (See Box 10-7 in the text.)
   • The American Society of Reproductive Medicine (ASRM)
   • RESOLVE, Inc.
   • International Counsel on Infertility Information Dissemination
   • American College of Obstetricians and Gynecologists (ACOG)
   Arrange for each student group to present their report to the class.

# SUGGESTED STUDENT LEARNING ACTIVITIES

1. *ATTEND* a meeting of a local chapter of RESOLVE, and interview one of its members. *WRITE* a report that includes the following:
   - Description of the formation of the organization and the chapter: who formed them, when, and why?
   - Purpose and mission of the organization and chapter
   - Process involved in publicizing the organization and chapter and encouraging people to join
   - Services offered to members of the organization and chapter and their families to help them find solutions to infertility and cope with the stressors involved in being infertile
   - Perceptions of the health care providers encountered and the health care system in terms of helping them during the diagnosis and treatment of infertility
   - Description of the meeting attended including the group dynamics observed
   - Suggestions for changes including additional services or activities; include rationale for changes

2. *WRITE* a three- to four-page paper concerning the ethical and legal issues surrounding the reproductive alternatives available to today's infertile couples. Include an annotated bibliography of references and Internet resources used in the preparation of the paper.

3. *SEARCH* the literature for nursing research studies related to impaired fertility—coping mechanisms, reactions, and nursing support measures found to be effective. Choose one study, and complete a bibliography card that includes the following:
   - Hypothesis; research question
   - Summary of the methodology used and key findings
   - Reliability of the study and its findings
   - Recommendations for further research
   - How the professional nurse can use the study's findings to enhance and improve the quality of health care provided to infertile couples

4. *INTERVIEW* a nurse who works with couples experiencing infertility. Write a summary of the information gathered during the interview, including the following:
   - Typical concerns expressed by the couples
   - Commonly used diagnostic procedures and treatment measures; nursing considerations for each
   - Support measures used by the nurse to assist couples as they react to their infertility and the diagnostic procedures and management strategies experienced
   - Strategies used to facilitate the couple's decision-making process
   - Reactions of couples to continuing inability to get pregnant or successful resolution of infertility with a pregnancy
   - Degree to which the nurse uses research findings to guide practice; areas of needed research identified by the nurse

# TOPICS FOR DISCUSSION

1. *Debate these issues:*
   - Should Medicaid cover the cost of infertility diagnosis and treatment for enrolled couples?
   - Should women who are unmarried or gay couples use currently available reproductive technology to have children?
   - Should reproductive technology be used to "engineer" the formation of children with specific genetic characteristics such as high intelligence, physical appearance, athletic ability, or special talents?
   - Should adoption and fertility technology (sperm and ovum donors) records be open so that children can trace their biologic parents?

2. *Address this question:* When should a woman make the decision to put her baby up for adoption, and how long should she have to change her mind? Support your response.

3. *Support this statement:* Nurses play a critical role in helping infertile couples make decisions about how to manage their infertility and to reach closure and acceptance if they cannot have children.

# MERLIN PROJECT

Search the Internet for sites designed to sell "eggs and sperm" so that individuals and couples can "design the child of their dreams" in terms of characteristics such as physical beauty and body appearance, intelligence, athletic ability, and talents. Write a report that includes the following:
- List of the sites
- Information about each site, including the following:
  - Sponsoring person(s), agency, or organization
  - Accessibility
  - Methods used to present the product or service offered
  - The process that an individual or couple needs to follow if wishing to take advantage of this service, including criteria, if any, that need to be met
  - Cost involved for the service
- Discussion of your views regarding this service and its use, including the ethical issues involved in the offering and use of these services and the long-term implications for the children created as a result of using this service

# Chapter 11

# Violence Against Women

## SUMMARY OF KEY CONCEPTS

The tragedy of violence against women is the subject of Chapter 11. The scope of the problem is described and the many myths surrounding violence against women are dispelled. The evolution of beliefs concerning the role of women and men in the reproductive process and sex role stereotyping are suggested as factors that have led to the escalation of violence against women. A discussion of the conceptual and cultural perspectives on violence is included. The three types of violence considered are battering, sexual abuse, and rape. Each type is viewed in terms of the adult female. The nursing process is used as the organizing framework for the care management of women who have been battered, sexually abused, or raped.

The discussion of battered women focuses on a number of concepts that foster student understanding of the problem and the people involved. Characteristics of the victim and the batterer are identified. Table 11-3 in the text presents both the myths and the facts regarding battering. Lenore Walker's landmark research provides the basis for the theory that battering is cyclical in nature, with three identifiable phases—tension-building state, acute battering incident, and kindness and contrite, loving behavior. The behaviors characteristic of each phase are identified, providing a focus for anticipatory guidance and teaching. The growing problem of battery during pregnancy is discussed. The student is informed of the cues indicative of an abusive relationship and of the approach to take when such a relationship is suspected, including variations from state to state in the legal mandate to report domestic violence.

Guidelines for the development of a helping relationship follow the ABCDES framework of sensitive nursing interventions suggested by Holtz and Furness (1993). The importance of anticipatory guidance is emphasized. A plan of care illustrates the use of the nursing process for the care management of a battered woman. The nursing diagnoses of risk for self-directed violence and social isolation are considered.

Sexual abuse focuses on the effects that it can have on the survivors of sexual abuse and assault, including incest and rape. Posttraumatic stress disorder, sexual dysfunction, depression, anxiety, and substance abuse are identified as major outcomes of sexual abuse. Characteristic behaviors of posttraumatic stress disorder are described, providing the student with the cues to look for that suggest a history of sexual abuse. Activities that can help survivors deal with the past trauma are identified and include participating in a recovery group, reducing isolation, improving self-esteem, and developing effective coping mechanisms.

A discussion of rape concludes the chapter. Explanation of the meaning of rape includes a discussion of the different types of rape. The three phases of rape-trauma syndrome are described. Assessment focuses on the need to obtain and preserve evidence as well as meet the physical, psychosocial, and emotional needs of the raped woman. Box 11-3 in the text outlines an adult sexual assault protocol. Care of the rape survivor is presented on three levels—immediate care, discharge process, and postdischarge follow-up.

## LEARNING OBJECTIVES

Define the key terms.
Describe the historic events that have perpetuated violence against women.
Contrast the theoretic premises underlying the victimization of women.
Discuss the incidence of battering in pregnant women.
Explain the cycle of violence and its use in assessment and intervention for battered women.
Develop a plan of care for a battered woman.
Identify behaviors associated with women who experienced sexual assault as children.
Discuss the nursing care for a survivor of childhood sexual abuse.
Discuss the dynamics of rape.
Describe the rape-trauma syndrome.
Develop a nursing plan of care for a woman in the acute phase of rape-trauma syndrome.
Describe the resources available to women experiencing abuse.
Identify topics of nursing research related to violence against women.

## OUTLINE OF CHAPTER CONTENT WITH COURSE GUIDELINES

| CONTENT | GUIDELINE |
|---|---|
| Historic perspective | B |
| Conceptual perspectives on violence | |
|   – Psychologic perspective | A |
|   – Sociological view | A |
|   – Biologic factors | A |
|   – Feminist perspective | A |
| Cultural considerations | A |
| Battered women | |
|   – Characteristics of women in battering relationships | A |
|   – Myths about battered women | A |
|   – Cycle of violence | A |
|   – Battery during pregnancy | A |
|   – Care management | A |
|   – Prevention | A |
|   – Plan of care—battered woman | A |
| Sexual abuse | A |
|   – Care management | A |
| Rape | A |
|   – Dynamics of rape | A |
|   – Rape-trauma syndrome | A |
|   – Care management | A |

# TEACHING STRATEGIES

1. Assign students to view a film that depicts a situation of violence against a woman. Involve the students in a discussion of the film that they viewed, including how the woman dealt with the violence experienced, how her support system reacted to the violence and to what degree they were able to offer her support, and how the community in which the woman lived provided the services needed. Use this discussion to encourage students to share their views regarding violence against women—their concept of the meaning of violence, the characteristics of women who experience violence and the persons who commit the violence, and the role of the nurse in prevention of violence and in the care of survivors.

2. Identify the agencies in your community that are available to aid women who face violence in their lives. Invite one or more of the directors from these agencies to discuss the approaches that they use to assist women and their children when they face violence.

3. Use case studies to illustrate the impact that battery, rape, and sexual abuse can have on women, their families, and the community.

4. Present statistical data that illustrates the prevalence of violence against women in our society in terms of the women's characteristics (e.g., age, race, education, and socioeconomic status). Compare the incidence of violence in your community, state, and the nation as a whole.

5. Divide students into groups. Assign each group to contact one of the resources for violence against women in Box 11-5 to determine the role that each plays in preventing violence and helping women who are the victims of violence. Provide time for each group to present their findings to the class. Involve all students in a discussion about how nurses working with battered and abused women can use these resources to enhance the quality and effectiveness of their care.

# SUGGESTED STUDENT LEARNING ACTIVITIES

1. *ASSESS* your community with respect to the incidence of violence against women and the services provided to support them.
   - *PREPARE* a report that includes the following:
     - Statistical data related to the incidence of battery, sexual assault, and abuse committed against women; data should reflect general incidence as well as incidence according to population groups
     - Comparison of your community's statistical picture with that of your state and the nation
     - Types and availability of support services for women who are victims of violence; include the services designed to teach women self-defensive measures
   - *COMPILE* this information into a pamphlet that could be distributed to women, giving them access to services for which they may have need.

2. *PREPARE* a three- to four-page report on the growing problem of violence against pregnant women. *DISCUSS* the incidence, risk factors, precipitating factors, consequences, and solutions and interventions. *INCLUDE* a bibliography of the references used in the preparation of the report.

3. *VISIT* a shelter for battered women in your community.
   - *INTERVIEW* the director of the shelter or one of the care providers. *GATHER* information concerning the following:
     - Services provided
     - Funding and payment
     - Rewards and frustrations of his or her role
     - Numbers and characteristics of the women who come for help
     - The respondent's view of the role that nurses should play in supporting the efforts of the shelter
   - *ASSESS* the environment of the shelter. To what degree does it meet the goal of providing comfort and protection for the battered woman and her children?
   - *SUGGEST* changes regarding the manner in which existing services are offered and the need for additional services; provide a rationale for each of your suggestions.

4. *SEARCH* the nursing literature for articles related to violence against women and the support measures that they require. *CHOOSE* one article, and complete a bibliography card that includes the following:
   - Summary of the article's key points
   - Personal reaction to the ideas presented in the article
   - How the professional nurse could use the information to enhance and improve health care

5. *VISIT* a rape trauma center in your community.
   - *INTERVIEW* the director of the center or one of the counselors. *GATHER* information concerning the following:
     - Services provided
     - Funding and payment
     - Rewards and frustration of his or her role
     - Numbers and characteristics of the women who come to the center for help
     - The respondent's view of the role that nurses should play in supporting the efforts of the center
   - *ASSESS* the environment of the center. To what degree does it meet the goal of helping women cope with the effects of a rape experience?
   - *SUGGEST* changes regarding the manner in which existing services are offered and the need for additional services; provide a rationale for each of your suggestions.

## TOPICS FOR DISCUSSION

1. *Discuss these questions:* What would you do if you suspect that one of your clients is being battered by her spouse or partner? What would you do if you suspect that a family member or friend is being abused?

2. *Support this statement:* The nursing profession should play an active role in preventing and reducing the violence that occurs against women.

3. *Consider this question:* Why are women so often the victims of violence and sexual abuse?

# MERLIN PROJECT

Use the Chapter 11 section of MERLIN as a starting point to search the Internet for web sites designed to provide information and support to women who have experienced sexual abuse or assault. Prepare a report that includes the following:

- List of sites
- Description of two sites that you found to be the most helpful in terms of the following:
  - Sponsoring person(s), agency, or organization
  - Clarity, accuracy, accessibility (ease of use), value, and depth of the information provided
  - Nature and quality of the support provided
  - Currency—frequency of site updates
  - Variety of links to other relevant web sites
  - Ability of persons visiting the site to obtain additional information and individualized support through services such as e-mail and chat rooms; manner in which confidentiality is protected
- Discussion about how the nurse could use these sites to inform and support women who have experienced sexual abuse or assault

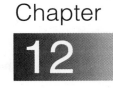

# Chapter
## 12
# Problems of the Breast

## SUMMARY OF KEY CONCEPTS

Chapter 12 introduces the student to health problems related to the breast, including benign and malignant tumors. Incidence, risk factors, clinical manifestations and diagnosis, therapeutic management, emotional impact, and nursing considerations are described. The nursing process is incorporated throughout the chapter as a guiding framework for the care management required by women diagnosed with breast problems.

The chapter begins with a definition of the key terms used in the text, namely neoplasm and benign and malignant tumors. Fibrocystic change is highlighted in the discussion of benign conditions of the breast. Benign breast conditions are described in terms of etiology, clinical manifestations, diagnosis, and therapeutic management. Care management of benign conditions of the breast uses a nursing process approach. Assessment stresses the importance of identifying risk factors for breast disorders, monitoring the breast condition, and documenting the woman's lifestyle habits, use of oral contraceptives, performance of breast self-examination (BSE), and emotional status. Highlighted nursing actions include demonstrating and stressing the importance of regular BSE and identifying the intervals and facets of regular breast screening, including professional breast examination and mammography. The importance of encouraging verbalization of fears and concerns, teaching regarding the components of the treatment regimen, including pain relief measures, referring women to support groups, and providing written educational materials is stressed.

The student is provided with a detailed discussion of breast carcinoma that begins with an overview of its incidence in the United States and the risk factors that are implicated in making a woman more vulnerable to this disease. The pathophysiology of breast cancer is described along with the typical clinical manifestations noted during physical examination and diagnostic testing. The typical procedure to reach a definitive diagnosis, define the prognosis, and determine the most advantageous course of treatment and the emotional impact that the diagnosis can have on both the woman and her family is described. A variety of treatment approaches—surgery and reconstruction, radiation, and adjuvant therapy using hormones and/or chemotherapy—are explained. Care management focuses on meeting the needs of a woman undergoing a modified radical mastectomy. Specific nursing measures are identified for the preoperative, immediate postoperative, and postdischarge periods. A plan of care illustrates the use of the nursing process in the care management of a postmenopausal woman with breast cancer. The nursing diagnoses of pain, risk for infection, and body image disturbance are developed.

# LEARNING OBJECTIVES

Define the key terms.

Discuss the pathophysiology of selected benign breast conditions and malignant neoplasms of the breasts found in women.

Discuss the emotional effect of benign and malignant neoplasms.

Develop a nursing plan of care for the woman with a lump in her breast.

Identify critical elements for teaching clients with selected procedures and medical-surgical management of benign or malignant neoplasms of the breast.

Identify topics for nursing research related to breast cancer.

# OUTLINE OF CHAPTER CONTENT WITH COURSE GUIDELINES

| CONTENT | GUIDELINE |
|---|---|
| Benign conditions of the breast | |
| – Fibrocystic changes | A |
| – Fibroadenomas | A |
| – Lipomas | A |
| – Mammary duct ectasia | B |
| – Intraductal papilloma | B |
| – Care management | A |
| Malignant conditions of the breast | |
| – Etiology | A |
| – Pathophysiology | A |
| – Clinical manifestations and diagnosis | A |
| – Prognosis | A |
| – Therapeutic management | A |
| – Surgery | A |
| – Breast reconstruction | A |
| – Radiation therapy | A |
| – Adjuvant therapy | A |
| Care management | |
| – Assessment and nursing diagnoses | A |
| – Expected outcomes of care | A |
| – Plan of care and interventions | A |
| – Emotional support after diagnosis | A |
| – Preoperative care | A |
| – Immediate postoperative care | A |
| – Discharge planning and follow-up care | A |
| – Evaluation | A |
| Plan of care | A |

# TEACHING STRATEGIES

1. Use biostatistical data to illustrate the scope of breast cancer in the United States and in selected countries worldwide. Present information related to who gets cancer, regions in the United States where incidence is high or low, and the most common treatment approaches used and their effectiveness.

2. Encourage students to discuss feelings regarding breast disorders including breast cancer and the impact that diagnosis and treatment can have on a woman's lifestyle, relationships, and body image.

3. Use case studies to describe breast cancer diagnosis and treatment and to illustrate the impact that a diagnosis of breast cancer can have on a woman and her family.

4. Invite women who have been treated for breast cancer to discuss how their cancer was discovered, the treatment approaches that they considered and chose, including how the decision was made, and the support measures from health care professionals and family that they found to be the most and least helpful.

5. Identify alternative therapies that have been found to be effective in treating the signs and symptoms that women with breast cancer experience as a result of the cancer and its medical treatment.

6. Assign students to survey the media (print, TV, radio) for advertisements and programs related to breast cancer—early detection and treatment. Involve students in a discussion of the impact that these presentations have had on their own views of breast cancer and the views of family and friends.

# SUGGESTED STUDENT LEARNING ACTIVITIES

1. *INTERVIEW* a "Reach for Recovery" volunteer. *WRITE* a report that describes the information gathered during the interview, including the following:
   - How the volunteer views her role during the process of adjustment by a woman and her partner and family to the impact of breast cancer and treatment
   - Services offered by this organization and the cost, availability, and when they are provided
   - The referral process that should be followed
   - How women, their partners, and their families react to the services offered
   - The role that nurses can play in fostering the efforts of this vital service

2. *SEARCH* the literature for nursing research studies related to women's reactions to cancer of the breast and its treatment and the nursing measures found to be effective in supporting these women and their families. *CHOOSE* one study, and complete a bibliography card that includes the following:
   - Hypothesis; research question
   - Summary of the methodology used and key findings
   - Reliability of the study and its findings
   - Recommendations for further research
   - How the professional nurse could use the findings to enhance and improve health care

3. *DESIGN* a pamphlet that can be given to a woman who has been diagnosed with breast cancer. The pamphlet should present information related to the effects of breast cancer, diagnostic procedures, and options for treatment, including lumpectomy, mastectomy, reconstruction, radiation, and chemotherapy. Measures to facilitate healing and recovery should be described, and support groups available in the community should be identified. Create an annotated bibliography of appropriate references and a list of resource available on the Internet.

4. *WRITE* a three- to four-page report on the role of alternative therapies as an adjunct to medical regimens for the treatment of breast cancer. Your report should include the following:
   - Description of methods found to be effective, the basis for the effectiveness, research findings regarding effectiveness if available, and the qualifications of those who developed the method or recommend its use
   - How you would use this information with women experiencing the effects of breast cancer and its treatment
   - An annotated bibliography of references used, including Internet resources

5. *INTERVIEW* a woman who has been diagnosed and treated for breast cancer.
   - *GATHER* information regarding the following:
     - The woman's description of the impact that breast cancer has had on her health and well-being and on her partner and family
     - Coping mechanisms that the woman and her partner and family used and are using to deal with the stressors encountered as a result of the diagnosis and treatment for breast cancer
     - The support measures, persons, and services that she and her partner and family found helpful and those that they found to be lacking or not helpful
     - Her impressions of the impact that the health care system and health care providers had on her health and well-being during the diagnosis and treatment for breast cancer
   - *DESCRIBE* how you would use this information to plan care that is effective not only related to the woman's physical needs but also related to the woman, her partner, and family's psychosocial and emotional needs. *INDICATE* how you would use this information to care for other women with this diagnosis.

## TOPICS FOR DISCUSSION

1. *Consider these questions:* How has society's fascination with the female breasts affected the response of women to the diagnosis and treatment for breast cancer? How has it affected the woman's partner and the couple's sexual relationship?

2. *Support this statement:* Nurses play an essential role in helping women and their partners cope effectively with the diagnosis and treatment for breast cancer.

3. *Address this question:* Should women try alternative therapies as one means of treating breast cancer?

4. *Debate these issues:*
   - Is it good, sensible business or is it unethical for insurance companies to refuse payment for experimental breast cancer treatments that have demonstrated some success but the success thus far is limited?
   - Outpatient mastectomies are a safe, cost-effective approach to breast cancer treatment.

## MERLIN PROJECT

Use MERLIN to assist you in searching the medical literature for journal articles related to treatment measures for breast cancer that have proven effectiveness and treatment measures that are still in the experimental stage, showing promise but not yet proven to be effective.
   - Create an annotated bibliography composed of five journal references, two that are related to experimental treatments.
   - Choose one journal article, and complete a bibliography card that includes the following:
     - Summary of the article's key points
     - Personal reaction to the ideas presented in the article
     - How you would use the information in the article to help a woman and her family make an informed decision regarding breast cancer treatments

# Chapter

## 13

# Structural Disorders and Neoplasms of the Reproductive System

## SUMMARY OF KEY CONCEPTS

Chapter 13 introduces the student to the health problems related to structural disorders and reproductive neoplasms, both benign and malignant. Incidence, etiology, risk factors, clinical manifestations and diagnosis, therapeutic management, emotional impact, and nursing considerations are described. The nursing process is incorporated throughout the chapter as a guiding framework for the care management required by women diagnosed with reproductive system problems. A variety of tables and boxes serve to emphasize and summarize important content for the student.

Alterations in pelvic support, urinary incontinence, and genital fistulas are the focus for the discussion concerning structural disorders of the reproductive tract. A variety of etiologic factors are identified, including trauma to the reproductive tract associated with childbirth, surgery and treatment, health problems such as infection and congenital anomalies, and the process of aging. Clinical manifestations and treatment approaches are included for each disorder. A nursing process approach is used as the organizing framework for the discussion of care management of women experiencing structural disorders of the reproductive tract.

The chapter continues with an extensive discussion of reproductive system neoplasms, including those of uterine, cervical, tubal, vaginal, vulvar, and ovarian origin. Leiomyomas (fibroid tumors), uterine polyps, ovarian cysts, and Bartholin cysts are presented as examples of benign reproductive system neoplasms. Clinical manifestations are described, as well as the treatment options available. The discussion of endometrial cancer focuses on hysterectomy as a treatment approach, and the discussion of cervical carcinoma focuses on a variety of treatment options with the choice dependent upon the invasiveness of the lesion. Special attention is paid to radiation therapy, both external and internal. An overview of the needs of women faced with the diagnosis of vulvar or ovarian cancer is presented. The impact on client and family of the poor prognosis that often accompanies a diagnosis of ovarian cancer is viewed in terms of the stages described by Kübler-Ross in her work on death and dying. A plan of care illustrates the use of the nursing process for the care management of a woman having a hysterectomy for endometrial cancer. Anxiety, fear, pain, risk for infection, body image disturbance, and risk for sexual dysfunction are the nursing diagnoses developed.

Cancer and pregnancy is the major focus of the final section of this chapter. The most frequently occurring types of cancer are reviewed, along with the issues that must be considered when the mode of treatment is determined, including risk to the fetus, timing of treatment, and the effect of delay on the woman's prognosis. Pregnancy after cancer treatment also is discussed. The chapter concludes with an overview of gestational trophoblastic disease. Etiology, risk factors, clinical manifestations, and typical care management approaches are explained.

## LEARNING OBJECTIVES

Define the key terms.
Describe the various structural disorders of the uterus and vagina.
Discuss the pathophysiology of selected benign and malignant neoplasms of the female reproductive tract.
Identify the common medical and surgical therapies for selected conditions.
Discuss the emotional impact of benign and malignant neoplasms.
Develop a nursing plan of care for a woman with endometrial cancer who has had a hysterectomy.
Explain diagnostic procedures in client-centered terms.
Explain treatments for preinvasive and invasive conditions.
Review health-promoting behaviors that reduce cancer risk.
Assess the impact of benign and malignant neoplasms on pregnancy.
Discuss the development and sequelae of gestational trophoblastic neoplasia.
Identify critical elements for teaching clients with selected benign or malignant neoplasms.
Identify topics for nursing research related to gynecologic neoplasia.

## OUTLINE OF CHAPTER CONTENT WITH COURSE GUIDELINES

| CONTENT | GUIDELINE |
|---|:---:|
| Structural disorders of the uterus and vagina | A |
| – Alterations in pelvic support | A |
| – Urinary incontinence | A |
| – Genital fistulas | A |
| – Care management | A |
| Benign neoplasms | A |
| – Ovarian cysts | A |
| – Uterine neoplasms | A |
| – Care management | A |
| – Assessment and nursing diagnoses | A |
| – Expected outcomes of care | A |
| – Plan of care and interventions | A |
| – Medical management | A |
| – Surgical management | A |
| – Preoperative care | A |
| – Postoperative care | A |
| – Discharge planning and teaching | A |
| – Evaluation | A |

*continued*

| CONTENT | GUIDELINE |
|---|:---:|
| – Vulvar neoplasms | B |
| Malignant neoplasms | A |
|   – Cancer of the endometrium | A |
|     – Incidence and etiology | A |
|     – Care management | A |
|       – Assessment and nursing diagnoses | A |
|       – Expected outcomes of care | A |
|       – Plan of care and interventions | A |
|         – Therapeutic management | A |
|         – Nursing care | A |
|         – Preoperative care | A |
|         – Postoperative care | A |
|         – Discharge planning and teaching | A |
|       – Evaluation | A |
|       – Plan of care | A |
|   – Ovarian cancer | A |
|     – Incidence and etiology | A |
|     – Clinical manifestation and diagnosis | A |
|     – Collaborative care | A |
|     – Nursing implications | A |
|   – Cancer of the cervix | A |
|     – Incidence and etiology | A |
|     – Clinical manifestations and diagnosis | A |
|     – Care management | A |
|       – Assessment and nursing diagnoses | A |
|       – Expected outcomes of care | A |
|       – Plan of care and interventions | A |
|         – Preinvasive lesions | A |
|         – Invasive cancer of the cervix | A |
|         – Recurrent and advanced cancer of the cervix | A |
|         – Nursing management | A |
|           – External radiation therapy | A |
|           – Internal radiation therapy | A |
|           – Pelvic exenteration | A |
|     – Evaluation | A |
| Other pelvic malignancies | |
|   – Cancer of the vulva | B |
|   – Cancer of the vagina | B |
|   – Cancer of the uterine tubes | B |
| Cancer and pregnancy | C |
|   – Types | C |
|   – Cancer therapy and pregnancy | C |
|   – Pregnancy after cancer treatment | C |
| Gestational trophoblastic disease | C |

# TEACHING STRATEGIES

1. Use biostatistical data to illustrate the scope of selected structural disorders and neoplasms of the reproductive system. Consider incidence of the disorders in terms of a woman's age and factors in her health history that could be involved in the etiology of these reproductive system disorders.

2. Discuss the care management of women experiencing cancer of the endometrium, cervix, and ovary using a variety of case studies. Involve students in the discussion by encouraging them to share client care situations that they have encountered related to cancer of the reproductive system.

3. Review the products that are available to help women cope with problems that they encounter as a result of structural disorders of the reproductive tract. Bring samples of these products to class. Involve students in a discussion regarding the impact that structural disorders and the need to use these products can have on a woman's lifestyle, including relationships with others. Describe support measures nurses can use to help women cope in a positive manner.

4. Identify health care agencies and services in your community designed to support and care for women with reproductive system disorders.

5. Organize a panel of women (and their partners if possible) who have experienced a variety of treatments for reproductive tract cancer, including surgery, radiation, chemotherapy, and complementary therapies, to discuss the impact that the cancer and treatment process had on their physical and emotional well-being. Encourage the women to share their perceptions of the health care that they received, especially from nurses—what support measures were helpful, what support measures were ineffective, and what support measures that they wish were offered.

6. Invite a hospice nurse to discuss the approach that he or she uses to support women who are dying of cancer and their families. Encourage students to share their feelings regarding death and caring for clients who are dying.

# SUGGESTED STUDENT LEARNING ACTIVITIES

1. *SEARCH* the literature for nursing research studies related to women's reactions to cancer of the reproductive tract and the treatment, including hysterectomy, and the nursing measures found to be effective in supporting these women and their families. *CHOOSE* one study, and complete a bibliography card that includes the following:
   - Hypothesis; research question
   - Summary of the methodology used and key findings
   - Reliability of the study and its findings
   - Recommendations for further research
   - How the professional nurse could use the findings to enhance and improve health care

2. *DEVELOP* a pamphlet that can be given to a woman who is recovering from an abdominal hysterectomy and bilateral salpingo-oophorectomy. The pamphlet should present information related to the effects of the surgery and treatment regimen, including alterations in physical status, emotions, and sexuality. Measures designed to facilitate healing and recovery should be emphasized. Create an annotated bibliography of appropriate references and a list of relevant Internet resources.

3. *WRITE* a three- to four-page report on the role of alternative therapies as a complement to medical regimens for the treatment of structural disorders and neoplasms of the reproductive system. Your report should include the following:
   - Description of methods found to be effective, the basis for the effectiveness, research findings regarding effectiveness if available, and the qualifications of those who developed the method or recommend its use
   - How you would use this information with women experiencing the effects of reproductive system problems and their treatment
   - An annotated bibliography of references used

4. *INTERVIEW* a woman who has been diagnosed and treated for invasive cervical cancer that requires hysterectomy and/or radiation therapy.
   - *GATHER* information regarding the following:
     - The woman's description of the impact that cervical cancer has had on her health and well-being and on her partner and family
     - Coping mechanisms that the woman and her partner and family used to deal with the stressors encountered as a result of the diagnosis of and treatment for cervical cancer
     - The support measures, persons, and services that she and her partner and family found helpful and those that she found to be lacking or not helpful
     - Her impressions of the impact that the health care system and health care providers had on her health and well-being during the diagnosis of and treatment for cervical cancer
   - *DESCRIBE* how you would use this information to plan care that is effective not only related to the woman's physical needs but also related to the woman, her partner, and family's psychosocial and emotional needs. Discuss how you would use this information when caring for other women with cervical cancer and their families.

## TOPICS FOR DISCUSSION

1. *Support this statement:* Nurses play a critical role in helping women and their partners cope effectively with the effects of abdominal hysterectomy, especially those related to sexuality and a woman's image as a female.

2. *Debate the issue:* Women should try alternative therapies as one means of treating ovarian cancer and coping with the effects of the cancer and its treatment.

3. *Consider these questions:*
   - What measures can nurses use to reduce the incidence of invasive cervical cancer?
   - How can nurses help a woman who is dying of ovarian cancer and her family work through the process of death and dying as defined by Elizabeth Kübler-Ross?
   - What can nurses do to help women deal with the embarrassment that they experience regarding the effects of stress incontinence and genital fistulas?

## MERLIN PROJECT

Organize students into three groups. Assign each group to use MERLIN as a starting point for an Internet search for resources that are designed to address the informational and support needs of women experiencing one of the following: incontinence, hysterectomy, and the physical and emotional effects of cancer of the reproductive tract and its treatment. Provide class or seminar time for each group to present its findings to the class. Require each group to prepare an annotated list of the most valuable Internet resources found in its search.

Chapter 13: Structural Disorders and Neoplasms of the Reproductive System    59

# Chapter 14

# Conception, Fetal Development, and Genetics

## SUMMARY OF KEY CONCEPTS

Chapter 14 introduces the student to the basic principles of human genetics, the process of conception and implantation, the development of the embryo and fetus, and the factors that can affect fetal development. A human development table and many illustrations clarify and summarize complex content.

A discussion of the stages of prenatal development (zygote, embryo, and fetus) follows a systems approach. The critical structures that support this development, namely the amniotic membranes and fluid, the yolk sac, the umbilical cord, and the placenta, are included in the discussion. An overview of multifetal pregnancies is included with an emphasis on twinning, both dizygotic and monozygotic.

The biologic basis of inheritance is described in terms of cell division, gametogenesis, and the function of genes and chromosomes. Chromosomal abnormalities are explored. A description of the patterns of genetic transmission includes the concepts of multifactorial and unifactorial inheritance. Nongenetic factors such as teratogens and their effect on the developing fetus are briefly discussed.

The chapter concludes by introducing the student to the concept of genetic counseling, including its purposes and services. A discussion of the management of genetic disorders focuses on the estimation and interpretation of risk and the ethical dimensions of genetic screening. The role of the nurse in genetic counseling is described with an emphasis on the nurse's importance in follow-up care and emotional support.

## LEARNING OBJECTIVES

Define the key terms.
Summarize the process of fertilization.
Explain basic principles of genetics.
Describe the development, structure, and functions of the placenta.
Describe the composition and functions of the amniotic fluid.
Identify three organs or tissues arising from each of the three primary germ layers.
Summarize the significant changes in growth and development of the embryo and fetus.
Identify the potential effects of teratogens during vulnerable periods of embryonic and fetal development.

Describe the Human Genome Project.

Describe the nurse's role in genetic counseling.

Examine ethical dimensions of genetic screening.

Identify topics for nursing research related to conception, fetal development, and genetics.

## OUTLINE OF CHAPTER CONTENT WITH COURSE GUIDELINES

| CONTENT | GUIDELINE |
|---|:---:|
| Conception | A |
| – Cell division | B |
| – Gametogenesis | B |
| – Fertilization | A |
| – Implantation | A |
| The embryo and fetus | A |
| – Primary germ layers | B |
| – Development of the embryo | B |
| – Membranes | A |
| – Amniotic fluid | A |
| – Yolk sac | B |
| – Umbilical cord | A |
| – Placenta—structure and functions | A |
| Fetal maturation | A |
| – Viability | A |
| – Circulatory system | A |
| – Hematopoietic system | B |
| – Hepatic system | B |
| – Gastrointestinal system | B |
| – Respiratory system | A |
| – Renal system | B |
| – Neurologic system | A |
| – Sensory awareness | B |
| – Endocrine system | B |
| – Reproductive system | B |
| – Immunological system | B |
| – Musculoskeletal system | B |
| – Integumentary system | B |
| Multifetal pregnancy | A |
| Nongenetic factors influencing development | A |
| Genetics and genetic counseling | A |
| – Importance of genetics in maternity care | A |
| – Genetic transmission | A |
| – Genes and chromosomes | A |
| – Chromosomal abnormalities | A |
| – Patterns of genetic transmission | A |

*continued*

| CONTENT | GUIDELINE |
|---|---|
| – Multifactorial inheritance | A |
| – Unifactorial inheritance | A |
| – Human Genome Project | B |
| Genetic counseling | A |
| – Purposes of genetic counseling | A |
| – Genetic counseling services | A |
| – Ethical considerations | A |
| – Management of genetic disorders | A |
| – Role of the nurse in genetic counseling | A |
| – Ethical dimensions of genetic screening | A |

## TEACHING STRATEGIES

1. Illustrate genetic concepts using a variety of diagrams and case studies that describe patterns of genetic transmission. Include relevant clinical experiences in the class discussion.

2. Use the work of Lennart Nilsson, including the book *A Child Is Born* (1990, Delacort Press) and the video *The Miracle of Life* (1983), to facilitate student understanding of the process of growth and development from conception to birth.

3. Arrange for students to view and examine a placenta, umbilical cord, and amniotic fluid and membranes after a birth that they have observed.

4. Invite a nurse working in a prenatal care setting to discuss how pregnant women and their families are educated regarding fetal development and the woman and family's role in ensuring fetal health and well-being.

5. Use media presentations collected from television programs, radio, magazines, and newspapers to identify current teratogens of concern. Involve the students in creating approaches that the nursing profession could use to alert the public of the danger and the need to avoid exposure.

6. Invite a nurse whose major role involves genetic counseling to discuss the impact that a diagnosis of an inherited disorder has on a couple and their family. Specific therapeutic communication and counseling techniques and emotional support measures used by the nurse should be included in the discussion.

7. Identify support groups and community services available to families experiencing genetic or congenital disorders.

## SUGGESTED STUDENT LEARNING ACTIVITIES

1. *CREATE* a chart that describes fetal development. The chart should be designed so that it can be used by a nurse who teaches pregnant women and their families.

2. COLLECT media presentations (e.g., newspapers, magazines, videos, and television and radio programs) that discuss teratogens and their impact on fertility and fetal development. DISCUSS how you could utilize this information when providing health care and guidance for women and men during their childbearing years.

3. INTERVIEW a nurse working in genetic counseling. PREPARE a report that includes the nurse's responses to the following:
   • Views regarding the purpose of genetic counseling and the role of the nurse as a genetic counselor
   • Philosophy of life and nursing and how each influenced his or her approach to genetic counseling and meeting the needs of couples seeking genetic counseling and management of a diagnosed genetic disorder
   • Description of the emotional needs of couples seeking genetic counseling and the support measures that the nurse has found to be most effective
   • Views regarding conducting research and using research findings to enhance his or her practice

4. SEARCH the nursing literature for articles related to genetic counseling, parental responses to a diagnosis of a congenital anomaly or genetic disorder, and the effects of teratogens on reproduction. CHOOSE one article, and complete a bibliography card that includes the following:
   • Summary of the article's key points
   • Personal reaction to the ideas presented in this article
   • How the professional nurse can use the article's ideas to enhance and improve the quality of health care

5. INTERVIEW a member of a support group for parents of children born with specific congenital malformations or genetic disorders (i.e., Down syndrome and spina bifida), and ATTEND one meeting. PREPARE a report that includes the following:
   • Description of the formation of the group: who formed the group, when, and why
   • Purpose and mission of the group
   • Process involved in publicizing the group and encouraging people to join
   • Services offered to the members of the group, their affected children, and other family members to help them cope with the effects of the congenital malformation or genetic disorder
   • Description of the meeting including the group dynamics observed
   • Changes that you would propose to enhance the purpose and mission of the group; state the rationale for each change that you propose

## TOPICS FOR DISCUSSION

1. *Consider this question:* Why is it important for nurses to examine their own beliefs, values, and attitudes regarding life, death, health, and well-being before becoming involved in genetic counseling?

2. *Consider this question:* Is genetic counseling relevant for couples who are pro-life?

3. *Support this statement:* A nurse working in prenatal health care should inform the public, especially childbearing families, about teratogens and their harmful effects.

4. *Consider this ethical dilemma:* Today genetic testing methods can detect the presence of a defective gene before pregnancy or a genetic or congenital disorder early in pregnancy. As a result, the potential exists to completely eliminate the occurrence of certain health problems such as Down syndrome and dwarfism. What are the moral and ethical ramifications of being able to encourage or even mandate persons with certain defects not to have children or to have an abortion if the defect already exists in their fetus?

# MERLIN PROJECT

Using a genetic or congenital disorder as a key word (e.g., Down syndrome, spina bifida, hemophilia), search the Internet for sites designed to inform and support families who are caring for a person (child or adult) with this disorder. Prepare a report that includes the following:

- List of sites found in your search
- Description of two of the sites in terms of the following:
  - Sponsoring person(s), agency, organization
  - Clarity, accuracy, accessibility (ease of use), value, and depth of information provided
  - Currency—frequency of site updates
  - Variety of relevant links to other sites
  - Ability of persons visiting the site to obtain additional information and individualized support through such services as e-mail and chat rooms
- Discussion of how the professional nurse working with families of a child or adult with the genetic or congenital disorder could use Internet resources such as those that you found to help these families cope in an effective manner and obtain the services needed by the affected family member

Chapter

# 15 Anatomy and Physiology of Pregnancy

## SUMMARY OF KEY CONCEPTS

Chapter 15 introduces the student to the expected physical adaptations that take place during pregnancy. A system-by-system approach is used to present the material clearly and concisely. Emphasis is placed on facilitating the student's ability to distinguish expected changes from those that would indicate an ineffective adaptation to pregnancy. The physiologic and mechanical bases for the adaptations to pregnancy are explored. The terms related to the concepts of gravidity and parity are defined. A four- and five-digit system used to describe a woman's history with regard to pregnancies and their outcome is included.

A discussion of pregnancy tests identifies not only the types of tests currently available but also the time frame involved with each test and its sensitivity. An overview of factors to consider when results of pregnancy tests are interpreted is included as part of the discussion.

## LEARNING OBJECTIVES

Define the key terms.
Determine gravidity and parity using the five- and four-digit systems.
Describe the various types of pregnancy tests.
Explain the expected maternal anatomic and physiologic adaptations to pregnancy.
Differentiate among presumptive, probable, and positive signs of pregnancy.
Identify the maternal hormones produced during pregnancy, their target organs, and their major effects on pregnancy.
Compare the characteristics of the abdomen, vulva, and cervix of the nullipara and multipara.
Identify topics for nursing research related to the anatomy and physiology of pregnancy.

# OUTLINE OF CHAPTER CONTENT WITH COURSE GUIDELINES

| CONTENT | GUIDELINE |
|---|:---:|
| Gravidity and parity | A |
| Pregnancy tests | A |
| Adaptations to pregnancy | A |
|   – Signs of pregnancy | A |
|   – Reproductive system and breasts | A |
|     – Uterus | A |
|     – Vagina and vulva | A |
|     – Breasts | A |
|   – General body systems | A |
|     – Cardiovascular system | A |
|     – Respiratory system | A |
|       – Basal metabolic rate | A |
|       – Acid-base balance | A |
|     – Renal system | A |
|       – Fluid and electrolyte balance | A |
|     – Integumentary system | A |
|     – Musculoskeletal system | A |
|     – Neurologic system | A |
|     – Gastrointestinal system | A |
|     – Endocrine system | A |

## TEACHING STRATEGIES

1. Explain gravidity and parity determinations by using case studies and obstetric histories of the clients for whom the students cared for in the clinical setting.

2. Bring to class a variety of pregnancy tests currently available for purchase by women. Divide the students into groups, and have each group assess one of the tests and report back to the class the results of their assessment of the assigned test in terms of cost, clarity of instructions, ease and convenience of use, and stated reliability of results. Involve students in the development of strategies to assist women to use the test if they have difficulty reading or are unable to understand the English language.

3. Illustrate each of the typical changes of pregnancy using diagrams and models from Childbirth Graphics and transparencies available with the text. Use a chart to describe how each body system adapts to pregnancy from one trimester to another.

4. Describe how women and their families experience the physiologic and anatomic adaptations associated with pregnancy, using prenatal case studies and the obstetric histories of clients for whom the students have cared in the clinical setting. Encourage students to share their clients' impressions regarding the impact that these adaptations had on their daily lives including relationships with others, role performance, body image, and self-esteem.

# SUGGESTED STUDENT LEARNING ACTIVITIES

1. *EVALUATE* the home pregnancy tests that are currently available by visiting your local pharmacy.
   - *DESCRIBE* your findings, including the number and types of tests available, the cost of the tests, the clarity and readability of the instructions that are included with the test, and stated accuracy rates and time periods for the confirmation of pregnancy (i.e., days after ovulation/fertilization, days before or after first missed menstrual period).
   - *OUTLINE* the instructions that you would give to women who plan to use these tests.
   - *DISCUSS* how home pregnancy tests could affect a woman's participation in early and ongoing prenatal care.

2. *DEVELOP* a chart that clearly and concisely presents the common adaptations that occur during pregnancy, their physiologic or mechanical cause, and the manner in which they are manifested in the pregnant woman. This chart should be designed for use as a teaching tool by a nurse who provides care for expectant couples.

3. *WRITE* a pamphlet designed to inform women about the anatomic and physiologic changes that occur during pregnancy, why they occur, and the signs and symptoms that she will experience, indicating effective adaptation to pregnancy or those that are warning signs for potential complications.

## TOPICS FOR DISCUSSION

1. *Consider this question*: How do home pregnancy tests affect a woman's participation in prenatal care—do they facilitate or inhibit early entry into care?

2. *Support this statement*: Nurses working with pregnant women and their families need to possess an in-depth knowledge of the anatomic and physiologic adaptations of a woman's body to pregnancy in order to enhance the health and well-being of pregnant women.

3. *Validate* the importance of early and ongoing prenatal care using the expected adaptations that occur during pregnancy to support your answer.

## MERLIN PROJECT

Use the Chapter 15 section of MERLIN as a starting point in a search of the Internet for web sites designed to inform pregnant women about the changes that they can expect to experience as they progress from one trimester to the next. Prepare a handout that will inform pregnant women about these sites. The handout would be distributed to women at a prenatal visit. The handout should include the following:
- List of at least three sites (the sites should be evaluated for the accuracy, currency, and value of the information provided as well as the qualifications of the sponsor)
- Description of each site in terms of following:
  - Internet address of the site
  - Sponsoring person(s), agency, organization
  - Information and services provided
  - How to fully access the information and services offered by the site
- Guidelines for the women to follow when accessing sites that are not on the list—how to evaluate the site to determine its reliability as a provider of information, services, and advice about pregnancy

# Chapter

# 16 Maternal and Fetal Nutrition

## Summary of Key Concepts

Chapter 16 provides the student with a comprehensive overview of concepts related to maternal and fetal nutrition before and during pregnancy and maternal nutrition during lactation. Nutrient needs and methods for assessment of nutritional status are discussed. The food guide pyramid is included for student reference.

The nutrient needs and recommended weight gain for a healthy pregnancy and fetal development are presented in the narrative of the text and then summarized in a variety of tables, boxes, and figures, thereby facilitating student learning and review. Nutrition is identified as a component of the web of influence that can affect the outcome of pregnancy. The rationale for increased need, sources for each nutrient, and nursing considerations are incorporated throughout the discussion. The student is provided with a method for determining individualized nutrient needs and pregnancy weight gain based upon calculation of a woman's body mass index (BMI). The hazardous consequences related to nutritional deficits and inappropriate weight gain are emphasized. An overview of nutritional issues that should be addressed when caring for pregnant women is provided.

Care management related to the nutritional needs during pregnancy and the postpartum period is the focus of the final section of the chapter. Nutritional assessment methods are provided along with descriptions of the factors critical to obtaining a holistic, nutritional picture of a pregnant woman. Students are introduced to the importance of recognizing cultural food patterns as they assess the nutritional status of their clients and plan appropriate interventions. Typical nutrition-related nursing diagnoses, expected outcomes, and interventions are identified. Methods helpful in coping with nutrition-related discomforts and in addressing cultural influences and the needs of vegetarians are described. A plan of care related to nutrition during pregnancy illustrates the care management approach as applied in a nutritional context. The nursing diagnoses of knowledge deficit, altered nutrition more than body requirements, and altered nutrition less than body requirements are developed.

## Learning Objectives

Define the key terms.
Explain recommended maternal weight gain during pregnancy.
State the recommended level of intake of energy sources, protein, and key vitamins and minerals during pregnancy and lactation.

Give examples of the food sources that provide the nutrients required for optimal maternal nutrition during pregnancy and lactation.

Examine the role of nutritional supplements during pregnancy.

List five nutritional risk factors during pregnancy.

Compare the dietary needs of adolescent and mature pregnant women.

Give examples of cultural food patterns and possible dietary problems for two ethnic groups or for two alternative eating patterns.

Assess nutritional status during pregnancy.

Apply the nursing process to maternal and fetal nutrition.

Identify topics for nursing research related to maternal and fetal nutrition.

## OUTLINE OF CHAPTER CONTENT WITH COURSE GUIDELINES

| CONTENT | GUIDELINE |
|---|---|
| Nutrient needs before conception | A |
| Nutrient needs during pregnancy | A |
| – Energy needs | A |
| – Weight gain | A |
| – Pattern of weight gain | A |
| – Hazards of restricting adequate weight gain | A |
| – Protein | A |
| – Fluid | A |
| – Minerals and vitamins | A |
| – Nutrient supplements | A |
| – Other nutritional issues during pregnancy | A |
| Nutrient needs during lactation | A |
| Care management | A |
| – Assessment and nursing diagnoses | A |
| – Expected outcomes of care | A |
| – Plan of care and interventions | A |
| – Adequate dietary intake | A |
| – Coping with nutrition-related discomforts of pregnancy | A |
| – Cultural influences | A |
| – Vegetarian diets | A |
| – Evaluation | A |
| Plan of care | A |

## TEACHING STRATEGIES

1. Divide students into groups. Assign each group to prepare a 2-day menu for a pregnant woman with a specific nutritional variable.
   - An adolescent who "lives on fast food"
   - A career woman whose mealtimes are erratic with many meals either skipped or eaten in restaurants or at her desk while working

Chapter 16: Maternal and Fetal Nutrition    69

- A Native American woman
- A Hispanic/Mexican-American woman
- A strict vegetarian

2. Invite a dietitian to discuss counseling techniques that he or she uses to help pregnant women follow a nutritious diet during pregnancy.

3. Contrast the nutrient requirements for a nonpregnant woman with those for a pregnant woman and for a woman who is lactating. Explain the consequences of inadequate nutrition before pregnancy, during pregnancy, and while lactating.

4. Use a variety of nutritional assessment tools and questionnaires to illustrate how such formats can be used to gather essential data for the nutritional management of women before they become pregnant, when they are pregnant, and when they are lactating.

5. Divide students into three groups. Assign each group to prepare a plan of care for each of the following nursing diagnoses (nutritional problems):
   - Altered nutrition: less than body requirements related to adolescent pregnancy and the concern regarding weight gain
   - Altered nutrition: more than body requirements related to knowledge deficit concerning nutritional needs during pregnancy.
   - Constipation related to decreased activity and inadequate fiber or fluid intake

   Arrange for a representative from each group to present their group's work as part of a panel discussion related to the management of nutrient needs during pregnancy.

## SUGGESTED STUDENT LEARNING ACTIVITIES

1. *ANALYZE* a female classmate's nutritional status and dietary patterns by using the nutrition questionnaire (Box 16-3) included in the chapter (or one supplied by professor) and by determining your classmate's BMI.
   - *COMPARE* the classmate's dietary patterns with the food guide pyramid.
   - *IDENTIFY* adjustments that would need to be made in her dietary patterns to meet the nutritional requirements for a healthy pregnancy and optimum fetal development.
   - *DETERMINE* the weight gain recommendation based on her BMI if she were pregnant.
   - *PLAN* a 1-day menu with your classmate that reflects her food preferences and the nutrient needs of pregnancy.

2. *ASSESS* the nutritional status and dietary patterns of one of your breastfeeding postpartum clients using the nutrition questionnaire in this chapter (or one supplied by professor) and the signs of good and poor nutrition identified in Table 16-3 in the text.
   - *COMPARE* the woman's status and patterns with the requirements for an adequate postpartum and lactation diet.
   - *IDENTIFY* a relevant nutrition-related nursing diagnosis along with expected outcomes and care measures.
   - *DESCRIBE* how you would evaluate attainment of expected outcomes.

3. *SEARCH* the nursing literature for articles related to a woman's nutritional needs during pregnancy and the nutrition-related discomforts often associated with pregnancy. *CHOOSE* one article, and complete a bibliography card that includes the following:
   - Summary of the article's key points
   - Personal reaction to the ideas presented in the article
   - How the professional nurse can use the article's ideas to enhance and improve a woman's nutritional status and dietary patterns before and during pregnancy and while breastfeeding

4. *CREATE* a poster, illustrating the nutritional requirements of pregnancy, that can be placed in the waiting room of a prenatal clinic informing pregnant women as they wait for their appointments.

5. *DESIGN* a nutrition pamphlet for a prenatal clinic that serves a predominantly Hispanic population. The pamphlet should focus on nutrient requirements of pregnancy and meal plans that reflect Hispanic traditions, food preferences, dietary patterns, and beliefs and practices related to nutrition during pregnancy. *DISCUSS* how you would change this pamphlet to meet the needs of another cultural group or the needs of persons who are following alternative diets (i.e., vegetarians).

6. *SURVEY* your community for nutritional services and resources available to pregnant and lactating women and their children. *PREPARE* a report that includes the following:
   - List of specific services and resources
   - Description of the provided benefits and the eligibility requirements for each service or resource listed
   - Analysis of the adequacy of the services and resources available in your community with specific suggestions to fill in any needs or gaps identified

## TOPICS FOR DISCUSSION

1. *Address this question:* What can nurses do to raise public awareness of the critical importance of good nutrition before, during, and after pregnancy?

2. *Support this statement:* Dollars spent in providing good nutrition for women before and during pregnancy represent dollars saved in terms of the cost of meeting the health care needs of infants affected by poor maternal nutrition.

## MERLIN PROJECT

Use MERLIN to help you log-on to the web site for the National Center for Education in Maternal-Child Health (NCEMCH). Search the site for publications that provide the latest information on nutrition requirements for pregnant and lactating women. Request one of the publications offered. Complete a short report about the publication that includes the following:
   - Summary of the key points covered in the publication
   - How you will use this information (and site) when caring for pregnant and breastfeeding women and their families

# Chapter

# 17

# Nursing Care During Pregnancy

## SUMMARY OF KEY CONCEPTS

Chapter 17 presents content relevant to the care management of pregnant women and their families during the antepartal period. A variety of boxes, tables, illustrations, and figures are included throughout the chapter to alert students to important content and to facilitate learning and review. Presumptive, probable, and positive indicators are identified as a basis for the diagnosis of pregnancy. Nägele's rule is provided as one method for determining a pregnant woman's estimated date of birth.

Adaptation to pregnancy is described concerning its impact on each family member. The discussion of maternal and paternal adaptation focuses on accepting the pregnancy, identifying with the role of the mother or father, reordering personal relationships, and establishing a relationship with the fetus. A box summarizes sibling preparation tips. An overview of grandparent adaptation is included in the description of adaptation to pregnancy.

The assessment process, as it is used during pregnancy, is viewed from both a maternal and a fetal focus. The health history interview, physical examination, and laboratory tests are discussed as the ongoing components of maternal assessment while fetal heart tones, fetal movement, and measurement of fundal height are the ongoing components of fetal assessment. The discussion of assessment highlights the unique focal points to consider during the initial visit and follow-up visits. The critical role that nurses play in the assessment process is emphasized. A box lists the potential complications for each trimester. Antepartal-related nursing diagnoses and expected outcomes are identified.

The student is introduced to a wide variety of nursing interventions including creating a care path about maternal and fetal change, educating clients for self-care during pregnancy, providing psychosocial support, and counseling couples regarding sexuality during pregnancy. A table presents the expected discomforts during each trimester of pregnancy in terms of their physiologic basis and self-care measures for relief. The concept of culture is further developed in this chapter with a discussion of cultural variations in prenatal care and expected maternal behaviors. Age-related differences are described for adolescent and older mothers. A brief discussion of multifetal pregnancy concludes the chapter.

Two plans of care are included in the chapter to illustrate the use of the nursing process to manage the health care of pregnant women and their families. The first plan of care relates to the discomforts of pregnancy and warning signs. The nursing diagnoses of knowledge deficit, altered nutrition: less than body requirements, fatigue, and constipation are developed. The second plan of care relates to an adolescent pregnancy and considers the nursing diagnoses of altered nutrition: less than body requirements, risk for injury, and social isolation.

# LEARNING OBJECTIVES

Define the key terms.

Describe the process of confirming pregnancy and estimating the date of birth.

Summarize the physical, psychosocial, and behavioral changes that usually occur as the mother and other family members adapt to pregnancy.

Discuss the benefits of prenatal care and problems of accessibility for some women.

Outline the patterns of health care provided to assess maternal and fetal health status at the initial and follow-up visits during pregnancy.

Describe the nursing assessments, diagnoses, interventions, and methods of evaluation that are typical when providing care for the pregnant woman.

Discuss education needed by pregnant women to understand physical discomforts related to pregnancy and to recognize signs and symptoms of potential complications.

Explain the impact of culture, age, parity, and number of fetuses on the response of the family to the pregnancy and on the prenatal care provided.

Identify topics for nursing research related to prenatal care.

# OUTLINE OF CHAPTER CONTENT WITH COURSE GUIDELINES

| CONTENT | GUIDELINE |
|---|---|
| Diagnosis of pregnancy | A |
| – Signs and symptoms | A |
| – Estimating date of birth | A |
| Adaptations to pregnancy | A |
| – Maternal adaptation | A |
| – Paternal adaptation | A |
| – Sibling adaptation | A |
| – Grandparent adaptation | B |
| Care management | |
| – Assessment and nursing diagnoses | A |
| – Initial visit | A |
| – Interview | A |
| – Physical examination | A |
| – Laboratory tests | A |
| – Follow-up visits | A |
| – Interview | A |
| – Physical examination | A |
| – Fetal assessment | A |
| – Laboratory tests | A |
| – Expected outcomes of care | A |
| – Plan of care and interventions | A |
| – Care paths | A |
| – Education about maternal and fetal changes | A |
| – Education for self-care | A |

*continued*

| CONTENT | GUIDELINE |
|---|:---:|
|     – Discomforts related to pregnancy | A |
|     – Sexual counseling | A |
|     – Psychosocial support | A |
|   – Evaluation | A |
| Plan of care | A |
| Variations in prenatal care | A |
|   – Cultural influences | A |
|   – Age | A |
|   – Multifetal pregnancy | A |
| Plan of care | A |

# TEACHING STRATEGIES

1. Show a video that depicts the assessment of women during pregnancy.

2. Arrange for a panel of nurses who work in prenatal care settings to discuss their approach to care management throughout pregnancy, including factors and incentives that influence participation in prenatal care, assessment tools and methods used, typical laboratory and diagnostic tests performed, and educational and family participation opportunities offered.

3. Identify the measures that nurses should use to promote the health of pregnant women and their families during pregnancy.

4. Discuss the physiologic, anatomic, and emotional basis for the typical discomforts encountered by women during each trimester of pregnancy. Use case studies to illustrate how these discomforts affect women and their families. Compare the measures used by these women to relieve the discomforts that they experienced with the measures recommended by health care professionals.

5. Arrange for adolescent and older primiparous women to participate in a panel discussion regarding the psychosocial impact that their pregnancy had on themselves, their partners, and families. Encourage the women to identify nursing care measures that would have facilitated their adaptation to pregnancy.

6. Invite a member of a Parents of Twins Chapter in your community to discuss the impact that a multifetal pregnancy and birth had on her and her family's life and the coping strategies that they found to be helpful.

# SUGGESTED STUDENT LEARNING ACTIVITIES

1. *INTERVIEW* two women who are pregnant or have recently given birth (one nullipara and one multipara). *PREPARE* a report that includes a description of the following:
   - The physical and emotional changes that the women experienced during their pregnancies and the types of stressors and the degree of stress that these women encountered as a result of the changes that they experienced

- The measures that the women found to be the most helpful and the least helpful in coping with the changes and the stressors that they experienced
- The role that nurses and family or support group members played or could have played in helping these women cope with the stressors in a positive manner
- Differences, if any, noted in the experiences, impressions, and coping mechanisms described by the nulliparous woman and the multiparous woman

2. *DESIGN* a pamphlet for pregnant women that describes, in a holistic manner, the expected changes that occur during each trimester of pregnancy. Also include self-care measures that pregnant women should use to promote health, cope with pregnancy discomforts, and prevent ineffective adaptations to the changes described.

3. *SEARCH* the nursing literature for articles related to the prenatal period, such as changes encountered by pregnant women and their families and effective nursing measures designed to help them cope with the changes and maintain health and well-being. *CHOOSE* one article, and complete a bibliography card that includes the following:
- Summary of the article's key points
- Personal reaction to the ideas presented in the article
- How the professional nurse can use the article's ideas to enhance and improve the quality of health care provided to pregnant women and their families

4. *DEVELOP* a creative approach to meeting the learning needs of pregnant women based on the following premise: Pregnant women have a multitude of individualized learning needs, yet time spent with a health care provider during a prenatal visit is limited, while time spent in the waiting room can be long, tedious, and even anxiety provoking.

5. *VISIT* your local library or bookstore and take note of the variety of literature (i.e., books, magazine articles) and videos related to pregnancy, childbirth, and preparation of siblings for the birth of a new baby. Considering the difficulty that a pregnant woman would have in deciding what to read or view, *CHOOSE* two of the items that you found to be the most appealing. *PREPARE* a report that describes your choices in terms of the following:
- Readability and clarity of presentation
- Accuracy, currency, and comprehensiveness of content presented
- Credentials of the authors
- Cost
- Manner in which you would use your choices to meet the learning needs of pregnant women and their families

6. *SURVEY* your community for the types of resources available to the pregnant woman and her family related to prenatal health care services, economic support, education classes about pregnancy and parenting, and child care services. *DESCRIBE* how you could make this information available to pregnant women and how you could use this information in your practice.

7. *SURVEY* your community for support groups for parents who have experienced a multifetal birth. *ATTEND* a meeting, and *INTERVIEW* a member of the group. *PREPARE* a report that includes the following:
- Description of the group's formation—who formed the group, when, and why?
- Purpose and mission of the group
- Processes involved in publicizing the group and encouraging people to join

- Services offered to the members of the group, their children, and other family members to help them cope with the stressors of multifetal birth
- Description of the meeting, including the group dynamics observed

8. *DEVELOP* an assessment tool that can be used to determine how a pregnant woman, the expectant father, and the family are adapting to pregnancy. Incorporate the chapter content when developing your tool.
   - *UTILIZE* this tool to assess clients in the prenatal clinical setting. (Friends or relatives who are pregnant could also be used.)
   - *ANALYZE* the data collected and identify appropriate nursing diagnoses.
   - *DESIGN* a plan that would facilitate this woman and her family's psychosocial adaptation to pregnancy.

9. *INVESTIGATE* the childbearing practices of a specific cultural group using a variety of sources including textbooks, journal articles, and media presentations.
   - *SUMMARIZE* the findings of your investigation.
   - *INTERVIEW* an expectant couple from the culture that you investigated.
   - *COMPARE* the findings from your investigation and your interview, and *DESCRIBE* the similarities and differences with regard to cultural beliefs and practices as they relate to childbearing.
   - *DISCUSS* the nursing implications derived from the information that you have gathered, including how it should influence the planning and implementation of care during pregnancy.

10. *INTERVIEW* several grandparents. *PREPARE* a report that includes the following:
    - Description of their feelings when they were told for the first time that they would be grandparents and the influence that society's views of grandparents may have had on their reactions
    - Their views regarding the role of grandparents as sources of support for their own children and caregivers for their grandchildren
    - Measures and strategies that they found helpful or would have found helpful in making the transition to the new role of grandparent

## TOPICS FOR DISCUSSION

1. *Discuss this question:* Recognizing that prenatal care is a critical factor in helping to ensure an optimal outcome to pregnancy, what can nurses do to encourage and facilitate the participation of pregnant women in early and ongoing prenatal care?

2. *Support this statement:* Nurses must provide pregnant women and their families with prenatal care that is sensitive to cultural beliefs and practices regarding pregnancy.

3. *Address these questions:*
   - How does society's view of the female body affect a pregnant woman and her partner's view of her changing body and their expressions of sexuality with each other?
   - How has today's view of the role of men and women in society impacted on their views of parenthood?
   - How does the view of aging in our society affect a person's adjustment to the role of grandparent?

4. *Consider this statement*: Employers have a responsibility to protect the health and well-being and safety of employees who are of childbearing age or who are pregnant.

5. *Debate this issue*: The community has a responsibility or does not have a responsibility to help parents to "parent effectively."

## MERLIN PROJECT

Use MERLIN to assist you in searching the medical literature for nursing research studies related to measures that have been found to be effective in helping pregnant women and their families cope with the physical and psychosocial changes and adaptations associated with pregnancy.

- Prepare an annotated bibliography of at least five nursing research studies.
- Choose one study, and complete a bibliography card that includes the following:
  - Hypothesis; research question
  - Summary of the methodology used and key findings
  - Reliability of the study and its findings
  - Recommendations for further research
  - How the professional nurse can use the study's findings to enhance and improve health care for women and their families during pregnancy
- Describe how you would use the findings of these research studies as a basis for evidenced-based practice.

# Chapter

## 18

# Childbirth Education

## SUMMARY OF KEY CONCEPTS

Chapter 18 introduces the student to three major health care delivery options available to women and their families who are anticipating pregnancy and childbirth, namely preconception care, childbirth education, and options for care including birth settings and care providers. The chapter begins with a discussion of preconception care that includes its purpose, value, and components. The critical role of the nurse in the provision of this health care service is emphasized.

The chapter continues with a description of childbirth education that includes historic perspectives, early methods, and current practices. Supportive strategies that this educational opportunity offers regarding pain management, family health and lifestyle management, couple relationship and sexuality concerns, infant care techniques, and needed family adjustments are identified and explained.

A description of the variety of care options currently available concludes the chapter. An overview of birth plans explains how this tool can be used by couples to accomplish an approach to their anticipated birth experience that meets their needs and wishes. Care provider options are reviewed with special emphasis on the emerging role of doulas. A variety of birth setting choices are described, including birth centers, LDR/LDRP rooms, and the homes of birthing couples. Criteria for use as well as advantages and disadvantages are incorporated into the description of each choice.

## LEARNING OBJECTIVES

Define the key terms.
Explain the importance of preconception care.
Identify the purpose of childbirth education.
Describe the role and benefits of a doula.
Discuss the different choices of care providers.
Describe four birth settings.
Compare methods of education for childbirth.
Identify topics for nursing research in childbirth education.

# OUTLINE OF CHAPTER CONTENT WITH COURSE GUIDELINES

| CONTENT | GUIDELINE |
|---|:---:|
| Preconception care | A |
| – Role of the nurse | A |
| Childbirth education | A |
| – History | B |
| – Early methods | B |
| – Current practices | A |
| – Strategies | A |
| Options for care | A |
| – Birth plan | A |
| – Care provider options | A |
| – Birth setting choices | A |
| – LDRs and LDRPs | A |
| – Birth centers | B |
| – Home birth | B |
| Components of childbirth education classes | A |
| – Pain management | A |
| – Promoting wellness and family health through education | A |
| – Prenatal/postnatal nutrition and lifestyle management | A |
| – Couple relationship and sexuality | A |
| – Infant care and feeding | A |
| – Infant stimulation and massage | B |
| – Family adjustment to parenthood | A |

## TEACHING STRATEGIES

1. Outline the components of preconception care. Illustrate the importance of preconception care by using case studies concerning women anticipating pregnancy who have a history of health problems such as diabetes mellitus, obesity, and smoking.

2. Illustrate the components and benefits of birth plans by bringing examples from several couples to class. Describe the process that the couples used to create the plans and their impressions of the efficacy of such plans, including the degree to which the plans were used in managing their childbirth experiences.

3. Identify the types of prenatal and parenting classes available in your community. Assign students to sit in on some of these classes and report back to the class about their observations and impressions.

4. Describe the types of birth setting choices available in your community. Encourage students to discuss their impressions of the birth settings that they encountered as part of their clinical experiences.

5. Invite a couple who has opted for and experienced home birth to discuss reasons for their choice and their impressions of the birthing experience.

## SUGGESTED STUDENT LEARNING ACTIVITIES

1. *DESIGN* a questionnaire that addresses the issue of preconception care in terms of what it is, its purpose and value, who should participate and when, what the components should be, and how much it should cost.
   - *DISTRIBUTE* the questionnaire to ten men and ten women of childbearing age.
   - *SUMMARIZE* in table form the responses obtained to each question.
   - *ANALYZE* the responses to the questionnaire and describe the following:
     - Overall awareness of men and women to this aspect of health care and the depth and accuracy of their knowledge
     - Differences noted between the responses of men and women—how did age, educational level, social background, and life experiences influence their responses?
     - Recommendations for health education based on the findings of your survey

2. *PREPARE* a class for young adult men and women that addresses the issue of preconception care.
   - *WRITE* a detailed outline of the content of the class.
   - *DESCRIBE* the teaching methodologies that you would use, including class format, demonstrations, audiovisual aids, role playing, and written materials.
   - *IDENTIFY* expected outcomes of the class.
   - *CONDUCT* the class, if possible, and evaluate the class and the expected outcomes.

3. *SEARCH* the nursing literature for articles related to the growing trend toward preconception care. *CHOOSE* one article, and complete a bibliography card that includes the following:
   - Summary of the article's key points
   - Personal reaction to the ideas presented in the article
   - How the professional nurse could use the information presented to enhance and improve preconception health care

4. *SURVEY* your community for parent and childbirth education classes available, and *CREATE* a table that describes these classes in terms of the following:
   - Type—content and to whom they are directed
   - Location—where they are offered and the setting used
   - Teacher(s) —persons or groups who offer the classes and their qualifications
   - Cost and method of payment
   - Timing—when they are offered

5. *VIEW* a film or video that depicts childbirth.
   - *EVALUATE* the film or video, focusing on its content (accuracy, comprehensiveness, currency), visual appeal, the qualifications of persons responsible for its production, and the manner of presentation. On the basis for your evaluation, would you recommend it for viewing by expectant couples? Support your answer.
   - *DESCRIBE* how you would use a film or video in a childbirth class.

6. *OBSERVE* a childbirth education class. *DESCRIBE* the class in terms of the following:
   - Content (topics covered, clarity, comprehensiveness) presented and teaching strategies (lecture, group discussion, demonstration, role play) used
   - Students—number; interaction with each other and with instructor
   - Teacher—effectiveness, expertise, ability to relate to students
   - Changes that you would recommend to enhance learning and improve the class; include the rationale for each change that you recommend

7. *INTERVIEW* your postpartum clients regarding the method of childbirth preparation that they used to cope with their labor experience. *PREPARE* a report that includes the following:
   - Description of the method that was used by each woman and her partner or coach
   - Perceptions of the method's effectiveness in meeting their goals for labor and birth and any changes that they would make if they had to do it all over again
   - Effectiveness of the health care providers managing their labor and birth in supporting their efforts to use the techniques learned in childbirth classes

## TOPICS FOR DISCUSSION

1. *Debate the issues:*
   - The availability of epidural anesthesia has had a negative effect on a woman's motivation to participate in childbirth classes and to use the pain management techniques learned.
   - Home births are a safe alternative to hospital births.

2. *Support the statements:*
   - Nurses play a critical role in encouraging men and women anticipating pregnancy to participate in preconception care.
   - Insurance companies should reimburse men and women for the costs of preconception care.

3. *Consider the question:* What are the responsibilities of nurses working with laboring couples with regard to supporting the couples' efforts to use the techniques that they learned in childbirth education classes?

## MERLIN PROJECT

Use MERLIN to assist you in searching the medical literature for nursing research studies related to the topic of the effectiveness of childbirth preparation as a method of maintaining control and managing pain during labor.
   - Prepare an annotated bibliography of at least five studies.
   - Choose one study, and complete a bibliography card that includes the following:
     - Hypothesis; research question
     - Summary of the methodology used and key findings
     - Reliability of the study and its findings
     - Recommendations for further research
     - How the professional nurse could use the findings to enhance and improve childbirth preparation classes
   - Discuss how you would use these studies to ensure adequate funding of childbirth preparation classes and encourage expectant couples to participate in these classes.

# 19 Labor and Birth Processes

## SUMMARY OF KEY CONCEPTS

Chapter 19 introduces the student to the process of labor, factors influencing progress, and the specialized terminology used to describe childbirth. A foundation is created upon which subsequent chapters in this unit are built. Tables and illustrations facilitate student learning and review.

The factors affecting labor, or the "five Ps," are described in terms of their effect on the progress of labor and on each other. Pregnancy adaptations that facilitate the process of labor, such as relaxed pelvic joints and softening of the passageway tissues, are included in the discussion. The student is made aware of the important role that the fetus plays in its own descent through the birth canal using the processes of molding, position changes, and cardinal movements of labor. The influences that primary and secondary powers and maternal position have on labor and birth are indicated.

The onset of labor is described regarding the signs that precede labor and the involvement of interrelated factors such as altered hormone levels, progressive uterine distention, and placental aging. An overview of the stages of labor, the events that occur in each stage, and the timing pattern that each stage encompasses is provided. The chapter concludes with a brief discussion of the fetal and maternal adaptations that occur during labor.

## LEARNING OBJECTIVES

Define the key terms.
Explain the five factors that affect the labor process.
Describe the anatomic structure of the bony pelvis.
Recognize the normal measurements of the diameters of the pelvic inlet, cavity, and outlet.
Review the anatomy and normal measurements of the fetal skull.
Explain the significance of molding of the fetal head during labor.
Describe the cardinal movements of the mechanism of labor.
Assess the maternal anatomic and physiologic adaptations to labor.
Describe fetal adaptations to labor.
Identify topics for nursing research related to factors that affect the labor process.

# OUTLINE OF CHAPTER CONTENT WITH COURSE GUIDELINES

| CONTENT | GUIDELINE |
|---|:---:|
| Factors affecting labor | A |
| – Passenger | A |
| – Size of fetal head | A |
| – Fetal presentation | A |
| – Fetal lie | A |
| – Fetal attitude | A |
| – Fetal position | A |
| – Passageway | A |
| – Bony pelvis | A |
| – Soft tissues | A |
| – Powers | A |
| – Primary powers | A |
| – Secondary powers | A |
| – Position of the laboring woman | A |
| Process of labor | A |
| – Signs preceding labor | A |
| – Onset of labor | A |
| – Stages of labor | A |
| – Mechanism of labor | A |
| Physiologic adaptation to labor | A |
| – Fetal adaptation | A |
| – Maternal adaptation | A |

# TEACHING STRATEGIES

1. Describe the process of labor using charts, diagrams, and graphs included in the text and/or available from Childbirth Graphics.

2. Describe fetal characteristics (head, lie, presentation, attitude, position) and pelvic characteristics using fetal and pelvic models. Demonstrate the mechanisms of labor using these models.

3. Arrange for students to view a video that depicts vaginal birth.

4. Describe principles of nursing documentation of a woman's progress through labor and birth using examples of a variety of charting formats from health care agencies in your community.

# SUGGESTED STUDENT LEARNING ACTIVITIES

1. *REVIEW* the labor and birth records of women at the agency where you have your obstetric clinical experience. *DESCRIBE* how the nurses, physicians, and midwives record the process of labor in terms of the following:
   - Factors affecting labor
   - Progress and process of labor
   - Maternal and fetal adaptations to labor

2. *PREPARE* a class for an expectant parents' group entitled "Factors that affect your progress in labor." *OUTLINE* the content that you would include in each of the following teaching methodologies:
   - Class lecture—information regarding the five Ps
   - Class discussion—the actions of the expectant couple that will facilitate or hinder the process of labor and birth
   - Audiovisual aids—pelvic and fetal model for the cardinal movements of childbirth; video or film illustrating the actions of the laboring couple and health care providers during childbirth; charts, diagrams, and illustrations depicting the five Ps

## TOPICS FOR DISCUSSION

1. *Consider this question*: How can teaching a pregnant woman and her partner or coach about the five Ps of labor enhance and facilitate the progress of labor?

2. *Support this statement*: Nurses working on a labor and birth unit should institute a protocol for management of the woman in labor that includes keeping the woman active for as long as possible, using a variety of positions for labor and birth, and changing the maternal position frequently.

## MERLIN PROJECT

Use MERLIN to assist you in searching the literature for nursing research studies related to the effects of various maternal positions on the process of labor and birth.
- Create an annotated bibliography of at least five nursing research studies.
- Choose one research study, and complete a bibliography card that includes the following:
  - Hypothesis; research question
  - Summary of the methodology used and key findings
  - Reliability of the study and its findings
  - Recommendations for further research
  - How the professional nurse can use the study's findings to enhance and improve the management of care for the laboring woman
- Describe how you would use these research studies to develop guidelines for laboring positions that are a reflection of evidence-based practice.

# Chapter

## 20

# Management of Discomfort

## SUMMARY OF KEY CONCEPTS

Chapter 20 introduces the student to the concept of management of discomfort as it applies to labor and birth. A three-part framework is used to present relevant content—the pain experience, nonpharmacologic and pharmacologic relief measures, and care management considerations.

The first part of this chapter deals with the experience of pain and discomfort during the process of childbirth. A concise description of physiologic and psychologic factors is included. The student is informed about the manner in which pain is experienced by the client in terms of physical signs and affective expressions. The need to consider the manner in which pain is perceived is emphasized along with factors that can influence pain response such as culture, anxiety and fear, previous experience, childbirth preparation, and support.

The chapter continues with an in-depth discussion of a variety of pain relief methods. Nonpharmacologic approaches for control of discomfort are described. Three childbirth preparation methods (Dick-Read, Lamaze, Bradley) are compared. Additionally, several relaxation and pain control measures are described, including focusing and feedback relaxation, music, breathing techniques, effleurage and counterpressure, water therapy, and TENS.

The discussion of pharmacologic methods begins with a review of the concepts of analgesia and anesthesia. Systemic analgesia is considered with the variety of medications available, including narcotics, mixed narcotic agonist-antagonist compounds, analgesic potentiators (ataractics), and narcotic antagonists. The discussion of nerve block analgesia and anesthesia incorporates descriptions of the major methods used today, such as local and pudendal blocks, spinal anesthesia, and epidural anesthesia and analgesia. Maternal and fetal effects and nursing considerations are identified. Specific considerations related to the administration of anesthesia to the woman who is obese and to the occurrence of maternal hypothermia related to vasodilation associated with administration of analgesia and anesthesia are identified. A brief overview of paracervical block, general anesthesia, and inhalation analgesia is provided.

The chapter concludes with a description of care management of the discomfort of labor using a nursing process framework. Attention is given to supporting the laboring woman and her partner and preparing them for pain relief procedures. Assessment findings are used as a basis for decision making concerning the type of pain relief measures that should be used. Nursing considerations related to informed consent, administration, safety, and general care are discussed. A plan of care related to the nonpharmacologic management of discomfort develops the nursing diagnosis of pain.

## LEARNING OBJECTIVES

Define the key terms.

Compare the various childbirth preparation methods.

Describe the breathing and relaxation techniques used for each stage of labor.

Identify nonpharmacologic strategies to enhance relaxation and decrease discomfort during labor.

Discuss the types of analgesia and anesthesia used during labor.

Compare the types of pharmacologic control used to relieve discomfort in the different stages of labor and for different methods of birth.

Discuss the use of naloxone (Narcan) and naltrexone (Trexan).

Relate each step of the nursing process to the pharmacologic management of labor discomfort.

Describe the nursing responsibilities for a woman receiving analgesia or anesthesia during labor.

Identify topics for nursing research related to pain management for labor and birth.

## OUTLINE OF CHAPTER CONTENT WITH COURSE GUIDELINES

| CONTENT | GUIDELINE |
|---|:---:|
| Discomfort during labor and birth | A |
| – Neurologic origins | B |
| – Perception of pain | A |
| – Expression of pain | A |
| – Factors influencing pain response | A |
| – Culture | A |
| – Anxiety and fear | A |
| – Previous experience | A |
| – Childbirth preparation | A |
| – Support | A |
| Nonpharmacologic management of discomfort | A |
| – Childbirth preparation methods | A |
| – Relaxation and breathing techniques | A |
| Pharmacologic management of discomfort | A |
| – Sedatives | B |
| – Analgesia and anesthesia | A |
| – Systemic analgesia | A |
| – Nerve block analgesia and anesthesia | A |
| – Local infiltration | A |
| – Pudendal block | A |
| – Spinal anesthesia | A |
| – Epidural block | A |
| – Epidural and intrathecal narcotics | A |
| – Paracervical block | C |
| General anesthesia | B |
| – Inhalation analgesia and anesthesia | B |

| CONTENT | GUIDELINE |
|---|---|
| Care management | A |
|   – Assessment and nursing diagnoses | A |
|   – Expected outcomes of care | A |
|   – Plan of care and interventions | A |
|     – Nonpharmacologic interventions | A |
|     – Informed consent | A |
|     – Timing of administration | A |
|     – Preparation for procedures | A |
|     – Administration of medication | A |
|     – Safety and general care | A |
|     – Special concerns | A |
|       – Anesthesia in the obese woman | B |
|       – Maternal hypothermia after analgesia and anesthesia | B |
|   – Evaluation | A |
| Plan of care | A |

## TEACHING STRATEGIES

1. Describe the physical, emotional, and cultural factors influencing the pain experience of childbirth. Involve students in a discussion of the concept of pain, including their experiences with pain and how they responded and their expectations regarding childbirth pain and how laboring women should respond to the pain that they are experiencing.

2. Describe the nonpharmacologic options for pain management available on the childbirth units in your community. Demonstrate a variety of these techniques to the students, and involve them in practicing these techniques with each other in role-playing situations. These techniques include position changes, breathing techniques, effleurage, imagery, acupressure, birthing balls, and counter pressure.

3. Identify childbirth preparation classes available in your community. Arrange for each student to attend at least one of these classes and observe the class activities and group dynamics. Provide class time for students to discuss their observations of the classes that they attended.

4. Use articles and research studies from the nursing literature to describe the effectiveness of nonpharmacologic and pharmacologic measures to manage childbirth pain. Contrast the perceptions of health care providers and laboring women regarding childbirth pain and the effectiveness of relief measures.

5. Describe protocols and nursing implications for each of the pharmacologic measures for pain relief during childbirth. Compare protocols recommended in the nursing literature with the protocols used in the agencies in your community.

# SUGGESTED STUDENT LEARNING ACTIVITIES

1. *REVIEW* the labor and birth records of your clients in the clinical setting to determine the types of nonpharmacologic and pharmacologic pain relief measures that were used. *DESCRIBE* the following:
   - Nonpharmacologic method(s) used and the documented effects (therapeutic and nontherapeutic)
   - Pharmacologic method(s) used and the documented effects (therapeutic and nontherapeutic)

   *INTERVIEW* each of the women for whom you cared to determine the following:
   - Their perception of the effectiveness of the methods used
   - How they would compare nonpharmacologic methods and pharmacologic methods in terms of effectiveness and acceptability
   - The influence that their partner or coach and primary health care provider had on the choice of pain relief measures and the effectiveness of the measures used

2. *DESCRIBE* the protocol for epidural block used by the agency where you have your obstetric clinical experience. *COMPARE* this protocol with the principles of administration described in this chapter. *DISCUSS* the scope of the nurse's role as determined by the hospital protocol for this pain relief method.

3. *SEARCH* the nursing literature for articles related to the topic of pharmacologic pain relief measures in childbirth and nursing actions that can enhance or hinder their effectiveness. Choose one article, and complete a bibliography card that includes the following:
   - Summary of the article's key points
   - Personal reaction to the ideas presented in the article
   - How the professional nurse can use the article's ideas to enhance and improve the quality of health care provided for the laboring woman

4. *CHOOSE* two cultural groups, and investigate the manner in which members of the culture perceive and express pain. Use the literature, personal experience, and interviews to obtain the required information. *PREPARE* a report that includes your findings and describes how these findings should influence the nursing care administered to laboring women representing these cultural groups.

5. *INTERVIEW* postpartum women before their discharge to determine their childbirth pain experience. *DESCRIBE* the following:
   - The women's prelabor expectations regarding how the pain of childbirth would be
   - The sources that the women used to formulate their expectations (i.e., personal experience, descriptions of friends and family members, the media)
   - Degree that the women's expectations were met
   - Types of pain relief measures that they used and the effectiveness of each

## Topics for Discussion

1. *Consider these questions:*
   - How does the media portray the pain experience associated with childbirth? What impact can these media portrayals have on pregnant women as they anticipate their labor and birth experience?
   - How is a nurse's care management of a laboring woman influenced by the manner in which the woman responds to the pain that she is experiencing?
   - What effect can a previous experience with pain during labor and birth have on future childbirths? What can nurses do to help a woman develop positive memories of pain and childbirth?

2. *Support this statement:* The availability of anesthetics that offer a nearly pain-free childbirth experience influences a woman's motivation to participate in nonpharmacologic pain relief measures.

## Merlin Project

Use MERLIN as a starting point to search the Internet for information regarding epidural analgesia and anesthesia as it is used for childbirth. Based on the findings of your search, develop guidelines for the use of epidural analgesia and anesthesia for labor and birth. The guidelines that you develop should include the following information:
- Criteria that candidates must meet before administration
- When the induction should take place in terms of progress made in labor
- Medications used, including dosage and frequency of increases in dosage
- Assessments required before induction, during administration, and after discontinuation
- Measures recommended to enhance effectiveness and prevent complications
- Annotated bibliography of references that you found on the Internet and used to develop the guidelines

# Chapter

## 21 Fetal Assessment

## SUMMARY OF KEY CONCEPTS

Chapter 21 introduces the student to fetal monitoring and its basis, methods, interpretation of findings, and nursing management responsibilities. A variety of tables, charts, checklists, and illustrations summarize and clarify chapter content. This approach serves to facilitate student learning and review. In addition, these resources are appropriate for use in a clinical setting.

The first part of the chapter presents background information on fetal assessment during childbirth. The rationale for monitoring is related to the nature of the stress experienced by a fetus during labor and how the fetus reacts to this stress as determined by the nature of its heart rate pattern—reassuring or nonreassuring. The techniques of intermittent auscultation and external and internal electronic monitoring are described. The description includes the advantages and disadvantages (limitations) of each method. The student is made aware of fetal heart rate (FHR) patterns in terms of their normal characteristics and the variations that could indicate actual or potential fetal compromise. The patterns included in the discussion are the baseline fetal heart rate (i.e., normal range, tachycardia, bradycardia, and variability), the periodic changes that occur with uterine contractions, and the episodic changes that are not associated with uterine contractions. Each pattern variation that is discussed is accompanied by a table that details its characteristics, causes, clinical significance, and appropriate nursing interventions.

The second part of the chapter uses a nursing process framework to describe the care management of laboring women who are being monitored. The discussion of assessment measures includes a checklist for FHR assessment and a checklist for fetal monitoring equipment. Other measures of assessment are described, including fetal blood sampling, fetal oximetry, and cord blood acid-base determination. The legal aspects related to fetal monitoring regarding guidelines and standards of nursing care and the nurse's responsibility are presented. Nursing interventions, including preventive measures, intrauterine resuscitation measures, and management measures for the laboring woman being monitored, are described. One box outlines a protocol for FHR monitoring and another box outlines care of a woman using electronic fetal monitoring. The importance of client and family teaching and documentation of findings is emphasized. Amnioinfusion and tocolytic therapy are identified as additional measures that can be used to prevent fetal compromise. The chapter concludes with a plan of care that illustrates the use of the nursing process with a laboring woman who is being electronically monitored. The nursing diagnoses of maternal anxiety and risk for fetal injury are developed.

# LEARNING OBJECTIVES

Define the key terms.

Identify typical signs of nonreassuring FHR patterns.

Compare FHR monitoring done by intermittent auscultation and external and internal electronic methods.

Explain baseline FHR and evaluate periodic changes.

Describe preventive measures that can be used to maintain FHR patterns within normal limits.

Differentiate between the nursing interventions used for managing specific FHR patterns, including tachycardia and bradycardia; increased and decreased variability; and late and variable decelerations.

Review the application of the monitor.

Review the documentation of the monitoring process necessary during labor.

Identify topics for nursing research related to fetal monitoring.

# OUTLINE OF CHAPTER CONTENT WITH COURSE GUIDELINES

| CONTENT | GUIDELINE |
| --- | :---: |
| Basis for monitoring | A |
| – Fetal response | A |
| – Fetal compromise | A |
| Monitoring techniques | A |
| – Intermittent auscultation | A |
| – Electronic monitoring | A |
| – External monitoring | A |
| – Internal monitoring | A |
| Fetal heart rate patterns | A |
| – Baseline FHR | A |
| – Periodic and episodic changes in FHR | A |
| – Accelerations | A |
| – Decelerations | A |
| Fetal blood sampling/fetal scalp stimulation | B |
| Fetal pulse oximetry | B |
| Care management | A |
| – Assessment and nursing diagnoses | A |
| – Expected outcomes of care | A |
| – Plan of care and interventions | A |
| – Electronic fetal monitoring | A |
| – Pattern recognition | A |
| – Nursing management of nonreassuring patterns | A |
| – Other methods of assessment and intervention | A |
| – Client and family teaching | A |
| – Documentation | A |
| – Evaluation | A |
| Plan of care | A |

# TEACHING STRATEGIES

1. Use illustrations and diagrams to depict how uteroplacental circulation is affected by uterine contractions. Describe how these changes affect the well-being of the fetus.

2. Describe fetal monitoring techniques using a fetoscope, ultrasound stethoscope, and brochures and samples of electronic monitoring equipment. Discuss the assessment protocols and the care measures required for each monitoring technique.

3. Arrange for students to tour a labor unit with a nurse who has expertise in electronic fetal monitoring (EFM) interpretation.

4. Use monitor tracings to illustrate the characteristics of reassuring and nonreassuring FHR patterns. Describe the nursing care management required when a nonreassuring FHR pattern occurs.

5. Use case studies to illustrate the nursing management of women in labor who are being monitored. Provide examples of nursing documentation of assessment findings, actions, and responses.

# SUGGESTED STUDENT LEARNING ACTIVITIES

1. *REVIEW* the electronic fetal monitoring protocol used during your clinical experience on a labor unit. *DESCRIBE* each of the following:
   - Methods and equipment used
   - Education required for nurses who are responsible for monitoring and interpreting tracings
   - Methods used to document findings and actions taken in response to fetal assessment findings
   - Nursing measures used with regard to assessing fetal responses to childbirth, preventing fetal compromise, and supporting the monitored woman and her family
   - Nursing actions taken when patterns indicative of fetal compromise appear
   - Women's reactions to monitoring
   - Effects of monitoring on a laboring woman's ability to remain active and change positions

2. *SEARCH* the nursing literature for articles related to nursing care management of the monitored woman and her fetus during childbirth. *CHOOSE* one article, and complete a bibliography card that includes the following:
   - Summary of the article's key points
   - Personal reaction to the ideas presented in the article
   - How the professional nurse could use the article's ideas to enhance and improve the care provided to the monitored woman during labor and the effectiveness and accuracy of fetal assessment

3. *DESIGN* a pamphlet related to fetal assessment methods used during childbirth that could be given to expectant couples. The pamphlet should inform as well as reduce the anxiety that might occur when unfamiliar equipment, often associated with illness, is used during what is expected to be a normal process.

## Topics for Discussion

1. *Debate this issue:* Should all laboring women be electronically monitored, given the fact that the majority of labors progress normally without signs of fetal compromise?

2. *Consider this nursing dilemma:* A nurse working with a laboring woman detects a FHR pattern that she interprets as nonreassuring. The nurse calls the woman's primary health care provider, who disagrees, stating "I am sure that she is doing just fine. Do not worry. Call me when she dilates to about 8 cm." The nurse remains concerned and still interprets the findings as nonreassuring. What action should the nurse take?

3. *Address this question:* How can electronic fetal monitoring inhibit the normal progress of labor? What can nurses do as advocates to counteract this effect?

## Merlin Project

Use MERLIN as a starting point to search the Internet for information related to standards that should guide fetal assessment methods during labor and nursing responsibilities related to assessment of the fetus, required interventions based on assessment findings, and documentation criteria. Based on information gathered in your Internet search, write a set of guidelines that nurses working in a childbirth setting could use to guide their practice. An annotated bibliography of references and Internet resources should be included as part of the guidelines.

Chapter

## 22

# Nursing Care During Labor

## SUMMARY OF KEY CONCEPTS

Chapter 22 focuses on the care management of women during labor and birth. A description of assessment during the first stage of labor emphasizes the importance of the initial contact with a woman in labor and includes information regarding distinguishing true labor from false labor. Students are informed about the critical importance of assessing psychosocial factors, cultural influences, and the nature of the stress experienced by both the mother and the father. The discussion of physical examination techniques emphasizes not only the factors to be assessed but also the need to adjust the frequency of data collection to the changing status of the maternal-fetal unit. A table summarizes the expected maternal progress during each phase of the first stage of labor, and a care path outlines assessment, physical care, and support measures for each phase of the first stage of labor. Laboratory and diagnostic tests relevant to this stage are described, including a review of membrane rupture and assessment of the characteristics of the amniotic fluid. A box is provided that summarizes available tests for rupture of membranes. Students are directed to be alert for warning signs that could indicate a potential complication of labor. Typical nursing diagnoses and expected outcomes for the first stage of labor are listed. A discussion of interventions begins with an overview of standards of care as they relate to the laboring woman. Emphasis is placed on the nurse's manner of approach when admitting the client and her partner/coach and on providing required physical care and support measures for the laboring woman and her family. A plan of care for the first stage of labor considers the nursing diagnoses of anxiety, pain, and risks for fluid volume deficit, infection, and altered urinary elimination.

The second stage of labor and the events and behaviors during its three phases are described. Critical assessment measures are emphasized, including the importance of identifying the signs indicative of the onset of this stage. A table summarizes the expected maternal progress during each phase of the second stage of labor, and a care path outlines assessment, physical care, and support measures for each phase of the second stage of labor. Nursing diagnoses and expected outcomes for the second stage of labor are listed. Students are introduced to the nursing management of childbirth (vertex) events in both controlled and emergency situations. Maternal behaviors, positions, and bearing-down efforts are described. Supportive nursing measures for both the mother and her partner/coach are presented. Childbirth in a birthing room is contrasted with childbirth in the traditional delivery room setting. An overview of perineal trauma related to childbirth includes a description of lacerations and episiotomies. A plan of care for the second stage of labor develops the nursing diagnosis of risk for ineffective individual coping.

The third stage of labor is described with an emphasis on signs of placental separation, maternal physical status, and potential problems. Nursing diagnoses and expected outcomes are identified. Nursing measures to assist with the expulsion of the placenta, to provide comfort, and to facilitate the attachment of family members to the newborn are described. Ineffective individual coping, fatigue, and risk for fluid volume deficit are the nursing diagnoses explored in the plan of care for the third stage of labor.

## LEARNING OBJECTIVES

Define the key terms.
Review the factors included in the initial assessment of the woman in labor.
Describe the ongoing assessment of maternal progress during the first, second, and third stages of labor.
State the physical and psychosocial findings indicative of maternal progress during labor.
Discuss aspects of fetal assessment during labor.
Identify signs of developing complications during the first, second, and third stages of labor.
Develop a comprehensive plan of care relevant to each stage of labor and birth.
Discuss the nurse's role in managing care for the woman and her significant others (support person[s], family) during each stage of labor and birth.
Examine the influence of cultural and religious beliefs and practices on the process of labor and birth.
Discuss the role of a woman's significant others (support person[s], family) in assisting her during labor and birth.
Outline nursing actions in preparation for birth.
Describe the role and responsibilities of the nurse in an emergency childbirth situation.
Identify the impact of perineal trauma on the woman.
Discuss the nurse's role in reducing the incidence of routine episiotomy.
Identify topics for nursing research related to nursing care during labor.

## OUTLINE OF CHAPTER CONTENT WITH COURSE GUIDELINES

| CONTENT | GUIDELINE |
|---|---|
| First stage of labor | |
| Care management | A |
| – Assessment and nursing diagnoses | A |
|   – Admission to labor unit | A |
|     – Admission data | A |
|     – Prenatal data | A |
|     – Interview | A |
|     – Psychosocial factors | A |
|     – Stress in labor | A |
|     – Cultural factors | A |
|     – Physical examination | A |
|       – General systems assessment | A |
|       – Leopold's maneuvers | A |
|       – Assessment of FHR and pattern | A |
|       – Assessment of uterine contractions | A |
|       – Vaginal examination | A |

*continued*

| CONTENT | GUIDELINE |
|---|:---:|
| – Laboratory and diagnostic tests | A |
| – Signs of potential problems | A |
| – Expected outcomes of care | A |
| – Plan of care and interventions | A |
| – Standards of care | B |
| – Physical nursing care during labor | A |
| – Support measures | A |
| – Father or partner during labor | A |
| – Support of grandparents | B |
| – Siblings during labor | B |
| – Doulas | A |
| – Emergency interventions | A |
| – Preparation for giving birth | B |
| – Birth setting | B |
| – Evaluation | A |
| Plan of care (first stage of labor) | A |
| | |
| Second stage of labor | |
| Care management | A |
| – Assessment and nursing diagnoses | A |
| – Expected outcomes of care | A |
| – Plan of care and interventions | A |
| – Prebirth considerations | A |
| – Maternal position | A |
| – Bearing down efforts | A |
| – Fetal heart rate (FHR) and pattern | A |
| – Support of father or coach | A |
| – Supplies, instruments, and equipment | B |
| – Birth in a delivery room or birthing room | B |
| – Mechanism of a vertex birth | A |
| – Immediate assessment and care of newborn | A |
| – Siblings during the second stage | B |
| – Perineal trauma related to childbirth | A |
| – Emergency childbirth | B |
| – Evaluation | A |
| Plan of care (second stage of labor) | A |
| | |
| Third stage of labor | |
| Care management | A |
| – Assessment and nursing diagnoses | A |
| – Expected outcomes of care | A |
| – Plan of care and interventions | A |
| – Family during the third stage | A |
| – Parent-newborn relationships | A |
| – Evaluation | A |
| Plan of care (third stage of labor) | A |

# TEACHING STRATEGIES

1. Describe the nursing care management of laboring women using a variety of case studies that depict nulliparous women, multiparous women, and prepared and unprepared women during labor. Use nursing research to identify currently recommended approaches to facilitate progress and enhance the health and well-being of the maternal-fetal unit during each stage of labor.

2. Invite a nurse who works on a labor unit in a hospital, a nurse who works in a birthing center, and a doula to discuss their approaches to physical and emotional care of laboring women and the measures that they use to support the coaches and families of these women.

3. Arrange for students to view videos that depict nursing care management of laboring women.

4. Compare the care management approaches used during childbirth and the resulting outcomes of obstetricians and nurse-midwives.

5. Describe the approaches to childbirth followed by a variety of cultural groups. Indicate how nursing care management approaches should incorporate these cultural variations.

6. Divide students into three groups. Assign the first group to develop a care management plan for the first stage of labor, the second group to develop a care management plan for the second stage of labor, and the third group to do the same for the third stage of labor. Encourage students to use the nursing literature as well as their own clinical experiences in labor when developing these plans. Provide time for each group to present their work to the entire class.

# SUGGESTED STUDENT LEARNING ACTIVITIES

1. *EXAMINE* the care management approach used on the labor unit where you have your clinical experience.
   - *DESCRIBE* the admission procedure followed.
   - *IDENTIFY* the measures used to enhance the progress of labor and ensure the safety of the maternal-fetal unit.
   - *DISCUSS* the supportive measures used to meet the emotional needs and reduce the stressors experienced by the laboring woman and her partner or coach, including the implementation of the couple's birth plan.
   - *EVALUATE* the care management approach used. Based on your evaluation, *IDENTIFY* changes that you would propose to improve the approach, and *INDICATE* the rationale for each proposed change.

2. *SEARCH* the nursing literature for articles that relate to the care management of women during labor and birth. *CHOOSE* one article, and complete a bibliography card that includes the following:
   - Summary of the article's key points
   - Personal reaction to the ideas presented in the article
   - How the professional nurse can use the article's ideas to enhance and improve the quality of health care provided to women and their families during labor

3. *INTERVIEW* your postpartum clients regarding their perception of the emotional support that they received during labor. *DESCRIBE* this support in terms of the following:
   - The nature of the support received and its effectiveness
   - The persons who provided the support and the degree to which they were supportive
   - What the women would like to see changed with regard to emotional support if they should have another labor experience

4. *COMPARE* the childbirth beliefs and practices of two cultural groups in your community.
   - *DESCRIBE* the similarities and differences noted in the beliefs and practices of the two cultural groups.
   - *SPECIFY* how the cultural information that you obtained should be used in providing culturally sensitive care to women and their families during their childbirth.

5. *OBSERVE* a vaginal birth. *DESCRIBE* your experience in terms of the following:
   - Location where the birth took place
   - Interaction of the laboring woman and her partner or coach with each other and with the health care providers attending the birth
   - Type and effectiveness of the childbirth positions and bearing-down efforts used
   - Immediate care of the woman and her newborn after birth
   - Your impressions of the experience, including any changes that you would propose to improve the quality of care and support provided to the laboring woman and her family; indicate the rationale for each change that you propose

6. *SEARCH* the literature for nursing research studies related to the most effective positions and bearing-down efforts for women to use during the second stage of labor and the nursing measures most useful in supporting the woman and her family during the second stage of labor. *CHOOSE* one study, and complete a bibliography card that includes the following:
   - Hypothesis; research question
   - Summary of the methodology used and key findings
   - Reliability of the study and its findings
   - Recommendations for further research
   - How the professional nurse could use the findings to enhance a woman's progress during the second stage of labor

## TOPICS FOR DISCUSSION

1. *Debate these issues:*
   - Episiotomy versus no episiotomy
   - Traditional versus nontraditional settings for childbirth
   - A nurse-midwife's approach to childbirth compared with an obstetrician's approach

2. *Consider this question:* Should children be present at their mother's labor and birth? If they are, what type of preparation programs should be made available, and what criteria should be met if children will be present during childbirth?

# MERLIN PROJECT

Use the Chapter 22 section of MERLIN as a starting point to search the Internet for web sites, journal articles, and research studies related to water birth as a childbirth option. Based on the results of your search, prepare a report that includes the following:

- Annotated list of web sites designed to inform pregnant women and health care providers about water birth
- Annotated list of articles and research studies that describe the effectiveness and implementation of water birth as an option for childbirth
- Description of the advantages and potential problems associated with water birth
- Protocol for a water birth that can be used on labor units when a laboring woman and her family wish to take advantage of this option; the protocol should include the following:
  - Criteria that clients must meet, including those related to maternal and fetal well-being and status of labor
  - When a woman should enter the water during labor; how long she can remain in the water; whether birth should occur in or out of the water
  - Type of tub, temperature of the water, and infection control measures

# Chapter

## 23 Postpartum Physiology

### Summary of Key Concepts

Chapter 23 provides students with an overview of the physiologic and anatomic changes that occur after birth. This overview, along with the content presented in Chapter 25, serves as a foundation for the care management of the postpartum woman and her family.

A system-by-system approach is used to describe the changes that occur during the period of recovery after birth. The changes are presented as reversals of the adaptations that occurred in response to pregnancy. Signs of effective reversal are contrasted with signs of ineffective reversal that signal potential problems. Time frames are included in the discussion to assist students in evaluating the normality of assessment findings. The chapter provides students with the knowledge and theory required for competent physical assessment of the postpartum woman. In addition, students will develop an awareness of the rationale for the recommended postpartum care measures and health teaching described in Chapter 24.

### Learning Objectives

Define the key terms.
Describe the anatomic and physiologic changes that occur during the postpartum period.
Identify characteristics of uterine involution and lochial flow, and describe ways to measure them.
List expected values for vital signs and blood pressure, deviations from normal findings, and probable causes of the deviations.
Identify research topics on postpartum physiology.

### Outline of Chapter Content with Course Guidelines

| CONTENT | GUIDELINE |
|---|---|
| Reproductive system and associated structures | A |
| – Uterus | A |
| – Involution process | A |
| – Contractions | A |
| – Afterpains | A |
| – Placental site | A |
| – Lochia | A |

| CONTENT | GUIDELINE |
|---|:---:|
| – Cervix | A |
| – Vagina and perineum | A |
| – Pelvic muscular support | A |
| Endocrine system | A |
| – Placental hormones | A |
| – Pituitary hormones and ovarian function | A |
| Abdomen | A |
| Urinary system | A |
| – Urine components | A |
| – Postpartal diuresis | A |
| – Urethra and bladder | A |
| Gastrointestinal system | A |
| Breasts | A |
| – Breastfeeding mother | A |
| – Nonbreastfeeding mother | A |
| Cardiovascular system | A |
| – Blood volume | A |
| – Cardiac output | A |
| – Vital signs | A |
| – Blood components | A |
| – Varicosities | A |
| Neurologic system | A |
| Musculoskeletal system | A |
| Integumentary system | A |
| Immune system | A |

## TEACHING STRATEGIES

1. Describe how each physiologic change or adaptation associated with pregnancy is reversed during the postpartum period.

2. Use photographs and/or video to illustrate selected changes, including the breasts, fundus, abdomen, lochia, perineum (i.e., episiotomy, lacerations, and hemorrhoids), and varicosities.

3. Involve students in a discussion regarding their postpartum clients and the manner in which the physiologic changes associated with the puerperium were assessed and exhibited.

## SUGGESTED STUDENT LEARNING ACTIVITIES

1. *PREPARE* and *IMPLEMENT* a teaching plan for a postpartum woman participating in an early discharge (24 hours after birth) program. The plan should be concise with emphasis on the critical self-assessment measures that distinguish signs of normal recovery from signs of inadequate recovery. Actions that must be taken if problems are encountered need to be a part of the plan. Teaching methods should take into consideration the expected physical and emotional status of a woman who has recently given birth.

2. *DESIGN* a poster that highlights the anatomic and physiologic changes that occur in a woman after birth. The poster should be designed for use by a nurse responsible for teaching postpartum women and preparing them for discharge.

## TOPICS FOR DISCUSSION

1. *Address this question:* Why should postpartum women and their families be fully informed about the expected anatomic and physiologic changes that occur as part of the recovery process after birth?

2. *Support this statement:* The nurse plays a critical role in promoting the safety of women who participate in an early discharge program and plan to return home within 12 to 24 hours after their vaginal birth.

## MERLIN PROJECT

Use the Chapter 23 section of MERLIN to assist you in a search of nursing and medical literature for articles related to the physiologic changes that occur during the puerperium. Appropriate articles should discuss what these changes are, how they occur, the significance of the changes, and methods to assess the progress of the changes.
- Prepare an annotated bibliography of at least five journal articles.
- Choose one article, and complete a bibliography card that includes the following:
  - Summary of the article's key points
  - Personal reaction to the ideas presented in the article
  - How the professional nurse can use the article's ideas to enhance and improve the quality of health care provided to postpartum women as they recover from pregnancy and childbirth

Chapter

## 24

# Assessment and Care During the Postpartum Period

## SUMMARY OF KEY CONCEPTS

Chapter 24 uses a care management framework to describe the health care of postpartum women and their families. Tables and boxes summarize important chapter content. An overview of the fourth stage of labor opens the chapter. Assessment for postpartum hemorrhage and progress of postanesthesia recovery is emphasized. A box highlights the important points to include while examining a woman's physical status during the first 1 to 2 hours after birth. The issue of discharge after birth is discussed in terms of timing, legal issues, and criteria to determine readiness for discharge.

The care management of the physical needs of postpartum women is the major focus of the first part of the chapter. Components of a continuing postpartum assessment including signs of potential physiologic complications, typical nursing diagnoses, and expected outcomes of care are identified. Nursing interventions related to physiologic needs are described, including prevention of infection and hemorrhage; promotion of comfort, rest, activity, and nutrition; promotion of bowel and bladder elimination; care of breasts and lactation suppression; and health promotion for future pregnancies and children.

The second part of the chapter covers the care management of the psychosocial needs of postpartum women and their families. Consideration is given to the assessment of the impact of the birth experience, maternal self-image, adaptation to parenthood, family functioning, and cultural diversity. Typical nursing diagnoses and expected outcomes are identified. A discussion of nursing interventions related to the psychosocial needs of the postpartum woman and her family focuses on cultural variations and discharge teaching regarding self-care, signs of complications, sexual activity, prescribed medications, and routine mother and baby checkups. Students are introduced to the importance of follow-up after discharge, which includes such measures as home visits, telephone follow-up, warm lines, support groups, and referral to community resources.

The chapter includes a plan of care that illustrates the care management of a woman who has had a spontaneous vaginal birth. The nursing diagnoses of risk for fluid volume deficit, pain, and risk for altered urinary elimination are developed. A care path for a 24-hour vaginal birth without complications is also included.

# LEARNING OBJECTIVES

Define the key terms.

Identify the priorities of maternal care given during the fourth stage of labor.

Identify common selection criteria for safe early postpartum discharge.

List the pros and cons of early postpartum discharge.

Give examples of physical and psychosocial nursing diagnoses pertaining to women in the postpartum period.

Identify expected outcomes for postpartum physical and psychosocial care.

Summarize nursing interventions to prevent infection and excessive bleeding.

Summarize nursing interventions to promote normal bladder and bowel patterns and care for the breasts of women who are breastfeeding or bottle-feeding.

Explain the influence of cultural expectations on postpartum adjustment.

Discuss the nurse's responsibilities regarding discharge teaching and preparation for home care.

Describe the nurse's role in these postpartum follow-up strategies: home visits, telephone follow-up, warm lines and help lines, support groups, and referrals to community resources.

Identify topics for nursing research related to postpartum care.

# OUTLINE OF CHAPTER CONTENT WITH COURSE GUIDELINES

| CONTENT | GUIDELINE |
|---|---|
| Fourth stage of labor | |
|   – Assessment | A |
|   – Postanesthesia recovery | A |
|   – Transfer from the recovery area | A |
| Discharge—before 24 hours and after 48 hours | A |
|   – Laws related to discharge | A |
|   – Future of early postpartum discharge | A |
|   – Criteria for discharge | A |
| Care management—physical needs | A |
|   – Assessment and nursing diagnoses | A |
|     – Ongoing physical assessment | A |
|     – Signs of potential complications | A |
|     – Routine laboratory tests | A |
|   – Expected outcomes of care | A |
|   – Plan of care and interventions | A |
|     – Prevention of infection | A |
|     – Prevention of excessive bleeding | A |
|     – Promotion of comfort, rest, ambulation, and exercise | A |
|     – Promotion of nutrition | A |
|     – Promotion of normal bowel and bladder patterns | A |
|     – Breastfeeding promotion and lactation suppression | A |
|     – Health promotion of future pregnancies and children | A |
|   – Evaluation | A |

| CONTENT | GUIDELINE |
|---|:---:|
| Care management—psychosocial needs | A |
|   – Assessment and nursing diagnoses | A |
|     – Impact of birth experience | A |
|     – Maternal self-image | A |
|     – Adaptation to parenthood and parent-infant interactions | A |
|     – Family structure and functioning | A |
|     – Impact of cultural diversity | A |
|     – Signs of potential complications | A |
|   – Expected outcomes of care | A |
|   – Plan of care and interventions | A |
|   – Evaluation | A |
| Discharge teaching | A |
|   – Self-care and signs of complications | A |
|   – Sexual activity/contraception | A |
|   – Prescribed medications | A |
|   – Routine mother and baby checkups | A |
|   – Follow-up after discharge | A |
|     – Home visits | A |
|     – Telephone follow-up | A |
|     – Warm lines | A |
|     – Support groups | A |
|     – Referrals to community resources | A |
| Plan of care | A |

## TEACHING STRATEGIES

1. Outline the required assessment protocol (areas to assess and frequency of assessment) of women during the fourth stage of labor. Discuss the rationale for the recommended protocol. Bring examples of recovery flow sheets and records used by local health care agencies to facilitate documentation of maternal health status during the fourth stage of labor.

2. Identify the physical and psychosocial stressors experienced by women and their families during the puerperium.

3. Discuss the nursing care management of vaginally delivered women and their families using case studies, especially those representing clients for whom the students cared during their clinical experiences. Encourage students to participate in the discussion by sharing their observations regarding the care that they administered to their clients.

4. Bring perineal care equipment and supplies to class (e.g., ice packs, peri bottles, sitz baths, topical preparations, and perineal pads). Describe and demonstrate the care measures used for healing, cleansing, and comfort of episiotomies, lacerations, perineal and labial edema, and hemorrhoids.

5. Identify specific pharmacologic measures used to relieve pain and stimulate bowel activity during the postpartum period. Encourage students to describe the medications that they administered to their postpartum clients.

6. Outline a discharge teaching plan for postpartum women and their families that emphasizes topics essential for the well-being of the new mother and her newborn. Compare recommendations for postpartum teaching with the teaching protocols used in the health care agencies in your community.

## SUGGESTED STUDENT LEARNING ACTIVITIES

1. *DESIGN* a fourth stage of labor assessment flow sheet that reflects the content presented in this chapter.
   - *USE* the flow sheet during your clinical experience with women in the recovery stage after birth.
   - *COMPARE* your flow sheet with the one used by the hospital where you have your obstetric experience.
   - *USE* the data collected on the flow sheet to identify appropriate nursing diagnoses. Based on the diagnoses identified, *DEVELOP* a plan of care for each woman assessed.

2. *SEARCH* the nursing literature for articles related to the topic of labor-delivery-recovery (LDR) and labor-delivery-recovery-postpartum (LDRP) rooms. Choose two of the articles, and prepare a report that describes the following:
   - The practice of single-room obstetric care as well as the response of women and nurses to this new approach for the delivery of health care in the postpartum period
   - Your impressions regarding this practice

3. *DEVELOP* a postpartum assessment form based on the content presented in Chapters 23, 24, and 25.
   - *USE* the assessment form that you developed to assess the physical and psychosocial needs of the postpartum women and families in your care.
   - *ANALYZE* the data collected. Based on this analysis, formulate appropriate nursing diagnoses, expected outcomes, and a plan of care.
   - *EVALUATE* the degree to which expected outcomes were attained.

4. *DESIGN* a pamphlet that could be given to postpartum women at discharge. The pamphlet should present in a clear and concise way the information that these women need to know in order to assess their status and care for themselves in such a manner that recovery is facilitated and complications prevented.

5. *INVESTIGATE* beliefs and practices of a cultural group that is part of the community in which you live, regarding the care of the postpartum woman and the care of the newborn.
   - *SUMMARIZE* the information gathered in your investigation, including references used.
   - *INTERVIEW* a woman representing the cultural group that you investigated to determine the extent to which she adheres to her culture's beliefs and practices regarding the care of a woman after she has given birth and the care of the newborn.
   - *DESCRIBE* how you would incorporate the cultural information gathered into a plan of care that respects the beliefs and practices of postpartum women from this culture.

## TOPICS FOR DISCUSSION

1. *Consider this question:* How do the priorities for health teaching differ when the perspectives of nurses are compared with the perspectives of women and their families who have given birth and are preparing for discharge with their new baby?

2. *Support this statement:* Problems can occur if nurses do not consider their postpartum clients' cultural beliefs and practices when preparing a plan of care and implementing it.

3. *Address this question:* What are the responsibilities of nurses and the nursing profession to ensure that the timing of discharge is appropriate and safe for each postpartum woman and her baby?

## MERLIN PROJECT

Use the Chapter 24 section of MERLIN to assist you in searching the medical literature for nursing research studies related to nursing interventions found to be effective in helping postpartum women and their families meet their physical and psychosocial needs.

- Create an annotated bibliography of at least five nursing research studies.
- Choose one article, and complete a bibliography card that includes the following:
  - Hypothesis; research question
  - Summary of the methodology used and key findings
  - Reliability of the study and its findings
  - Recommendations for further research
  - How the professional nurse can use the study's findings to enhance and improve the quality of health care provided to postpartum women and their families
- Discuss how the research studies that you found in your search could be used as a basis for evidenced-based practice during the postpartum period.

# Chapter

## 25 Transition to Parenthood

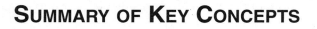

## SUMMARY OF KEY CONCEPTS

Chapter 25 presents the psychosocial impact created by the incorporation of a new member into the family unit as a result of childbirth. Emphasis is placed upon the parenting process, including the manner in which parents attach to and communicate with their newborn. Many tables and boxes summarize key chapter content, thereby facilitating student learning and review.

Students are informed about the need of parents to develop their ability in the skill and knowledge component and the valuing and comfort component of the parenting role. Both parental role components are critical for the infant's physical and emotional growth and development. The process of parental acquaintance, bonding, and attachment to the newborn and the measures that nurses can use to foster this process are described.

Communication between the parents and their new child involves a variety of sensory techniques (e.g., touch and eye-to-eye contact), and the parents need to tune-in to the initiating and reciprocal cues offered by the infant. Early and extended contact and the change that occurs in the parental role with childbirth are discussed.

The fourth trimester is a period of adjustment to parenthood. It involves both an early period during which care giving and nurturing skills are attained and a consolidation period in which roles are negotiated and tasks and commitments are stabilized.

Maternal adjustment to the parenthood role is contrasted with paternal adjustment to the parenthood role. Maternal adjustment is described according to three phases: dependent (taking in), dependent-independent (taking hold), and interdependent (letting go). A discussion of postpartum blues ("baby blues") and postpartum depression is included as part of the description of maternal adjustment. Paternal adjustment is described as a three-stage process. A discussion of the father-infant relationship and the impact of fatherhood is included. Factors that influence parental responses include age, social support, culture, socioeconomic conditions, personal aspirations, and parental sensory impairment (visual and hearing impaired parents). An overview of sibling and grandparent adaptation to the newborn is included as part of the discussion regarding parental adjustment.

The chapter concludes with a description of the care management approach as it applies to the family during the first weeks at home with their newborn. Assessment methods, nursing diagnoses, and expected outcomes are identified for this period of time. Interventions are suggested, including instructions for the first few days at home, infant care, and anticipatory guidance for the newborn. Boxes provide information regarding resources for new parents, tub bathing, safety precautions, quieting techniques, teaching newborns and infants, benefits of infant massage, immunizations, and signs of illness. Two tables highlight infant growth and development and sensory stimulation during the first 3 months of infancy. A plan of care for home care follow-up during the transition to parenthood is included at the conclusion of the chapter. The nursing diagnoses of sleep pattern disturbance and risks for altered family processes, ineffective breastfeeding, and impaired home maintenance management are explored.

## LEARNING OBJECTIVES

Define the key terms.
Discuss transition as a concept central to the discipline of nursing.
Describe the two components of the parenting process.
Discuss five preconditions that influence attachment.
Describe sensual responses that strengthen attachment.
Differentiate the three periods in parental role change after childbirth.
Discuss the six parental tasks and responsibilities.
Identify infant behaviors that facilitate and inhibit parental attachment.
Identify behaviors of the three phases of maternal adjustment.
Discuss paternal adjustment.
Discuss ways to facilitate parent-infant adjustment.
Discuss the effects of the following on parental response: parental age (adolescence and over 35 years), social support, culture, socioeconomic conditions, personal aspirations, and sensory impairment.
Describe sibling adjustment.
Describe grandparent adaptation.
Discuss nursing care management for assisting transition to parenthood.
Identify topics for nursing research related to family dynamics during the transition to parenthood.

## OUTLINE OF CHAPTER CONTENT WITH COURSE GUIDELINES

| CONTENT | GUIDELINE |
|---|---|
| Transition | B |
| Parenting process | A |
| – Skill and knowledge component | A |
| – Valuing and comforting component | A |
| Parental attachment, bonding, and acquaintance | A |
| – Assessment of attachment behaviors | A |
| Parent-infant contact | A |
| – Early contact | A |
| – Extended contact | A |
| Communication between parent and infant | A |
| – Touch | A |
| – Eye-to-eye contact | A |
| – Voice | A |

*continued*

| CONTENT | GUIDELINE |
|---|:---:|
| – Odor | A |
| – Entrainment | B |
| – Biorhythmicity | B |
| – Reciprocity and synchrony | B |
| Parental role after childbirth | A |
| – Transition to parenthood | A |
| – Parental tasks and responsibilities | A |
| – Maternal adjustment | A |
| – Dependent phase (taking-in) | A |
| – Dependent-independent phase (taking-hold) | A |
| – Postpartum blues | A |
| – Interdependent phase (letting-go) | A |
| – Paternal adjustment | A |
| – Father-infant relationship | A |
| – Impact of fatherhood | A |
| – Infant-parent adjustment | A |
| – Rhythm | B |
| – Repertoires of behavior | B |
| – Responsivity | B |
| Factors influencing parental responses | |
| – Age | A |
| – Social support | A |
| – Culture | A |
| – Socioeconomic conditions | A |
| – Personal aspirations | A |
| Parental sensory impairment | B |
| – Visually impaired parent | B |
| – Hearing impaired parent | B |
| Sibling adaptation | A |
| Grandparent adaptation | B |
| Care management: practical suggestions for the first weeks at home | A |
| – Assessment and nursing diagnoses | A |
| – Expected outcomes of care | A |
| – Plan of care and interventions | A |
| – Instructions for first days at home | A |
| – Infant care | A |
| – Anticipatory guidance regarding the newborn | A |
| – Evaluation | A |
| Plan of care | A |

## TEACHING STRATEGIES

1. Show videos and/or photographs that depict the reciprocal communication patterns between the parent and newborn. Discuss how nurses can foster this process of communication and the progress of attachment.

2. Use case studies to illustrate the impact that a newborn can have on a family and how each family member changes and adapts to this impact.

3. Divide students into groups. Assign each group to contact one of the resources for new parents listed in Box 25-5 in the text. Arrange for students to report their findings to the class and discuss how they would use the resource's services when planning care for new parents.

4. Arrange for a panel of new parents—mothers and fathers—to describe their experiences caring for their newborn during the first few weeks at home after birth. Encourage them to identify how nurses helped or could have helped them meet the challenges that they faced regarding newborn care.

## SUGGESTED STUDENT LEARNING ACTIVITIES

1. *ASSESS* the mothering behaviors of two new mothers—a primipara and a multipara. These new mothers can be clients, friends, or family members.
   - *ANALYZE* the data that you collected, identifying behaviors that are adaptive or ineffective.
   - *DESCRIBE* the nursing care measures that you would use to reinforce adaptive behaviors and help the woman change ineffective ones.
   - *COMPARE* the "mothering" styles of the two mothers who you observed.

2. *DEVELOP* an assessment tool that can be used to determine the quality of the developing family-newborn relationship. The tool should reflect application of the concepts presented in Chapters 23 and 24. Each family member involved in the process should be considered.
   - *USE* the tool that you developed to assess one or more of your postpartum families.
   - *ANALYZE* the data that you collected; *IDENTIFY* appropriate nursing diagnoses and expected outcomes, and *CREATE* a plan of care.
   - *EVALUATE* your clinical site with regard to the provisions that it has made to facilitate the adjustment of parents, siblings, and grandparents to the newborn.
   - *SUGGEST* relevant changes based on the results of your evaluation; include the rationale for each change that you propose.

3. *SEARCH* the literature for research studies related to the nurse's role in fostering the development of a healthy family-newborn relationship. *CHOOSE* one study, and complete a bibliography card that includes the following:
   - Hypothesis; research question
   - Summary of the methodology used and its findings
   - Reliability of the study and its findings
   - Recommendations for further research
   - How the professional nurse can use the findings to help parents foster a healthy relationship with their newborn

4. *INTERVIEW* new parents (clients, family members, friends) regarding their adjustment to parenthood. *PREPARE* a report that includes the following information from your interview:
   - Their description of their "dream" or "fantasy" child as compared with their actual child and the manner in which they came to terms with any differences that they identified
   - Behaviors reflective of the phases or stages of maternal and paternal adjustment

- Factors that helped or hindered their adjustment to the new baby, including actions of each other, health care providers, family members, and friends; policies of the health care agency where they gave birth; and information obtained in parenting classes and reading
- Their description regarding how they communicate with their newborn and how the newborn communicates with them
- Their description of sibling and grandparent adaptation and how it affected parental adjustment to the new baby
- Strategies that they used to foster sibling adaptation to the newborn and the degree to which these strategies were successful

5. *OBSERVE* several parent-infant interactions. *IDENTIFY* the following:
   - Infant and parent behaviors that facilitated communication
   - Infant and parent behaviors that inhibited communication
   - Cultural influences on the parental behaviors toward the newborn

6. *CONSIDER* the unique needs of visually or hearing impaired parents.
   - *DEVELOP* teaching plans regarding newborn care that takes into consideration parental sensory impairment.
   - *DESCRIBE* measures that could be used to help them care for their infants, such as support of significant others, special devices, self-help or support groups, and community resources.

7. *USE* the "AM I BLUE?" assessment tool included in this chapter (Fig. 25-8) with two women who have recently given birth. These women can be clients, friends, or family members.
   - *ANALYZE* the results to determine the level of blues that they may be experiencing—none, mild, moderate, or severe.
   - *DEVELOP* a plan of care for each woman that will help her and her family prevent or minimize the postpartum blues or cope with the blues in a healthy manner.

## TOPICS FOR DISCUSSION

1. *Consider this question:* What impact can early discharge (within 24 hours or less of birth) have on a family's adjustment to a new baby, the development of parenting skills, and progress of parent-infant attachment?

2. *Support this statement:* Nursing interventions are critical in helping parents during pregnancy and after discharge to foster the development of healthy, well-adjusted families.

## MERLIN PROJECT

Imagine that you are a nurse working on a postpartum mother-baby unit. You have been asked to prepare a handout for new parents on Internet resources designed to inform and support women and men as they make the transition to parenthood and assume the responsibilities of caring for their newborn. Compile a list of web sites, including the following information for each site listed:
- Address and sponsor of the site
- Summary of the information and support services provided
- Guidelines for using the site for maximum effectiveness
- Services such as relevant links, e-mail, and chat rooms that will allow the user of the site to obtain additional information and individualized support

Chapter

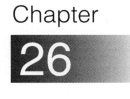

# Physiology and Physical Adaptations of the Newborn

## SUMMARY OF KEY CONCEPTS

Chapter 26 introduces the student to the newborn and the manner in which he or she adapts to life outside the uterus. The transition period after birth is described in terms of the periods of reactivity and the newborn behaviors typical of each.

The biologic characteristics of the newborn are presented in a system-by-system format. Changes for each system that occur after birth, characteristics and functional capacity, comparison with mature functioning on the adult level, and signs of risk for problems are identified. This format facilitates the student's ability to distinguish signs that indicate normal adaptation from those that indicate ineffective adaptation and potential problems. In addition, it provides the student with the theoretic basis for the nursing measures used to care for newborns.

The newborn's biologic characteristics and appropriate procedures and methods for data collection are organized into a physical assessment framework. Two tables concisely summarize the physical assessment of the newborn. One of the tables outlines the physical assessment of the newborn, contrasting normal findings and variations with those findings that indicate deviations from the normal range and the presence of possible problems. A second table highlights newborn reflexes, including methods used to elicit each reflex, and a description of the characteristic response to the stimulus. This approach provides the student with the knowledge and tools required to assess the newborn in a safe and systematic manner while in the clinical setting.

The chapter concludes with a discussion of the newborn's behavioral characteristics, including factors that influence behavior, such as sleep-wake states, sensory capabilities, and the manner in which the newborn responds to environmental stimuli. The discussion emphasizes the uniqueness of each newborn and the manner in which his or her behavioral characteristics influence his or her development and reciprocal responses from others.

# LEARNING OBJECTIVES

Define the key terms.

Describe the changes in the biologic system of the neonate during the transition to extrauterine life.

Identify the sequence to follow in assessment of the newborn.

Gather appropriate neonatal health history information from the prenatal and intrapartal periods.

Recognize deviations from normal physiologic findings during examination of the newborn.

Compare and contrast the four types of heat loss in a neonate and how to prevent heat loss.

Describe the behavioral adaptations of the newborn, including sleep-wake states and periods of reactivity.

Identify the sensory/perceptual functioning of the neonate.

# OUTLINE OF CHAPTER CONTENT WITH COURSE GUIDELINES

| CONTENT | GUIDELINE |
|---|:---:|
| Biologic characteristics | |
| – Respiratory system | A |
| – Circulatory system | A |
| – Thermogenic system | A |
| – Renal system | A |
| – Gastrointestinal system | A |
| – Hepatic system | A |
| – Immune system | A |
| – Integumentary system | A |
| – Reproductive system | A |
| – Skeletal system | A |
| – Neuromuscular system | A |
| Physical assessment | |
| – General appearance | A |
| – Vital signs | A |
| – Baseline measurements of physical growth | A |
| – Skin texture, color, opacity | A |
| – Head and neck | A |
| – Chest | A |
| – Abdomen | A |
| – Back and anus | A |
| – Genitalia | A |
| – Extremities | A |
| – Neurologic assessment | A |
| Behavioral characteristics | |
| – Sleep-wake states | A |
| – Other factors influencing behavior of newborns | B |
| – Sensory behaviors | A |

| CONTENT | GUIDELINE |
|---|---|
| – Response to environmental stimuli | B |
|    – Temperament | B |
|    – Habituation | B |
|    – Consolability | B |
|    – Cuddliness | B |
|    – Irritability | B |
|    – Crying | B |

## TEACHING STRATEGIES

1. Compare physiologic function of the newborn with physiologic function of an adult. Describe how these differences should influence the nursing care management of newborns.

2. Arrange for students to view a video that depicts newborn assessment and the unique characteristics of newborns.

3. Describe typical newborn characteristics and normal variations. Encourage students to share their observations of the characteristics of the newborns for whom they cared during their clinical experiences.

4. Describe the infant behaviors typical of each sleep and wake state. Discuss the approach that the nurse and parents should use to adapt to each state when caring for infants.

5. Use the Brazelton Neonatal Behavioral Assessment Scale (BNBAS) to illustrate how newborns respond to their environments and how these responses can be used to facilitate infant development and parent-infant attachment.

## SUGGESTED STUDENT LEARNING ACTIVITIES

1. *DESIGN* a newborn assessment form based on newborn characteristics and function presented in this chapter.
   - *USE* this assessment form during your clinical experience caring for newborns.
   - *ANALYZE* the data collected for each newborn assessed. Based upon this analysis, *IDENTIFY* the nursing diagnoses present and the expected outcomes. *FORMULATE* a plan of care appropriate to the nursing diagnoses of each newborn. (NOTE: Use Chapters 27 and 28 to assist you in completing this part of the activity.)
   - *USE* the data collected as a basis for individualized teaching sessions with the parents of each newborn. The goals of the teaching session would be to:
     - Familiarize the parents with the normal newborn characteristics exhibited by their baby and how these characteristics influence the care required by the newborn
     - Demonstrate to the parents how they can assess their baby to distinguish signs of normal function from those that indicate potential problems requiring follow-up by a health care provider

2. *DEVELOP* a parenthood education class related to newborn behavioral characteristics and parental activities designed to foster optimum newborn growth and development. The goals of the class would be to help parents become more aware of the following:
   - The uniqueness of their newborn in terms of sleep-wake states and responses to environmental stimuli
   - The capacity of their newborn to sense stimuli in their environment and respond to them
   - The types of stimuli and activities that parents can provide to foster the development of their newborn

## TOPICS FOR DISCUSSION

1. *Support these statements:*
   - Nurses play a critical role in helping new parents get to know their newborns.
   - Parental knowledge about the physical and behavioral characteristics of the newborn facilitates the process of parent-infant attachment.

2. *Consider these questions:*
   - What effect will participation in an early discharge program have on the level of knowledge that parents require regarding their newborn and the ability of the nurse to provide them with this knowledge?
   - How can sibling adjustment be enhanced by teaching children about the characteristics and behaviors of their new baby brother or sister?

## MERLIN PROJECT

Use MERLIN to assist you in searching the medical literature for nursing journal articles related to newborn biologic and behavioral characteristics, the manner in which nurses assess these characteristics, and how learning about these characteristics can help parents to foster the growth and development of their newborns. *CHOOSE* one article, and complete a bibliography card that includes the following:
   - Summary of the article's key points
   - Personal reaction to the ideas presented in the article
   - How the professional nurse could use the information presented to more accurately and efficiently assess newborns and teach parents about the biologic and behavioral characteristics of their newborns

Chapter

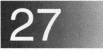

27

# Assessment and Care of the Newborn

## SUMMARY OF KEY CONCEPTS

Chapter 27 focuses on the care management of normal newborns during the period of time from birth through the first 2 hours and then from 2 hours after birth until discharge. This chapter builds on the content related to physiology and physical adaptations of the newborn that was covered in Chapter 26. Several boxes, tables, and illustrations highlight and emphasize important aspects of newborn care management.

The student is made aware of the importance of the nurse's role in newborn assessment in terms of the initial assessment after birth, gestational assessment, physical examination, and assessment for physical injuries and physiologic problems. Common laboratory and diagnostic tests and the normal ranges for a newborn and procedures appropriate for specimen collection are identified.

Nursing diagnoses and expected outcomes of care relevant to the newborn are listed. A protective environment for the newborn is described in terms of providing adequate lighting and warmth, eliminating hazards, including those arising from the presence of pathogenic microorganisms, and implementing security measures. Emphasis is placed on the critical role that the nurse plays in supporting the newborn's adaptation to extrauterine life. Consideration is given to maintaining a stable body temperature and an adequate oxygen supply and airway patency. Emergency boxes and illustrations concerning infant CPR and relieving airway obstruction are included in the chapter. Principles and methods related to infant feeding, positioning and holding, cord care, hygiene, and safety focus not only on what a nurse needs to know and do but also on parental responsibilities in each area. Bathing of the newborn receives special attention in the text and in the Home Care Box. The infant's social needs are briefly mentioned. A discussion of nursing responsibilities with regard to therapeutic interventions focuses on eye prophylaxis, intramuscular injections, therapy for hyperbilirubinemia, and circumcision. The student is introduced to the priority topics for discharge planning and teaching as they relate to the parents of a newborn.

The chapter includes a care path related to neonatal adaptation to extrauterine life and a plan of care that illustrates the use of the nursing process to manage the care of the normal newborn. Several nursing diagnoses are explored, including the risks for ineffective airway clearance, altered body temperature, infection, injury, and family coping—potential for growth.

# LEARNING OBJECTIVES

Define the key terms.

Identify purpose and components of the Apgar score.

Compare and contrast the characteristics of preterm, term, postterm, and postmature neonates.

Assess the gestational age and birth weight of newborns.

Rate infants using the physical maturity scale and neuromuscular maturity scale.

Explain what is meant by a safe environment.

Discuss phototherapy and the guidelines for teaching parents about this treatment.

Explain the purposes for and methods of circumcision, the postoperative care of the circumcised infant, and parent teaching information regarding circumcision.

Review procedures for doing a heel stick, collecting urine specimens, assisting with venipuncture, and restraining the newborn.

Review the anticipatory guidance nurses provide the parents before discharge.

Identify topics for nursing research related to assessment and care of the newborn.

# OUTLINE OF CHAPTER CONTENT WITH COURSE GUIDELINES

| CONTENT | GUIDELINE |
|---|:---:|
| Care management—from birth through the first 2 hours | |
| – Initial assessment and nursing diagnoses | A |
|   – Apgar score | A |
|   – Initial physical assessment | A |
| – Nursing diagnoses | A |
| – Expected outcomes of care | A |
| – Plan of care and interventions | A |
|   – Stabilization and resuscitation | A |
|   – Maintaining body temperature | A |
|   – Immediate interventions | A |
| – Evaluation | A |
| Care management—from 2 hours after birth until discharge | |
| – Assessment and nursing diagnoses | A |
|   – Assessment of gestational age | A |
|   – Assessment of common problems in the newborn | A |
|    – Physical injuries | A |
|    – Physiologic problems | A |
|    – Laboratory and diagnostic tests | A |
|    – Pain physiology | A |
| – Nursing diagnoses | A |
| – Expected outcomes of care | A |
| – Plan of care and interventions | A |
|   – Protective environment | A |
|   – Supporting parents in the care of their infant | A |

| CONTENT | GUIDELINE |
|---|---|
| – Therapeutic and surgical procedures | A |
| – Intramuscular injection | A |
| – Therapy for hyperbilirubinemia | A |
| – Circumcision | A |
| – Discharge planning and teaching | A |
| – Evaluation | A |
| Plan of care | A |

## TEACHING STRATEGIES

1. Discuss the care management of the newborn during the immediate postbirth period. Use the policies and procedures of agencies in your community and case studies to illustrate Apgar scoring and immediate assessment protocols, identification procedures, and prophylactic care measures.

2. Discuss the process of bonding and attachment as it applies to a newborn and the parents and family during the immediate period after birth. Describe the measures that nurses could use to facilitate or promote bonding and attachment behaviors. Encourage students to describe the observations that they made regarding bonding and attachment when working with newborns and their families immediately after birth.

3. Arrange for students to shadow a nurse who is responsible for the care management of a newborn during the immediate postbirth period. Provide class time for students to describe their experiences.

4. Describe the care management of newborns from 2 hours after birth until discharge by means of case studies, including those that involve newborns and their families cared for by the students during their clinical experiences. Encourage students to share their observations regarding newborn care during this period of time.

5. Demonstrate newborn care measures such as bathing, diapering, cord and circumcision care, restraining, specimen collections, and administration of medications using a "realistic" newborn doll or a newborn in the clinical setting.

6. Identify the essential components of discharge planning and teaching. Describe the content of a basic teaching plan and the difficulties that nurses might encounter in its implementation, especially in terms of time with an early-discharge program. Bring to class a variety of teaching aids including models, videos, books, and pamphlets that can be used to enhance a teaching plan and facilitate learning. Encourage students to devise creative approaches to teaching parents about their newborns.

7. Identify parent support groups, classes, and home care agencies available in your community to assist new parents as they take on the responsibility to care for and nurture their new baby.

# SUGGESTED STUDENT LEARNING ACTIVITIES

1. *DESIGN* a newborn assessment form according to the critical newborn adaptations to extrauterine life that can be used during the first 2 hours after birth.
   - *USE* this assessment form when caring for newborns during the immediate postbirth period.
   - *ANALYZE* the data collected for each newborn assessed. On the basis of this analysis, develop a protocol that nurses can follow to facilitate a newborn's transition to extrauterine life.

2. *OBSERVE* the newborn environment during your clinical experience. *WRITE* a report that includes each of the following points:
   - Types of environments used for newborns, such as a neonatal nursery, transition or admission nursery, the mother's room, and an intensive care nursery (ICN)
   - The manner in which environmental factors are regulated, infection is controlled, and safety and security are maintained
   - Changes that you would propose with regard to the newborn environment; include rationale for each proposed change
   - Measures that you used to regulate environmental factors, control infection, and maintain safety and security

3. *SEARCH* the nursing literature for articles related to single room maternity care (SRMC) or mother-baby (couplet) care as an approach to health management of the new family. Choose one article, and complete a bibliography card that includes the following:
   - Summary of the key concepts presented in the article
   - Degree of satisfaction with this approach to health care delivery from both the client and nurse's point of view
   - Your reaction to this approach
   - How the professional nurse could use the information in the article to enhance and improve health care for the newborn and his or her family

4. *VISIT* your local library or bookstore, and take note of the variety of literature (i.e., books, magazine articles) and videos related to newborn care and parenting. Considering the difficulty that new parents would have in deciding what to read or view, choose two of the items that you found to be the most appealing. *DESCRIBE* your choices in terms of the following:
   - Readability and clarity of presentation
   - Accuracy, currency, and comprehensiveness of content presented
   - Credentials of the authors
   - Cost
   - Manner in which you would use your choices to meet the learning needs of new parents

5. *DESIGN* a pamphlet for new parents that highlights a newborn's characteristics and his or her care needs. Also include the impact that this infant will have on the entire family and the coping strategies that the parents could use to facilitate the adaptation of each family member to the baby.

6. *DETERMINE* the gestational age of a newborn using the Newborn Maturity Rating and Classification form (Fig. 27-1) included in the chapter. *COMPARE* your findings with the gestational age of the newborn as determined by the estimated date of birth (EDB) or sonography.

7. *PREPARE* a 2-hour class for new parents that focuses on the essential care needs of newborns for the first few days after birth. The class would be presented before discharge as part of a home care program. *INCLUDE* the following:
   - Outline and rationale of class content
   - Teaching strategies that you would use, such as lecture, demonstrations, discussion, handouts, and audiovisual presentations
   - Follow-up methods to evaluate learning and discuss concerns

8. *INVESTIGATE* the infant care beliefs and practices of one cultural group in your community.
   - *SUMMARIZE* the information gathered in your investigation, including references used.
   - *INTERVIEW* parents representing the cultural group that you investigated to determine the extent to which they adhere to their culture's beliefs and practices regarding the care of infants.
   - *DESCRIBE* how you would incorporate the cultural information gathered into a plan of care that respects the infant care beliefs and practices of parents from this culture.

## TOPICS FOR DISCUSSION

1. *Support these statements:*
   - The cultural background of parents should be considered when caring for newborns and teaching parents about newborn care and characteristics.
   - The nurse has a responsibility to ensure the safety, security, and well-being of newborns before and after they are discharged.

2. *Consider this question:* How should couplet (mother-baby) care be individualized to meet the unique needs of new families?

3. *Debate the issue:* Are circumcisions necessary to preserve the health of a male and eventually his female sexual partner **OR** are circumcisions performed primarily on the basis of tradition?

## MERLIN PROJECT

Use MERLIN to access the Centers for Disease Control and Prevention (CDC) and National Center for Health Statistics (NCHS) web sites to gather statistical information related to gestational age (preterm, term, postterm, postmature), intrauterine growth (LBW, IUGR, SGA, AGA, LGA), and infant morbidity and mortality.
   - Create a table that illustrates your findings, including rate of occurrence and characteristics of the mothers and families of these infants.
   - Prepare a report that describes your proposals for health services that will help reduce the rates of gestational and growth problems and infant morbidity and mortality. Include the rationale for your proposals.

# Chapter

## 28

# Newborn Nutrition and Feeding

## SUMMARY OF KEY CONCEPTS

Chapter 28 introduces students to infant nutrient requirements and care management as it relates to infant nutrition and feeding. The benefits of breastfeeding for infants, mothers, families, and society are delineated. The process for making an informed decision when choosing an infant feeding method is described according to the factors influencing the decision and the role of the nurse in guiding the process.

A description of newborn feeding readiness cues and the nutrients required for optimal growth includes comparisons among breast milk, cow's milk, and formulas with respect to nutrient content and their composition and compatibility with the infant's digestive system. Students are informed about the influence of culture on infant feeding practices.

Lactation, as a method of infant feeding, is described in extensive detail. Numerous illustrations, photographs, boxes, and tables highlight critical content and can be used by students to teach breastfeeding women and their families. The physiologic processes involved in normal lactation are discussed, including milk production and the uniqueness of human milk.

The care management of the breastfeeding mother and infant follows a nursing process framework. Factors to consider when assessing infant and mother before and during breastfeeding and for ongoing assessment and the indicators of effective breastfeeding during the first week are identified. Typical nursing diagnoses and expected outcomes related to breastfeeding are listed. Consideration is given to the nurse's role in formulating a plan of care. A description of effective breastfeeding techniques includes positioning, latch-on, let-down reflex, feeding patterns, engorgement, pumping, and weaning. Nurses and lactation consultants are essential to the success and continuation of breastfeeding. Maternal care emphasizes the effect of nutrition, weight loss, activity and rest, breast care, sexuality, contraception, and use of medications on the lactation process. Common maternal-infant problems, special considerations related to breastfeeding, and the identification of appropriate measures to solve each problem are discussed. A plan of care related to breastfeeding develops the nursing diagnosis of ineffective breastfeeding.

A discussion of formula feeding follows a format similar to breastfeeding. Care measures for mother and infant, formula preparation, and feeding techniques are included. A box highlights the critical teaching points for formula preparation and feeding.

# LEARNING OBJECTIVES

Define the key terms.

List newborn feeding-readiness cues.

Describe current recommendations for feeding infants.

Discuss benefits of breastfeeding for infants, mothers, families, and society.

Explain the nurse's role in helping families to choose an infant feeding method.

Describe nutritional needs of infants.

Describe the anatomy and physiology of breastfeeding.

Explain the species specificity of human breast milk and its uniqueness for the infant.

Identify nursing interventions to facilitate and promote successful breastfeeding.

List signs of adequate intake in the breastfed infant.

Develop a nursing plan of care for the breastfeeding mother and infant.

Identify common problems associated with breastfeeding and nursing interventions to help resolve them.

List the types of commercial infant formula, advantages of each, and appropriate methods of preparation.

Discuss client teaching for the formula-feeding family.

Identify topics for nursing research related to newborn nutrition and feeding.

# OUTLINE OF CHAPTER CONTENT WITH COURSE GUIDELINES

| CONTENT | GUIDELINE |
|---|---|
| Recommended infant nutrition | A |
| Breastfeeding rates | C |
| Benefits of breastfeeding | A |
| Choosing an infant feeding method | B |
| Cultural influences on infant feeding | B |
| Feeding readiness | A |
| Nutrient needs | A |
| Overview of lactation | |
|   – Milk production | A |
|   – Uniqueness of human milk | B |
| Care management of the breastfeeding mother and infant | |
|   – Assessment and nursing diagnoses | A |
|   – Expected outcomes of care | A |
|   – Plan of care and interventions | A |
|     – Positioning | A |
|     – Latch-on | A |
|     – Milk ejection or let-down | A |
|     – Frequency and duration of feedings | A |
|     – Indicators of effective breastfeeding | A |
|     – Special considerations | A |
|     – Supplements, bottles, and pacifiers | A |
|   – Evaluation | A |

*continued*

| CONTENT | GUIDELINE |
|---|:---:|
| Role of the nurse in promoting successful lactation | A |
| – Follow-up after hospital discharge | A |
| Formula feeding | A |
| – Reasons for formula feeding | A |
| – Parent education | A |

## TEACHING STRATEGIES

1. Identify the nutrient and fluid needs of the infant. Discuss the signs indicative of adequate newborn nutrition and hydration.

2. Describe the process of lactation. Identify maternal, newborn, and environmental factors that could facilitate or hinder the process.

3. Use case studies, including those involving women for whom students have cared during their clinical experiences, to illustrate the care management of breastfeeding women and bottle-feeding women. Identify reasons that these women cited for their choice of feeding method.

4. Demonstrate breastfeeding and bottle-feeding techniques (e.g., latch-on, removal, positions of mother and infant, and burping) using illustrations and/or a "realistic" newborn doll.

5. Discuss the approaches that employed breastfeeding women can use to continue breastfeeding after returning to work. Bring to class a variety of breast pumps. Demonstrate the use of a breast pump, and discuss their cost and availability. Describe the process of safe milk storage.

6. Arrange for students to view a breastfeeding video.

7. Invite a lactation consultant to discuss the typical problems encountered by breastfeeding women and the solutions that she has found to be helpful.

8. Identify breastfeeding support services available in your community.

9. Bring to class a variety of commercially prepared formulas. Discuss nutritional content, method of preparation, and cost of each type of formula. Compare breast milk with commercially prepared formulas with regard to nutritional balance and ability to facilitate infant development and growth.

## SUGGESTED STUDENT LEARNING ACTIVITIES

1. *INTERVIEW* parents 1 week after discharge regarding the feeding of their newborn. *PREPARE* a report that includes information regarding the following:
   - When they made the decision concerning the method that they would use to feed their baby
   - How they made their decision, including factors that influenced their decision
   - What sources they used to learn the information that they needed to know about how to feed their baby using their method of choice

- Their perception of the nurse's effectiveness in helping them to learn how to feed their baby correctly
- The level of confidence that they feel and demonstrate in terms of their skill in feeding the baby

2. *SURVEY* your community for the types of breastfeeding support services available (e.g., La Leche groups, breastfeeding classes, and lactation consultation practices).
   - *DESCRIBE* the services available, including cost, location, services offered, qualifications of those offering the services, and population served.
   - *COMPILE* the information, and devise a method of distribution to women who would have need for such services.

3. *EVALUATE* the types of commercially prepared infant formulas that are currently available. To obtain this information, visit stores in your local area that sell infant formulas.
   - *COMPARE* brands as to nutrient value.
   - *ASSESS* the clarity and readability of the instructions given for those types of formulas that require some preparation. Are the instructions illustrated for parents who cannot read or are they written in a different language for parents who do not understand English?
   - *COMPARE* the cost based on brands (i.e., generic versus name brands), the forms in which it is sold (i.e., ready-to-use, powder, and concentrate), and the age of the infant at 1 month, 4 months, and 6 months.
   - *SUMMARIZE* in chart from the data you collected.
   - *DISCUSS* the type of formula that you would recommend to a family on a limited budget; *GIVE* the rationale for your recommendation.

4. *INTERVIEW* a nurse who works as a lactation consultant. The interview should cover topics such as the following:
   - Educational background and certification status
   - Role description and philosophy of nursing
   - Degree of acceptance by other nurses, physicians, other health care providers, and breastfeeding women and their families
   - Common lactation problems encountered and solutions found to be effective
   - Manner in which she uses nursing research findings when providing care
   - Method of payment for services

5. *INVESTIGATE* the infant feeding practices of two cultural groups in your community.
   - *DESCRIBE* the beliefs and practices concerning the recommended method of feeding, care of mother and infant, weaning, and the offering of solid foods.
   - *COMPARE* each culture, noting similarities and differences.
   - *DISCUSS* how this information should be used when planning care for women and infants representing the cultures identified.

6. *VISIT* your local library or bookstore, and take note of the variety of literature (i.e., books and magazine articles), computer programs, and videos related to infant feeding methods. Choose one book, magazine article, or video that you find to be the most appealing, and describe it in terms of the following:
   - Readability and/or clarity of presentation
   - Accuracy, currency, and comprehensiveness of content presented

- Credentials of the authors
- Cost
- Manner in which you would use your choice to meet the learning needs of new parents

## TOPICS FOR DISCUSSION

1. *Consider these questions:*
   - What effect does a mother's career role have on the method of feeding chosen? How will this career affect breastfeeding if that is her choice?
   - What effect does our society's image of the female breast have on a woman's choice to breast-feed, her partner's reaction to breastfeeding, and her ability to breastfeed outside her home?
   - What effect does early discharge have on a primiparous woman's ability to develop skill and confidence with breastfeeding?

2. *Support this statement:* Prenatal breastfeeding classes have a positive impact on breastfeeding success after the baby is born.

## MERLIN PROJECT

1. Use MERLIN to assist you in searching the medical literature for nursing research studies related to effective nursing measures designed to support the breastfeeding mother and prevent and manage common breastfeeding problems including nipple soreness, engorgement, and maternal and/or newborn difficulty with adjustment to breastfeeding.
   - Create an annotated bibliography of at least five nursing research studies.
   - Choose one study, and complete a bibliography card that includes the following:
     - Hypothesis; research question
     - Summary of the methodology used and key findings
     - Reliability of the study and its findings
     - Recommendations for further research
     - How a lactation consultant could use the findings to improve the breastfeeding care and support that she provides to breastfeeding women and their newborns
   - Discuss how you would use the findings of these research studies to create an evidence-based protocol for mother-baby nurses to follow when they manage the care of breastfeeding women. Explain why such a protocol is an important factor in successful, long-term breastfeeding.
2. Use MERLIN to assist you in finding the Update for Healthy People 2000 Report. Write a report that includes the following:
   - Summary of the goals for breastfeeding in the United States
   - Degree to which the goals have been met
   - Characteristics of women who breastfeed and how long they breastfeed
   - Programs that you would propose to:
     - Target populations that are least likely to breastfeed
     - Increase the duration of breastfeeding

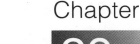

# Assessment for Risk Factors

## SUMMARY OF KEY CONCEPTS

In Chapter 29, students are introduced to the problem of high risk pregnancy—its scope and the factors and methods used to determine the presence and degree of risk.

Statistical data illustrate the scope of the problem. Rates for maternal and perinatal morbidity and mortality and trends within population groups are included. Tables delineate biophysical, psychosocial, sociodemographic, and environmental risk factors. The concept of regionalization of health care services as a means of providing adequate cost-effective care to both low and high risk pregnant women is discussed.

A variety of biophysical, biochemical, and electronic testing methods are described. Test descriptions include indications for use, associated risk, methodology, interpretation of findings, and nursing measures related to the preparation and support of women undergoing these tests and their families.

## LEARNING OBJECTIVES

Define the key terms.
Explore the scope of high risk pregnancy.
Discuss regionalization of health care services.
Examine risk factors identified through history, physical examination, and diagnostic techniques.
Describe diagnostic techniques and the implications of findings.
Explain diagnostic techniques to clients and their families.
Identify topics for nursing research related to assessment of high risk pregnancy.

# OUTLINE OF CHAPTER CONTENT WITH COURSE GUIDELINES

| CONTENT | GUIDELINE |
|---|:---:|
| Definition and scope of the problem | A |
| – Maternal health problems | A |
| – Fetal and neonatal health problems | A |
| – Regionalization of health care services | C |
| – Assessment of risk factors | A |
| Antepartum testing and biophysical assessment | A |
| – Daily fetal movement count | A |
| – Ultrasonography | A |
| – Doppler blood flow analysis | B |
| – Biophysical profile | A |
| – Magnetic resonance imaging | B |
| Biochemical assessment | A |
| – Amniocentesis | A |
| – Percutaneous umbilical blood sampling | B |
| – Chorionic villus sampling | A |
| – Maternal assays | A |
| Electronic fetal monitoring | A |
| – Indications | A |
| – Fetal response to hypoxia or asphyxia | A |
| – Nonstress test (fetal activity determination) | A |
| – Fetal acoustic stimulation | A |
| – Contraction stress test | A |
| Nursing role in antepartal assessment for risk | A |

# TEACHING STRATEGIES

1. Describe, through information from the media and biostatistical data, the problem of high risk pregnancy in your community as compared with your state and the nation.

2. Create a chart that illustrates how health care services for pregnant women, their infants, and families are organized in your community.

3. Use the case histories of clients cared for by the students in the clinical setting to provide specific examples of high risk factors representing each category. Encourage the students to describe how their clients' risk factors affected them and their families and how the factors were managed during the clients' prenatal care.

4. Compare diagnostic test protocols implemented by the health care agencies in your community with the protocols described in the text.

5. Arrange for students to observe antepartal testing during their clinical experiences. Involve students in a discussion of their observations, including why the tests were performed, client and family reactions, and nursing care measures.

6. Use transparencies and videos to illustrate the techniques involved in performing antepartal fetal monitoring.

7. Illustrate results of nonstress tests and contraction stress tests using monitor tracings from actual tests performed.

8. Invite a nurse involved in antepartal testing to discuss the measures that he or she uses to prepare women and their families for antepartal tests and to care for them during and after the tests.

9. Identify support services that are available in your community to assist high risk pregnant women and their families.

## SUGGESTED STUDENT LEARNING ACTIVITIES

1. *DESCRIBE* the fetal assessment measures used by the hospital where you have your clinical experience. *PREPARE* a report that includes the following:
   - Protocols followed
   - Nursing responsibilities and input with regard to the protocols used
   - Degree and nature of client preparation and support
   - Legal implications, including need for informed consent
   - Comparison of the data gathered with information presented in this chapter
   - Changes that you would propose, if any, in this agency's practices with regard to high risk antepartal testing; include rationale for each change that you propose

2. *INTERVIEW* a postpartum woman (client, friend, or family member) who experienced a high risk pregnancy. *GATHER* data related to the following:
   - Factors that placed her pregnancy in the high risk category
   - Physical and psychosocial stressors that she identified as outcomes of her high risk status; indicate the degree of stress
   - Types of antepartal testing that she experienced, her reaction to the testing, and her family's reaction
   - Supportive measures provided by nurses and other health care providers that helped her and her family cope with the stressors that she identified and with the antepartal testing that she experienced; indicate the degree of support that each measure represented
   - Additional measures that she and her family would have appreciated

3. *SEARCH* the nursing literature for articles related to high risk pregnancies—identification of risk, monitoring of progress, and general care management measures. *CHOOSE* one article, and complete a bibliography card that includes the following:
   - Summary of the article's key points
   - Personal reaction to the ideas presented in the article
   - How the professional nurse can use the article's ideas to enhance and improve the quality of health care provided to high risk pregnant women and their families

4. *INVESTIGATE* the high risk pregnancy situation in your community. *PREPARE* a report that includes the following:
   - The types of high risk problems that are the most common
   - The incidence of these problems, including a breakdown according to area, population, and age
   - Type and accessibility of services provided to prevent as well as treat high risk pregnancies—before, during, and after pregnancy
   - Degree that regionalization of pregnancy services—Level I, Level II, and Level III services—are used in your community; indicate the agencies designated for each category

## TOPICS FOR DISCUSSION

1. *Address this question:* Should antepartal testing be used for reasons other than the assessment of fetal health and well-being (e.g., selecting the "perfect child" according to characteristics, gender, or absence of genetic health problems of any kind)?

2. *Support this statement:* The nurse plays a critical role as advocate and supporter of the high risk pregnant woman and her family before, during, and after antepartal testing used to assess the health and well-being of the future baby.

## MERLIN PROJECT

Use MERLIN to assist you in an Internet-based investigation of the high risk pregnancy situation in the United States today. Prepare a report that includes the following:
   - The types of high risk problems that are the most common
   - The incidence of these problems, including a breakdown according to the area of the country, aggregate or group, and characteristics of women experiencing high risk pregnancy
   - Type and accessibility of services provided to prevent as well as treat high risk pregnancies—before, during, and after pregnancy
   - Degree that regionalization of pregnancy services—Level I, Level II, and Level III services—is used in the United States

Chapter

# 30

# Hypertensive Disorders in Pregnancy

## Summary of Key Concepts

The focus of Chapter 30 is the hypertensive disorders of pregnancy, their classifications, distinguishing characteristics, and approaches to treatment.

Hypertensive disorders, a leading cause of maternal, fetal, and newborn morbidity and mortality, are classified according to their relationship to pregnancy—gestational or those induced by pregnancy (transient hypertension, preeclampsia, eclampsia, HELLP syndrome) and those present before pregnancy (chronic hypertension with or without superimposed preeclampsia/eclampsia). Characteristics that distinguish each classification are fully described in the text and highlighted in tables and boxes, thereby facilitating the students' ability to assess their clients for the presence, severity, and progress of these disorders. Furthermore, students are assisted to understand the basis of the typical manifestations of pregnancy-induced hypertension (PIH) by contrasting the normal maternal physiologic changes that occur with pregnancy with the ineffective maternal physiologic changes that result in pregnancy-induced hypertensive disorders. Current theories and research related to causative factors are presented.

Care management of women with preeclampsia and eclampsia uses the nursing process as an organizing framework. Assessment methods include interview, physical examination, and laboratory tests. Risk factors are delineated to assist in the identification of women most vulnerable to the development of PIH. Typical nursing diagnoses and expected outcomes of care are provided. Interventions focus on the prenatal, intrapartum, and postpartum periods, as well as considerations for home and hospital care. Medical and nursing measures are guided by the severity of the problem from mild to severe preeclampsia and to eclampsia. A number of highlight boxes assist the student in planning interventions and health teaching. The discussion of severe preeclampsia emphasizes pharmacologic protocols and seizure precautions and care.

Two plans of care are included in the chapter. The first presents a woman with mild preeclampsia who is being managed at home. The nursing diagnoses of risk for injury, fear/anxiety, and diversional activity deficit are developed. The second plan of care presents a woman with severe preeclampsia being managed in the hospital. The nursing diagnoses of altered tissue perfusion and risks for injury to the mother, fluid volume excess, impaired gas exchange, decreased cardiac output, and injury to the fetus are developed.

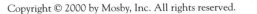

# LEARNING OBJECTIVES

Define the key terms.
Differentiate between PIH and chronic hypertension.
Review etiologic theories of PIH.
Describe the pathophysiology of PIH.
Evaluate maternal, fetal, and newborn morbidity and mortality attributable to PIH.
Identify assessment techniques for PIH.
Differentiate between the management of the woman with mild preeclampsia and the woman with severe preeclampsia.
Describe HELLP syndrome, including appropriate nursing actions.
Identify the priorities for management of eclamptic seizures.
Evaluate the use of anticonvulsant and antihypertensive therapies.
Identify topics for nursing research related to hypertensive disorders in pregnancy.

# OUTLINE OF CHAPTER CONTENT WITH COURSE GUIDELINES

| CONTENT | GUIDELINE |
|---|:---:|
| Hypertension in pregnancy | |
|   – Significance and incidence | A |
|   – Morbidity and mortality | A |
|   – Classification | A |
|     – Preeclampsia | A |
|     – Eclampsia | A |
|     – HELLP syndrome | A |
|     – Chronic hypertension | A |
|     – Transient hypertension | A |
|   – Etiology | A |
|     – Pathophysiology | A |
|     – HELLP syndrome | A |
| Care management | |
|   – Assessment and nursing diagnoses | A |
|     – Interview | A |
|     – Physical examination | A |
|     – Laboratory tests | A |
|   – Nursing diagnoses | A |
|   – Expected outcomes of care | A |
|   – Plan of care and interventions | A |
|     – Preeclampsia | A |
|       – Home care | A |
|     – Severe preeclampsia and HELLP syndrome | A |
|       – Hospital care | A |
|       – Magnesium sulfate | A |
|       – Control of blood pressure | A |

| CONTENT | GUIDELINE |
|---|---|
| – Eclampsia | A |
|    – Immediate care | A |
|   – Postpartum nursing care | A |
| – Evaluation | A |
| Plans of care | A |

## TEACHING STRATEGIES

1. Use statistical data to describe the incidence of hypertensive disorders in pregnancy. Compare local, state, and national incidences.

2. Create a profile of pregnant women who are likely to experience hypertensive disorders.

3. Contrast expected cardiovascular changes associated with pregnancy with those associated with PIH. Compare typical assessment findings for each hypertensive disorder.

4. Use case studies, especially those related to the students' clinical experiences, to explain the care management of pregnant women with hypertensive disorders.

5. Compare the magnesium sulfate protocol of the health care agencies in your community with the protocols suggested in the text and by professional associations such as ACOG and AWHONN.

6. Describe the options available locally and nationally for home care and hospital care (specialty obstetric critical care units) for pregnant women with hypertensive disorders.

7. Invite a nurse involved in the care of high risk pregnant women and a woman who has experienced a high risk pregnancy to participate in a class discussion concerning the experience and management of hypertensive disorders during pregnancy.
   - The nurse should discuss the care management approaches that are used when caring for these pregnant women and their families at home and in a hospital setting.
   - The woman should discuss her personal recollections of the impact that her high risk pregnancy had on her and her family and of the care management approaches that were helpful or not helpful in assisting them to cope in a positive way with the stressors associated with her high risk status.

## SUGGESTED STUDENT LEARNING ACTIVITIES

1. *DESCRIBE* the protocol used for the administration of magnesium sulfate therapy to treat women with severe preeclampsia in the hospital where you have your clinical experience.
   - *SUMMARIZE* the protocol used, including nursing input into its creation and nursing responsibilities when it is implemented.
   - *COMPARE* your findings with the information presented in this chapter.
   - *DESCRIBE* any changes that you would propose in the protocol. Include the rationale for each of your proposed changes.

2. *SURVEY* your community for the resources that would be available to assist low-income pregnant women to cope with bed rest at home as part of the care management for preeclampsia.

3. *INTERVIEW* a woman whose pregnancy was complicated by preeclampsia.
   - *GATHER* information regarding the following:
     - The woman's description of the impact that this pregnancy related health problem had on her pregnancy, on herself, and on her family
     - Coping mechanisms that the woman and her family used to deal with the stressors encountered as a result of the health problem that she experienced during her pregnancy
     - The support measures, persons, and services that she and her family found to be helpful and those that they found to be lacking or not helpful
     - Additional support measures that she and her family would have appreciated
     - Her impressions of the impact that the health care system and health care providers had on her health and well-being during pregnancy, childbirth, and the puerperium
   - *DESCRIBE* how you would use this information to plan care that is effective not only related to the woman with preeclampsia's physical needs but also related to the woman and her family's psychosocial and emotional needs.

## TOPICS FOR DISCUSSION

1. *Support these statements:*
   - Nurses play a critical role in the early detection of and prompt treatment for preeclampsia.
   - Home care is a safe and effective alternative to hospital care when pregnant women are diagnosed with mild preeclampsia. State the rationale for your response. Indicate the criteria that should be used to determine whether or not a woman is a candidate for home care.

2. *Consider these questions:*
   - How can the safety of the maternal-fetal unit be ensured when the woman with preeclampsia is treated in her home?
   - How can the nurse address the emotional needs of the critically ill pregnant woman and her family?

## MERLIN PROJECT

Use MERLIN to assist you in searching the medical literature for research studies related to the care management of women with preeclampsia, including the impact that bed rest can have on the pregnant woman.
   - Create an annotated bibliography of at least three studies.
   - Choose one study, and complete a bibliography card that includes the following:
     - Hypothesis; research question
     - Summary of the methodology used and key findings
     - Reliability of the study and its findings
     - Recommendations for further research
   - Describe how you would use the research findings to provide evidenced-based care to the pregnant woman with preeclampsia.

## Chapter

# 31

# Antepartal Hemorrhagic Disorders

## SUMMARY OF KEY CONCEPTS

Chapter 31 presents the student with a detailed overview of disorders that can result in antepartal maternal hemorrhage. The disorders are categorized according to their occurrence during pregnancy, either early or late. Each disorder is described in terms of its pathophysiology, incidence, etiology and risk factors, clinical manifestations, maternal and fetal effects, and care management. The care management for several of the disorders is discussed within the nursing process framework. Assessment factors and methods, nursing diagnoses, expected outcomes of care, and a variety of interventions are identified and described. Home care issues are raised as part of the discussion. Numerous tables, boxes, and illustrations accompany the discussion of the disorders, thereby facilitating student learning and review.

Spontaneous abortion, incompetent cervix, ectopic pregnancy, and hydatidiform mole are the disorders explored as the causes for early pregnancy bleeding. The discussion of late pregnancy bleeding focuses on the placental disorders of placenta previa and abruptio placenta. A plan of care is included that illustrates the use of the nursing process for the care management of a woman experiencing placenta previa. The nursing diagnoses of decreased cardiac output and risks for injury to the fetus and infection are developed.

The chapter concludes with a concise overview of the clotting disorders that can complicate pregnancy. The primary focus of the overview is disseminated intravascular coagulation (DIC).

## LEARNING OBJECTIVES

Define the key terms.
Compare and differentiate abruptio placentae and placenta previa.
Discuss clotting disorders in pregnancy, with emphasis on disseminated intravascular coagulation.
Discuss differences in plans of care for the woman with an unruptured ectopic pregnancy versus a ruptured ectopic pregnancy.
Review the physiology of a hydatidiform mole and the risk factors for the woman's immediate health future.

Summarize the role of the nurse in the health care team approach to the treatment of bleeding disorders.

Identify topics for nursing research related to antepartal maternal hemorrhagic disorders.

## OUTLINE OF CHAPTER CONTENT WITH COURSE GUIDELINES

| CONTENT | GUIDELINE |
|---|---|
| Early pregnancy bleeding | A |
| – Spontaneous abortion (miscarriage) | A |
| – Incompetent cervix | A |
| – Ectopic pregnancy | A |
| – Hydatidiform mole | B |
| Late pregnancy bleeding | A |
| – Placenta previa | A |
| – Premature separation of placenta | A |
| – Plan of care—placenta previa | A |
| – Cord insertion and placental variations | B |
| Clotting disorders in pregnancy | A |
| – Normal clotting | A |
| – Clotting problems | A |
| – Disseminated intravascular coagulation (DIC) | B |
| – Von Willebrand's disease | C |

## TEACHING STRATEGIES

1. Use statistical data to describe the incidence of disorders responsible for antepartal hemorrhage. Compare local, state, and national incidences.

2. Create profiles of women who are at risk for the disorders that can lead to early and late antepartal hemorrhage.

3. Use case studies, especially those related to the students' clinical experiences, to explain the nursing care management of pregnant women with bleeding disorders. Compare the case studies with the recommended care management in the textbook.

4. Describe options available locally and nationally for home care and hospital care for pregnant women with bleeding disorders.

5. Create a chart that compares clinical findings and care management approaches for the most common disorders responsible for early (spontaneous abortion, ectopic pregnancy) and late (placenta previa, abruptio placentae) antepartal hemorrhage.

6. Invite couples who have experienced a pregnancy loss related to one of the bleeding disorders described in the chapter to discuss the impact that this event had on their lives and the degree to which nurses helped them cope with the loss. Encourage the couples to share the nursing actions that were helpful or not helpful and what support measures they hoped for but did not receive.

# SUGGESTED STUDENT LEARNING ACTIVITIES

1. *SEARCH* the literature for nursing research studies related to parental responses to a sudden, late pregnancy loss associated with such disorders as placenta previa and abruptio placentae and the nursing support measures found to be effective. *CHOOSE* one study, and complete a bibliography card that includes the following:
   - Hypothesis; research question
   - Summary of the methodology used and key findings
   - Reliability of the study and its findings
   - Recommendations for further research
   - How the professional nurse could use the findings to enhance and improve supportive care of a woman and her family who have experienced a sudden, late pregnancy loss

2. *INTERVIEW* a woman who experienced a spontaneous abortion (miscarriage).
   - *GATHER* information regarding the following:
     - The feelings and emotions of the woman and her family regarding the abortion (miscarriage)—when it was happening and afterwards
     - Coping mechanisms that the woman and her family used to deal with the loss of the pregnancy and the anticipated child
     - The woman's thoughts and feelings at the present time with regard to the lost child, when the expected date of birth occurs, and on the anniversary date of the pregnancy loss; include the feelings of her family
     - Support measures, persons, and services that she and her family found to be helpful and those that they found to be lacking or not helpful
     - Support measures that they would have liked to have received but did not
   - *DESCRIBE* how you would use the information gathered to offer supportive care to other women and their families who are experiencing a spontaneous abortion (miscarriage).

3. *SEARCH* the nursing literature for articles related to the care management of hemorrhagic disorders that occur during pregnancy. *CHOOSE* one article, and complete a bibliography card that includes the following:
   - Summary of the article's key points
   - Personal reaction to the ideas presented in the article
   - How the professional nurse could use the information presented to enhance and improve health care

# TOPICS FOR DISCUSSION

1. *Consider these questions:*
   - What types of support services should hospitals provide to assist couples who have experienced a loss of pregnancy? What should the role of the nurse be in establishing these services and supporting the couples affected?
   - What, if anything, can nurses do to reduce the incidence of spontaneous abortions (miscarriages) and ectopic pregnancies?

2. *Support these statements*:
   - The nurse plays a critical role in providing emotional support to a woman experiencing late pregnancy bleeding and her family.
   - Home care is a safe and effective alternative to hospital care for women who are diagnosed with threatened abortion and placental previa. State the rationale for your response. Indicate the criteria that should be used to determine if the woman would be a candidate for home care.

# MERLIN PROJECT

Use MERLIN to access the CDC and the NCHS to gather statistical information regarding the scope of the problem of the antepartal bleeding disorders identified in Chapter 31. Create a chart that includes the following:
   - Incidence of each of the types of bleeding disorders in your state and in the nation as a whole
   - Characteristics of women who develop each of these disorders
   - Impact of each of the disorders on maternal and fetal/newborn morbidity and mortality
   - Types of treatment modalities used—home care and hospital care

# Chapter

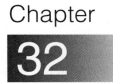

32

# Endocrine and Metabolic Disorders

## SUMMARY OF KEY CONCEPTS

Endocrine and metabolic disorders, with an emphasis on pregestational and gestational diabetes mellitus, are the focus of Chapter 32. Care management and the latest research findings concerning these disorders and their medical management provide the student with the knowledge required to apply the nursing process when caring for women whose pregnancy is complicated by these disorders. Statistical data and risk factors are included for each disorder.

The chapter begins with an in-depth discussion of diabetes mellitus and its effect on pregnancy and pregnancy's effect on the diabetes mellitus. A brief overview of the pathogenesis of diabetes mellitus and the metabolic changes that occur during pregnancy are provided and serve as the foundation for the discussion of diabetes during pregnancy. The classification of diabetes mellitus using the system recommended by the Expert Committee on the Diagnosis and Classification of Diabetes Mellitus is explained. The student is introduced to the concept of preconception counseling as a critical factor in achieving the goal of a healthy maternal and newborn outcome to a pregnancy complicated by pregestational diabetes. The maternal, fetal, and newborn risks and complications are clearly delineated. Care management of the pregnant diabetic woman is presented using a nursing process framework. The changing status and needs of the diabetic woman as she progresses through the antepartum, intrapartum, and postpartum periods are described. A variety of teaching boxes is provided to assist the student when managing the care of a pregnant diabetic woman during the antepartum period. A plan of care illustrates the use of the nursing process for a pregnancy complicated by insulin-dependent diabetes. The nursing diagnoses of knowledge deficit, risk for fetal injury, and anxiety are developed. The discussion of gestational diabetes mellitus considers the method of diagnosis and maternal and fetal risks. The nursing process is used as the guiding framework for the care management of a woman with gestational diabetes mellitus at each stage of pregnancy.

The discussion of hyperemesis gravidarum includes accepted theories concerning its cause. Risk factors are identified and serve as a guide for assessment, along with the physiologic impact of the disorder. The nursing process format is used as the organizing framework for care management of a woman experiencing hyperemesis gravidarum. A plan of care is provided that considers the three major nursing diagnoses of fluid volume deficit, altered nutrition: less than body requirements, and anxiety.

The chapter concludes with an overview of the impact that thyroid disorders (hyperthyroidism and hypothyroidism) and maternal phenylketonuria can have on pregnancy.

# LEARNING OBJECTIVES

Define the key terms.

Differentiate the types of diabetes mellitus and their respective risk factors in pregnancy.

Summarize the effects of pregnancy on insulin requirements.

Discuss maternal and fetal risks or complications associated with diabetes in pregnancy.

Discuss care management for the pregnant woman with pregestational or gestational diabetes.

Discuss care management for the woman with hyperemesis gravidarum.

Discuss care management for the woman with thyroid dysfunction.

Describe the effects of maternal phenylketonuria on pregnancy outcome.

Identify topics for nursing research related to diabetes in pregnancy and other endocrine disorders.

# OUTLINE OF CHAPTER CONTENT WITH COURSE GUIDELINES

| CONTENT | GUIDELINE |
|---|---|
| Diabetes mellitus | A |
| – Pathogenesis | A |
| – Classification | A |
| – Metabolic changes associated with pregnancy | A |
| Pregestational diabetes mellitus | A |
| – Preconception counseling | A |
| – Maternal risks and complications | A |
| – Fetal and neonatal risks and complications | A |
| Care management | A |
| – Assessment and nursing diagnoses | A |
| – Interview | A |
| – Physical examination | A |
| – Laboratory tests | A |
| – Expected outcomes of care | A |
| – Plan of care and interventions | A |
| – Antepartum | A |
| – Diet | A |
| – Monitoring blood glucose levels | A |
| – Insulin therapy | A |
| – Exercise | A |
| – Urine testing | A |
| – Fetal surveillance | A |
| – Complications requiring hospitalization | A |
| – Determination of birth date and mode of birth | B |
| – Intrapartum | A |
| – Postpartum | A |
| – Evaluation | A |
| – Plan of care | A |
| Gestational diabetes mellitus | A |
| – Maternal-fetal risks | A |

| CONTENT | GUIDELINE |
|---|:---:|
| Care management | A |
|   – Assessment | A |
|     – Screening for gestational diabetes mellitus | A |
|   – Interventions | A |
|     – Antepartum | A |
|     – Intrapartum | A |
|     – Postpartum | A |
|   – Evaluation | A |
| Hyperemesis gravidarum | A |
|   – Etiology | A |
|   – Clinical manifestations | A |
|   – Collaborative care | A |
|     – Initial care | A |
|     – Home care | A |
|   – Plan of care | A |
| Thyroid disorders | B |
|   – Hyperthyroidism | B |
|   – Hypothyroidism | B |
| Maternal phenylketonuria | C |

## TEACHING STRATEGIES

1. Describe how the expected metabolic changes during pregnancy can affect pregnant women with pregestational diabetes mellitus and can lead to the development of gestational diabetes.

2. Review the assessment methods used to monitor pregnant women with pregestational diabetes and to diagnose and monitor women with gestational diabetes. Demonstrate use of a glucose monitor for blood testing and a dipstick for testing urine for acetone.

3. Describe the stressors experienced by pregnant women with pregestational and gestational diabetes and their families.

4. Use case studies to describe the nursing care management of pregnancies complicated by diabetes mellitus. Compare the care management of these clients with the care management recommendations in the literature.

5. Compare and contrast the risks involved with and the care management required by a pregnant woman diagnosed with hyperthyroidism and by a pregnant woman diagnosed with hypothyroidism.

6. Use case studies to illustrate the care management of a pregnant woman diagnosed with hyperemesis gravidarum in her home and in the hospital.

7. Identify agencies in your community that are able to assist the pregnant woman with hyperemesis gravidarum during home care.

# Suggested Student Learning Activities

1. *DESIGN* a pamphlet that will assist women with newly diagnosed gestational diabetes to understand the disorder that they are experiencing and its impact on themselves, their pregnancy, and their fetus. The pamphlet should also address the self-care required to maintain glucose control and prevent the complications associated with gestational diabetes.

2. *SEARCH* the literature for articles related to the care management of pregnant women with one of the metabolic or endocrine disorders discussed in this chapter. *CHOOSE* one article, and complete a bibliography card that includes the following:
   - Summary of the article's key points
   - Personal reaction to the ideas presented in the article
   - How the professional nurse could use the information presented to enhance and improve health care

3. *PREPARE* a health teaching program for a group of women with pregestational diabetes who are experiencing their first pregnancy. The program should include content relevant to diabetes in pregnancy as well as stress-reduction techniques and group support measures. Include the teaching methods and visual aids that you would use as part of the program you developed.

4. *INTERVIEW* a woman whose pregnancy was complicated by hyperemesis gravidarum or gestational diabetes.
   - *GATHER* information regarding the following:
     - The woman's description of the impact that this pregnancy related health problem had on her pregnancy, on herself, and on her family
     - Coping mechanisms that the woman and her family used to deal with the stressors encountered as a result of the health problem that she experienced during her pregnancy
     - The support measures, persons, and services that she and her family found to be helpful, those that they found not to be helpful or lacking, and those that they wish had been provided
     - Her impressions of the impact that the health care system and health care providers had on her health and well-being during pregnancy, childbirth, and the puerperium
   - *DESCRIBE* how you would use this information to plan care that is effective not only related to the woman's physical needs but also related to the woman and her family's psychosocial and emotional needs.

# Topics for Discussion

1. *Support this statement:* Nurses play a critical role in the early detection and prompt treatment of gestational diabetes.

2. *Address these questions:*
   - How can the safety of the maternal-fetal unit be ensured when the woman with hyperemesis gravidarum is treated in her home?
   - What can nurses who work with young women of childbearing age with diabetes mellitus do to help the women experience a healthy pregnancy?

# MERLIN PROJECT

1. Use MERLIN to assist you in searching the medical literature for nursing research studies regarding the characteristics of women who experience hyperemesis gravidarum and measures found to be effective in the care management of these women.
   - Create an annotated bibliography of three nursing research studies.
   - Choose one study, and complete a bibliography card that includes the following:
     - Hypothesis; research question
     - Summary of the methodology used and key findings
     - Reliability of the study and its findings
     - Recommendations for further research
   - Describe how you would use the findings of these studies to develop an evidenced-based protocol to guide the care management of women diagnosed with hyperemesis gravidarum.
2. Use MERLIN to access the CDC and the NCHS to gather statistical information regarding gestational diabetes and hyperemesis gravidarum. Create a chart that includes the following:
   - Incidence of each disorder in your state and in the nation as a whole
   - Characteristics of women who develop these disorders
   - Impact of each disorder on maternal and fetal/newborn morbidity and mortality
   - Types of treatments used to treat each disorder

Chapter

# Medical-Surgical Problems in Pregnancy

## SUMMARY OF KEY CONCEPTS

Chapter 33 describes the impact that medical and surgical problems can have on pregnancy and the impact that pregnancy can have on these disorders. The most current research findings concerning care management and maternal and fetal effects are included for each disorder. Special emphasis is placed on the cardiopulmonary and hematologic problems that complicate pregnancy.

The discussion of cardiovascular disorders centers around the classification system of organic heart disease developed by the New York Heart Association. Care management of pregnant women is presented within a nursing process framework and is applied to each stage of pregnancy—antepartum, intrapartum, and postpartum. The student is made aware of the critical need for nurses to assess pregnant women with cardiovascular disorders for signs of cardiac decompensation and to use measures to reduce the stress that is placed on the heart. Planning and identification of expected outcomes consider the significant needs of women representing each class of heart disease—Class I, II, III, and IV. Pharmacologic measures to enhance cardiac function and prevent complications are described. The impact of these medications on pregnancy and the fetus and newborn are included in the description. A plan of care illustrates the application of the nursing process for the pregnant woman with cardiac disease. The nursing diagnoses of activity intolerance, risk for altered tissue perfusion, and decreased cardiac output are developed.

Anemia, the most common medical disorder of pregnancy, is discussed in terms of its effect on pregnancy and its outcome. Expected physiologic changes in the oxygen carrying capacity of the blood during pregnancy are contrasted with the pathologic changes inherent in such hematologic disorders as iron deficiency anemia, folic acid deficiency anemia, sickle cell hemoglobinopathy, and thalassemia.

The superimposition of pulmonary disorders on the normal adaptations that occur during pregnancy is described, with bronchial asthma, adult respiratory distress syndrome (ARDS), and cystic fibrosis as examples. The discussion of medical problems continues with consideration of gastrointestinal (cholelithiasis and cholecystitis, inflammatory bowel disease, appendicitis, intestinal obstruction, hernia), integumentary, neurologic (epilepsy, multiple sclerosis, Bell's palsy), and autoimmune (rheumatoid arthritis, systemic lupus erythematosus, myasthenia gravis) disorders.

An overview of the major factors related to the maternal-fetal unit that must be considered when a pregnant woman requires surgery is included. Care management of the pregnant woman undergoing surgery is discussed with an emphasis on preoperative and postoperative nursing actions and preparation essential for discharge.

## LEARNING OBJECTIVES

Define the key terms.
Describe the management of cardiovascular disorders in pregnant women.
Identify nursing interventions for the pregnant woman with a cardiovascular disorder.
Discuss anemia during pregnancy.
Explain the care of pregnant women with pulmonary disorders.
Review the effect of gastrointestinal disorders on gastrointestinal function during pregnancy.
Review the effects of neurologic disorders on pregnancy.
Describe the care of women whose pregnancies are complicated by autoimmune disorders.
Explain basic principles of care for a pregnant woman having abdominal surgery.
Identify topics for nursing research on medical-surgical problems in pregnancy.

## OUTLINE OF CHAPTER CONTENT WITH COURSE GUIDELINES

| CONTENT | GUIDELINE |
|---|---|
| Cardiovascular disorders | A |
| Care management: antepartum | A |
| – Assessment and nursing diagnoses | A |
| – Interview | A |
| – Physical examination | A |
| – Laboratory tests | A |
| – Expected outcomes of care | A |
| – Plan of care and interventions | A |
| – Resuscitation of the pregnant woman | A |
| – Heart surgery during pregnancy | A |
| – Evaluation | A |
| Intrapartum | A |
| – Physical examination | A |
| Postpartum | A |
| – Nursing diagnoses | A |
| Plan of care | A |
| Associated cardiovascular disorders | B |
| – Peripartum cardiomyopathy | B |
| – Rheumatic heart disease | B |
| – Mitral valve stenosis | B |
| – Infective endocarditis | C |
| – Eisenmenger's syndrome | C |

*continued*

| CONTENT | GUIDELINE |
|---|:---:|
| – Mitral valve prolapse | A |
| – Marfan's syndrome | B |
| – Cerebrovascular accidents | A |
| – Anemia | A |
|   – Iron deficiency anemia | A |
|   – Folic acid deficiency anemia | B |
|   – Sickle cell hemoglobinopathy | A |
|   – Thalassemia | B |
| Pulmonary disorders | A |
|   – Asthma | A |
| – Adult respiratory distress syndrome | C |
| – Cystic fibrosis | B |
| Integumentary disorders | B |
| Neurologic disorders | B |
|   – Epilepsy | A |
|   – Multiple sclerosis | B |
|   – Bell's palsy | C |
| Autoimmune disorders | B |
|   – Rheumatoid arthritis | B |
|   – Systemic lupus erythematosus | B |
|   – Myasthenia gravis | C |
| Gastrointestinal disorders | B |
|   – Cholelithiasis | A |
|   – Cholecystitis | A |
|   – Inflammatory bowel disease | B |
|   – Appendicitis | A |
|   – Intestinal obstruction | B |
|   – Abdominal hernias | B |
| Surgery during pregnancy | A |
|   – Care management | A |
|     – Hospital care | A |
|     – Home care | A |

## TEACHING STRATEGIES

1. Describe how the expected cardiovascular changes during pregnancy can affect pregnant women with cardiac disorders and can lead to the development of cardiac decompensation.

2. Review assessment methods to monitor pregnant women with cardiac disorders for signs of cardiac decompensation and pulmonary edema.

3. Describe the stressors experienced by pregnant women with cardiac disorders and their families. Explain the importance of women and their families actively participating in the care management plan.

4. Use case studies to describe the nursing care management of pregnancies complicated by cardiac disorders. Compare the care management of these clients with care management standards described in the literature.

5. Use case studies to illustrate the care management of selected medical disorders and surgical problems presented in this chapter. Encourage students to share experiences that they may have had in caring for women whose pregnancies were complicated by these disorders.

6. Divide students into groups. Assign each group to research a specific medical problem that can complicate pregnancy and develop a care management protocol for the medical problem. Arrange for a representative from each group to present the care management protocol developed by their group.

7. Explain how the expected changes associated with pregnancy increase the woman's risk for iron deficiency anemia. Identify prevention and treatment measures.

## SUGGESTED STUDENT LEARNING ACTIVITIES

1. *DEVELOP* an assessment tool that can be used to facilitate the planning and implementation of care for pregnant women with cardiovascular disorders, from the time of their first prenatal visit through their recovery in the postpartum period. The tool should reflect content presented in this chapter and facilitate the collection of appropriate baseline data and the early detection of cardiac decompensation.

2. *INTERVIEW* a woman whose pregnancy was complicated by one of the medical disorders discussed in this chapter.
   - *GATHER* information regarding the following:
     - The woman's description of the impact that this disorder had on her pregnancy, on herself, and on her family
     - Coping mechanisms that the woman and her family used to deal with the stressors encountered as a result of the high risk status of her pregnancy
     - The support measures, persons, and services that she and her family found to be helpful and those that they found to be lacking or not helpful
     - Her impressions of the impact that the health care system and the health care providers had on her health and well-being during pregnancy, childbirth, and the puerperium
   - *DESCRIBE* how you would use this information to plan care that is effective not only related to the woman's physical needs but also related to the woman and her family's psychosocial and emotional needs.

3. *SEARCH* the nursing literature for articles related to the care management of the medical and surgical disorders described in this chapter as they relate to pregnancy. *CHOOSE* one article, and complete a bibliography card that includes the following:
   - Summary of the article's key points
   - Personal reaction to the ideas presented in the article
   - How the professional nurse could use the information presented to enhance and improve health care

# TOPICS FOR DISCUSSION

1. *Consider this question:* What can nurses, who work with women of childbearing age with cardio-vascular problems, do to help these women make an informed decision regarding becoming pregnant and to help them experience a healthy pregnancy should pregnancy be their choice?

2. *Support this statement:* Nurses play a critical role in fostering the importance of preconception care for women of childbearing age with a medical disorder that can complicate a potential pregnancy.

# MERLIN PROJECT

Use MERLIN to assist you in contacting the web site for the American Heart Association (AHA). Explore the site and prepare a report that includes the following:
- Summary of the information available regarding cardiac disease and pregnancy
- Description of the types of services provided for health care professionals and services provided for pregnant women with cardiac disorders and their families
- Discussion about how a professional nurse working with women with cardiac problems could use the AHA site and its services to enhance the care that they provide to women before they become pregnant and once they are pregnant

Chapter

# 34 Obstetric Critical Care

## SUMMARY OF KEY CONCEPTS

Chapter 34 focuses on three major topics related to the high risk pregnant woman and her family—obstetric critical care, hemodynamic monitoring, and trauma. Numerous boxes, tables, procedures, and figures highlight and clarify complex content that is further explained in the text of the chapter.

The first part of the chapter introduces the student to the new and evolving advanced practice nursing specialty of obstetric critical care. The rational for establishing this area of specialty practice and for the care of critically ill pregnant women in an obstetric critical care unit is emphasized. Criteria that pregnant women should meet to qualify for obstetric critical care are explained. An overview of the cardiorespiratory changes of pregnancy, anatomy and physiology of circulation, and cardiac output provides the foundation for the discussion of hemodynamic monitoring as it is used for the critically ill pregnant woman. Methods of invasive hemodynamic monitoring are discussed, including indications for use, method and procedures used, expected values for the woman who is pregnant, and potential complications associated with use. Three case studies are included to illustrate the use and interpretation of hemodynamic monitoring for the critically ill pregnant woman. The case studies are organized in such a way that the students could focus on the case and write their interpretation of assessment findings. Then they could compare their evaluation with the evaluation provided by the author.

Trauma during pregnancy is discussed in the second part of the chapter. The significance and incidence of trauma as it relates to the pregnant woman and the effect of trauma on the maternal-fetal unit are explained. Various mechanisms of trauma are identified. Care management is described in terms of the primary survey as part of immediate stabilization and the secondary survey, which includes electronic fetal monitoring, fetal-maternal hemorrhage, ultrasound, and radiation exposure. The components of physical assessment of the pregnant woman who has experienced trauma are outlined in a box.

The chapter concludes with an overview of the concept of family-centered obstetric critical care. It recognizes the importance of providing care not only to the critically ill pregnant woman but also to her family. The components of family-centered care are discussed with an emphasis on the need for family members to visit the pregnant woman and the need to foster parent-infant contact and attachment.

# LEARNING OBJECTIVES

Define the key terms.

Discuss factors that have contributed to the development of the specialty of critical care obstetrics.

Describe conditions that may place a pregnant woman in a critically ill state.

Discuss factors that affect the provision of obstetric critical care when a pregnant woman becomes critically ill.

Describe significant cardiovascular, pulmonary, and hematologic alterations during pregnancy that affect critical care for the pregnant woman.

Review cardiac anatomy and physiologic features, including location of chambers, valves, major blood vessels, and path of circulation.

List the four determinants of cardiac output and relate the clinical significance of each.

Describe the parameters measured and normal values for pulmonary artery monitoring.

Describe the parameters measured and normal values for arterial pressure monitoring.

Discuss treatment strategies based on interpretation of hemodynamic profiles.

Discuss implications of trauma on mother and fetus during pregnancy.

Identify physiologic alterations of pregnancy that affect stabilization and treatment of the pregnant client who has undergone trauma.

Describe immediate assessment and stabilization measures for the pregnant victim of trauma.

Describe components of the primary and secondary surveys for the pregnant woman who has undergone trauma.

Discuss inclusion of the components of family-centered maternity care for the critically ill pregnant woman.

Identify topics for nursing research about critical care obstetrics.

# OUTLINE OF CHAPTER CONTENT WITH COURSE GUIDELINES

| CONTENT | GUIDELINE |
| --- | --- |
| Obstetric intensive care unit | A |
| Provision of obstetric critical care | A |
| Equipment and expertise | A |
| Indications for obstetric critical care | A |
| Cardiorespiratory changes of pregnancy | A |
| – Cardiovascular changes | A |
| – Colloid osmotic pressure | A |
| – Respiratory changes | A |
| – Hematologic changes | A |
| – Systemic vascular resistance | A |
| Hemodynamic monitoring | A |
| – Anatomic and physiologic characteristics of circulation | A |
| – Cardiac output | A |
| – Invasive hemodynamic monitoring | B |
| – Pulmonary artery catheter | B |
| – Arterial pressure catheter | B |
| – Pressure lines | B |

| CONTENT | GUIDELINE |
|---|---|
| – Data collection | B |
| – Oxygenation | B |
| – Central venous pressure lines | B |
| – Interpretation of hemodynamic data (cases) | B |
| – Pulmonary edema | A |
| Trauma during pregnancy | A |
| – Significance | A |
| – Maternal physiologic characteristics | A |
| – Fetal physiologic characteristics | A |
| – Mechanisms of trauma | A |
| – Immediate stabilization | A |
| – Primary survey | A |
| – Secondary survey | A |
| – Electronic fetal monitoring | A |
| – Fetal-maternal hemorrhage | A |
| – Ultrasound | A |
| – Radiation exposure | A |
| – Perimortem cesarean delivery | B |
| – Physical assessment | A |
| Family-centered obstetric critical care | A |

## TEACHING STRATEGIES

1. Identify how the adaptations that occur during pregnancy influence the assessment and care management of pregnant women who are critically ill or have undergone trauma.

2. Use case studies to illustrate the assessment and care management of the critically ill pregnant woman and a woman who has undergone trauma in an automobile accident.

3. Discuss the benefits of an obstetric critical care unit. Identify specific units and their location, especially one that might be in your community or nearby.

4. Invite a nurse involved in the care of critically ill pregnant women to discuss the challenges of his or her role and its responsibilities. Encourage this person to identify the measures that he or she uses to support these women and their families.

## SUGGESTED STUDENT LEARNING ACTIVITIES

1. *SEARCH* the nursing literature for articles related to obstetric critical care and trauma during pregnancy. *CHOOSE* one article, and complete a bibliography card that includes the following:
   - Summary of the article's key points
   - Personal reaction to the ideas presented in the article
   - How the professional nurse could use the information presented to enhance and improve health care

2. *INTERVIEW* a woman who required obstetric critical care during her pregnancy.
   - *GATHER* information regarding the following:
     - The woman's description of the impact that her critical status had on herself and her family
     - Coping mechanisms that the woman and her family used to deal with the stressors and fears encountered as a result of her critical status
     - The support measures, persons, and services that she and her family found to be helpful, those that they found not to be helpful or lacking, and those that they wished had been provided
     - Her impressions of the impact that the health care system and health care providers had on her health and well-being
   - *DESCRIBE* how you would use this information to plan care that is effective not only related to the woman's physical needs but also related to the woman and her family's psychosocial and emotional needs.

3. *INTERVIEW* a nurse working in an emergency room and a nurse working in an obstetric critical care unit of a large metropolitan hospital.
   - *DETERMINE* how both of these nurses approach the care of a pregnant woman who has experienced trauma and the manner in which it differs from how they approach the care of a trauma client who is not pregnant.
   - *COMPARE* their responses to the information presented in the chapter. Based on your comparison, what changes would you suggest? Give the rationale for each change that you propose.

## TOPICS FOR DISCUSSION

1. *Consider these questions:*
   - Why should tertiary centers designated for the care of critically ill pregnant women establish obstetric critical care units to provide this care?
   - How should pregnancy affect the care management approach used when the woman is critically ill or has experienced trauma?
   - What services can the health care system provide to prevent health problems from escalating to the point where a woman will require critical care?

2. *Support this statement:* An essential role responsibility of nurses working with critically ill pregnant women is to provide emotional support for the women and for their families.

## MERLIN PROJECT

Use the Chapter 34 section of MERLIN as a starting point in a search of the Internet for hospitals that have an obstetric critical care unit as one of their services. Contact at least three of these hospitals, and obtain information about these units. Prepare a report that includes the following:
- List of the hospitals that have obstetric critical care units
- Description of each of the obstetric critical care units contacted in terms of the following:
  - Mission and philosophy of care
  - Capacity including nurse-client ratio
  - Qualifications of the health care professions providing care
  - Types of health problems that they treat
  - Cost of care
  - Average length of stay
  - Extension of services to home care after discharge
  - Support services offered to the clients and their families

Chapter

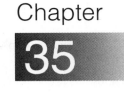

# Mental Health Disorders and Substance Abuse

## SUMMARY OF KEY CONCEPTS

Chapter 35 introduces the student to the impact that mental health disorders and substance abuse have on pregnancy and childbearing. The discussion of mental health disorders emphasizes the principal disturbances of anxiety and mood disorders during pregnancy and postpartum depression with and without psychotic features and panic disorders during the postpartum period. An exploration of the incidence, predisposing and risk factors, and typical behaviors associated with each mental health disorder is included in the discussion. The nursing process is the framework used for the care management of women experiencing these disorders. Implications for treatment in the home, the community, and the hospital are described. Psychotropic medications that are useful in treating the mood disorders are addressed in terms of their effect on the mother, her disorder, and the fetus, if given antepartally, or the infant, if used while breastfeeding. Boxes list the most commonly used antidepressant and antipsychotic drugs. A plan of care illustrates the use of the nursing process when managing the care of a woman with postpartum depression. The nursing diagnoses of risk for injury to newborn and client and ineffective family coping are developed.

Substance abuse is viewed regarding prevalence, risk factors, barriers to treatment, and legal considerations. The discussion focuses on the substances of alcohol, marijuana, cocaine, opiates, methamphetamine, and phencyclidine and their impact on pregnancy, the fetus, and the newborn. A table highlights the physiologic and psychologic signs exhibited by the user of these substances. The care management of pregnant women with substance abuse problems is discussed. The CAGE questionnaire and the T-ACE test used for recognition of alcohol abuse are included in a box and discussed in the text. A plan of care related to substance abuse during pregnancy illustrates how the nursing process can be used to manage care. Nursing diagnoses of altered nutrition: less than body requirements and ineffective individual coping are developed.

## LEARNING OBJECTIVES

Define the key terms.
Discuss emotional complications during pregnancy, including management of anxiety disorders and mood disorders.
Discuss substance abuse during pregnancy, including dual diagnosis, prevalence, risk factors, legal considerations, treatment programs, barriers to treatment, and care management.

*Chapter 35: Mental Health Disorders and Substance Abuse* 153

Differentiate among postpartum emotional complications, including incidence, risk factors, signs and symptoms, and management.

Summarize the role of the nurse in assessing and managing care of women with emotional complications during pregnancy and postpartum.

Identify topics for nursing research on mental health disorders and substance abuse in pregnancy.

## OUTLINE OF CHAPTER CONTENT WITH COURSE GUIDELINES

| CONTENT | GUIDELINE |
|---|:---:|
| Mental health disorders during pregnancy | A |
| – Anxiety disorders | A |
| – Mood disorders | A |
| Substance abuse during pregnancy | A |
| – Prevalence | A |
| – Risk factors | A |
| – Barriers to treatment | A |
| – Legal considerations | A |
| – Cigarette smoking and caffeine consumption | A |
| – Alcohol | A |
| – Marijuana | A |
| – Cocaine | |
| – Opiates | B |
| – Methamphetamines | B |
| – Phencyclidine | A |
| Care Management | A |
| – Assessment and nursing diagnoses | A |
| – Expected outcomes of care | A |
| – Plan of care and interventions | A |
| – Treatment programs for alcohol- and drug-dependent women | A |
| – Evaluation | A |
| Plan of care—substance abuse | A |
| Postpartum psychologic complications | A |
| – Mood disorders | A |
| – Postpartum depression without psychotic features | A |
| – Postpartum depression with psychotic features | A |
| – Bipolar disorders | A |
| – Etiology | A |
| Care management | A |
| – Assessment and nursing diagnoses | A |
| – Expected outcomes of care | A |
| – Plan of care and interventions | A |
| – On the postpartum unit | A |
| – In the home and community | A |
| – Psychiatric hospitalization | B |
| – Psychotropic medications | A |
| – Postpartum onset of panic disorder | A |
| – Care management | A |
| – Evaluation | |
| Plan of care—postpartum depression | |

# TEACHING STRATEGIES

1. Discuss how changes associated with pregnancy and the postpartum period precipitate mental health disorders. Use cases studies to illustrate the assessment and care management of women who are experiencing postpartum depression with and without psychotic features.

2. Create a profile of women who are more likely to develop postpartum psychologic complications.

3. Compare assessment findings typical of postpartum blues and postpartum depression with and without psychotic features.

4. Discuss safety considerations for the woman, newborn, and family if the woman is experiencing a postpartum psychologic complication.

5. Identify methods that nurses can use to alert postpartum women and their families to the signs and symptoms associated with postpartum blues and depression and to the measures that can be used to prevent and treat these disorders.

6. Describe measures that can be used to facilitate the maternal and newborn attachment when the mother is experiencing a postpartum psychologic complication.

7. Invite a nurse or a psychologist involved in the care of postpartum women with psychogenic disorders to discuss the care management approach that he or she uses when working with these women and their families.

8. Use case studies to illustrate the impact that substance abuse can have on pregnancy and the fetus and newborn. Identify agencies that are available in your community to provide services to assist pregnant women who abuse alcohol and/or drugs.

9. Invite a nurse who works at a substance abuse treatment center for pregnant women to discuss the care management approach that he or she uses when working with these women and their families.

10. Discuss the importance of preconception care as a method of identifying and treating women with substance abuse problems before they become pregnant.

# SUGGESTED STUDENT LEARNING ACTIVITIES

1. *WRITE* a two- to three-page paper concerning one of the following issues affecting pregnant women, their health, and health care in the United States today:
   - Postpartum mood disorders as a rationale for maternal violence against self or newborn
   - Management of substance abuse when the client is a pregnant woman
   - Impact of early discharge, single parenthood, and maternal age on the incidence of postpartum blues and depression

   Your paper should include a description of current societal views, as well as your own views, concerning the issue. Your paper should reflect viewpoints from the media (newspapers, magazines, television, radio) and professional sources (journals, textbooks, workshops) on the issue. Cite the references that you used in preparation of this paper.

2. *DESIGN* a support program for postpartum mothers to help them deal with the demands and responsibilities of family, newborn, and career. The program should provide anticipatory guidance, strategies for dealing with the demands and responsibilities, and active support from other postpartum women.

3. *ASSESS* the effect of substance abuse and dependence as it relates to the pregnant women in your community.
   - *COLLECT* data concerning the following:
     - Scope of the problem, including incidence according to population groups
     - Community resources available to assist pregnant women to deal with their abuse/dependence problem
   - *SUMMARIZE* the data collected and compare with national norms.
   - *VISIT* one of the community agencies identified. *DESCRIBE* the services that this agency provides and the approach used in providing these services.

4. *SEARCH* the nursing literature for articles related to the early detection and treatment of pregnant women with substance abuse problems. *CHOOSE* one article, and complete a bibliography that includes the following:
   - Summary of the article's key points
   - Personal reaction to the ideas presented in the article
   - How professional nurses working with pregnant women with substance abuse problems could use the article's ideas to enhance and improve the quality of health care they provide

## TOPICS FOR DISCUSSION

1. *Consider the question:* Should maternal abuse of drugs or alcohol be considered a form of child abuse and a basis for criminal prosecution? Give the rationale for your opinion and your suggestions for approaches to the problem.

2. *Debate the issue:* Postpartum depression with psychotic features can be used as a legal defense when a postpartum woman is accused of harming her infant.

3. *Support these statements:*
   - The nurse plays a critical role as an advocate in ensuring appropriate care for pregnant women experiencing mental health disorders or substance abuse problems.
   - The community has a responsibility to provide appropriate services specifically designed to help pregnant woman who abuse drugs.

# MERLIN PROJECT

1. Use MERLIN to assist you in searching the medical literature for nursing research studies related to postpartum psychologic disorders.
   - Create an annotated bibliography of five nursing studies.
   - Choose one study, and complete a bibliography card that includes the following:
     - Hypothesis; research question
     - Summary of methodology used and key findings
     - Reliability of the study and its findings
     - Recommendations for further research
   - Describe how you would use the findings of these studies to develop an evidenced-based protocol for the prevention and treatment of postpartum psychologic disorders.
2. Use MERLIN to access the CDC and the NCHS web sites. Gather statistical data regarding substance abuse during pregnancy and postpartum psychologic disorders. Create a chart for each problem area that includes the following:
   - Incidence in your community, state, and the nation as a whole
   - Characteristics of women who experience these problems
   - Impact of the problem on pregnancy and the postpartum recovery, including ability to care for and nurture her newborn and her family
   - Based on the statistical information that you gathered, cite several measures that you would propose to facilitate the prevention or early detection and treatment of these problems.

# Chapter

## 36

# Preterm Labor and Birth

## SUMMARY OF KEY CONCEPTS

The focus of Chapter 36 is the identification and management of preterm labor and birth and preterm premature rupture of the membranes. The nursing process is the organizing framework for the care management of women experiencing preterm labor and birth.

A variety of etiologic and risk factors traditionally implicated in the occurrence of preterm labor and birth are identified. Students are informed that knowledge of risk factors alone is not sufficient to identify women who will experience preterm labor because at least 50% of all women who ultimately give birth prematurely have no identifiable risk factors. The point is emphasized—to be effective, preterm birth prevention programs must be made available to all pregnant women, not just those identified as high risk for preterm labor and birth. Care management focuses on the timely diagnosis of preterm labor and the most commonly used measures to prevent or treat preterm labor, including lifestyle modifications, suppression of preterm labor, promotion of lung maturity, and management of inevitable preterm birth. Nursing considerations related to the identification and care of women in preterm labor are fully described in the text and highlighted in numerous boxes. A plan of care illustrates the use of the nursing process for preterm labor. The nursing diagnoses of knowledge deficit, risk for maternal and fetal injury, fear/anxiety, and diversional activity deficit are developed.

An overview of premature rupture of the membranes includes a brief discussion of incidence, etiologic factors, and home versus hospital care management approaches.

## LEARNING OBJECTIVES

Define the key terms.
Understand the difference between preterm birth and low birth weight.
Identify the risk factors for preterm birth.
Understand current interventions to prevent preterm birth.
Describe the appropriate client education for pregnant women regarding preterm birth.
Discuss the use of tocolytics and antenatal glucocorticoids in preterm prevention.
Discuss the nursing care of women confined to home for prevention of preterm birth.
Describe the deleterious effects of bed rest on pregnant women.
Define preterm premature rupture of membranes.
Identify the nursing care strategies for women with preterm premature rupture of membranes.
Identify topics for nursing research related to preterm labor and birth.

# OUTLINE OF CHAPTER CONTENT WITH COURSE GUIDELINES

| CONTENT | GUIDELINE |
|---|---|
| Preterm labor and birth | |
| – Preterm birth versus low birth weight | A |
| – Incidence and etiology | A |
| – Physiology of preterm birth | A |
| Care management | |
| – Assessment and nursing diagnoses | A |
| – Expected outcomes of care | A |
| – Plan of care and interventions | A |
| – Prevention | A |
| – Lifestyle modifications | A |
| – Early recognition and diagnosis | A |
| – Suppression of uterine activity | A |
| – Promotion of fetal lung maturity | A |
| – Home care | A |
| – Management of inevitable preterm birth | A |
| – Evaluation | A |
| Plan of care | A |
| Preterm premature rupture of the membranes | A |
| – Incidence and etiology | A |
| – Care management: home versus hospital care | A |

# TEACHING STRATEGIES

1. Use biostatistical data to illustrate the scope of and trends in preterm labor and birth in your community, state, and the nation as a whole.

2. Use case studies to describe the care management of women and their families experiencing preterm labor and birth.

3. Describe the psychosocial and emotional impact of preterm labor and birth on the pregnant woman and her family.

4. Discuss the nursing responsibilities during labor suppression using tocolytics. Compare labor suppression protocols of local health care agencies with current professional standards and research.

5. Identify home care agencies available in your community that provide care to women experiencing preterm labor. Describe the services offered. Arrange for students to accompany professional nurses on home visits to women experiencing preterm labor. Provide an opportunity for these students to present their observations of the visit to the class.

# SUGGESTED STUDENT LEARNING ACTIVITIES

1. *REVIEW* the protocols for the suppression of preterm labor developed and used on the labor unit where you have your clinical experience. *PREPARE* a report that includes the following:
   - Description of the protocols used
   - Comparison of the protocols used with the standards and norms presented in this chapter
   - Description of the role of the nurses on this unit with regard to the development of the protocols and their implementation with women experiencing a preterm labor
   - Description of emotional support measures provided to the women undergoing the labor suppression treatment regimen and their families
   - Identification of changes that you would propose in terms of the care management of these clients; include the rationale for each of the changes that you propose

2. *SEARCH* the nursing literature for articles related to the care management of women at risk for and experiencing preterm labor. *CHOOSE* one article, and complete a bibliography card that includes the following:
   - Summary of the article's key points
   - Personal reaction to the ideas presented in the article
   - How the professional nurse can use the article's ideas to enhance and improve the quality of health care provided to women at risk for or experiencing preterm labor.

3. *SURVEY* your community for the availability of services related to the home care management of women at risk for or experiencing preterm labor.
   - *DESCRIBE* the types of services available, their cost, accessibility, typical population using the service, and nursing input into the management of the services.
   - *INTERVIEW* one of the nurses involved in providing care to the women using this service to determine the nurse's view regarding his or her role, including type of care provided, typical client responses, effectiveness of the service, use of nursing research, or ideas for nursing research based on their experiences.

4. *INTERVIEW* a woman who experienced a preterm labor and birth to determine her perception of the event.
   - *PREPARE* a report that includes the woman's description of the following:
     - Her performance during childbirth
     - Stressors that she experienced
     - Support measures and persons she found to be helpful and those she found not to be helpful or lacking—how helpful these measures and persons were to her family or support persons
     - Additional support measures that she would have liked to have had available to her and her family
     - How this experience could affect future pregnancies and births
   - *DESCRIBE* how you would use this information when planning more sensitive care for laboring women, especially those experiencing labors and births that are at risk.

# TOPICS FOR DISCUSSION

1. *Consider this question:* What can nurses do to reduce the incidence of preterm labor and birth?

2. *Support this statement:* The home is an appropriate and safe site for the care management of women experiencing signs of preterm labor.

3. *Debate the issue*: Effectiveness of bed rest versus limited activity as a component of the care management of women experiencing signs of preterm labor.

# MERLIN PROJECT

1. Use MERLIN to assist you in searching the medical literature for nursing research studies related to the effectiveness of bed rest in suppressing preterm labor and delaying preterm birth.
   - Create an annotated bibliography of at least five research studies.
   - Choose one research study, and complete a bibliography card that includes each of the following:
     - Hypothesis; research question
     - Summary of the methodology used and key findings
     - Reliability of the study and its findings
     - Recommendations for further research
   - Discuss your impressions of the research findings and whether bed rest is an intervention to be recommended. What alternatives to bed rest would you propose based on the findings in the studies?

2. Use MERLIN to access the CDC and NCHS to gather statistical information regarding preterm labor and birth. Create a chart that includes the following:
   - Incidence of preterm labor and birth in your community, state, and the nation as a whole
   - Characteristics of women who experience preterm labor and birth
   - Impact of preterm birth on the health and well-being of the newborn
   - Types of methods used to suppress preterm labor and prevent preterm birth

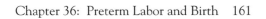

# Chapter

## 37 Labor and Birth Complications

## SUMMARY OF KEY CONCEPTS

The focus of Chapter 37 is the identification and management of labor and birth that deviates from expected standards and norms. Consideration is given to dystocia, postterm pregnancy and birth, and obstetric emergencies. The nursing process is the organizing framework for the care management of women experiencing labor and birth complications.

Dystocia—long, difficult, or abnormal labor—is explained in terms of how the five essential factors of labor contribute to its occurrence. The interdependent nature of the five factors—powers, passage, passenger, position of the mother, and psychologic response—is stressed. The common deviations for each power are described and include contributing factors, characteristic signs and symptoms, impact on the maternal fetal unit, and typical care management. The defining criteria for abnormal labor patterns are categorized according to the affected phase of cervical dilation (prolonged latent, protracted active, and secondary arrest), progress of descent of the presenting part (protracted, arrest, and failure of descent), and the duration of the labor process (precipitous labor). A variety of tables, boxes, and figures clarify the aspects of dysfunctional labor and the criteria and treatment approaches for abnormal labor patterns. The use of therapeutic rest, measures to enhance labor progress and provide support, oxytocin, and cesarean births are the primary focus of the discussion of management techniques for dystocia. Guidelines for the use of cervical ripening agents, amniotomy, and oxytocin administration are outlined. Forceps-assisted and vacuum-assisted birth are described in terms of indications, techniques, effects on the woman and her newborn, and nursing considerations. The discussion of cesarean birth explores incidence, indications, surgical techniques, complications and risks, prenatal preparation, and care measures during the preoperative, intraoperative, and postoperative periods. A care path for a 48- to 72-hour postoperative length of stay enhances the discussion. The option of vaginal birth after cesarean (VBAC) is described. A plan of care illustrates the use of the nursing process in managing the care of a dysfunctional labor secondary to inertia. The nursing diagnoses of risks for injury to mother and/or fetus and maternal/fetal infection, pain, and anxiety/ineffective coping are developed.

An overview of postterm pregnancy and birth includes identification of maternal and fetal risks and a description of typical care management. Four obstetric emergencies are highlighted at the end of the chapter. The etiologic factors, clinical manifestations, and typical care management of shoulder dystocia, prolapsed umbilical cord, rupture of uterus, and amniotic fluid embolism are discussed. Emergency boxes and a variety of illustrations clarify key concepts related to these emergencies.

## LEARNING OBJECTIVES

Define the key terms.

Identify the assessments for women experiencing different types of abnormal labor.

Formulate nursing diagnoses based on the assessment of abnormal labor.

Describe the nursing management of a trial of labor, the induction and augmentation of labor, forceps-assisted birth, vacuum-assisted birth, cesarean birth, and vaginal birth after a cesarean birth.

Discuss the criteria for evaluating the nursing care of women experiencing labor and birth complications.

Describe the care management of women experiencing a postterm pregnancy.

Discuss obstetric emergencies and their appropriate management.

Identify topics for nursing research related to labor and birth complications.

## OUTLINE OF CHAPTER CONTENT WITH COURSE GUIDELINES

| CONTENT | GUIDELINE |
|---|:---:|
| Dystocia | A |
| – Dysfunctional labor | A |
| – Hypertonic uterine dysfunction | A |
| – Hypotonic uterine dysfunction | A |
| – Secondary powers | A |
| – Alterations in pelvic structure | A |
| – Pelvic dystocia | A |
| – Soft tissue dystocia | A |
| – Fetal causes | A |
| – Anomalies | A |
| – CPD | A |
| – Malposition | A |
| – Malpresentation | A |
| – Multifetal pregnancy | A |
| – Position of the mother | A |
| – Psychologic responses | A |
| – Abnormal labor patterns | A |
| Care management | A |
| – Assessment and nursing diagnoses | A |
| – Expected outcomes of care | A |
| – Plan of care and interventions | A |
| – Version | B |
| – Trial of labor | A |
| – Induction of labor | A |
| – Cervical ripening methods | A |
| – Amniotomy | A |
| – Oxytocin | A |

*continued*

| CONTENT | GUIDELINE |
|---|---|
| – Augmentation of labor | A |
| – Forceps-assisted birth | B |
| – Vacuum-assisted birth | B |
| – Cesarean birth | A |
| – Vaginal birth after cesarean | A |
| – Evaluation | A |
| – Plan of care | A |
| Postterm pregnancy, labor, and birth | A |
| – Care management | A |
| Obstetric emergencies | |
| – Shoulder dystocia | B |
| – Prolapsed umbilical cord | B |
| – Rupture of uterus | B |
| – Amniotic fluid embolism | B |

# TEACHING STRATEGIES

1. Divide students into three groups. Provide each group with a case study representing a labor and birth complication: dystocia—hypertonic uterine dysfunction with prolonged latent phase; post-date pregnancy requiring stimulation of labor using cervical ripening and oxytocin induction; and cesarean birth related to failure of descent and fetal distress. Assign students to create a nursing care management plan for their case study using current nursing literature and research and their own clinical experiences. Select one student from each group to present the group's plan to the class.

2. Describe the impact of dystocia, postdate pregnancy, and obstetric emergencies on the pregnant woman and her family.

3. Describe nursing care management during labor stimulation (augmentation and induction). Compare labor stimulation protocols of local health care agencies with current standards and research.

4. Use charts and diagrams to illustrate patterns of dystocia. Contrast these patterns with labor and birth that reflects expected patterns.

5. Describe care management approaches for dystocia using case studies. Contrast a medically managed approach with an approach that emphasizes more natural, creative, and less invasive measures. Use research findings to illustrate the effectiveness and impact of each approach.

6. Use statistical data to describe the incidence, risk factors, and impact of dystocia, postdate pregnancy, and obstetric emergencies.

# SUGGESTED STUDENT LEARNING ACTIVITIES

1. *REVIEW* the protocols for the augmentation and induction of labor that have been developed and used on the labor unit where you have your clinical experience. *PREPARE* a report that includes the following:
   - Description of the protocols used
   - Comparison of the protocols used with the standards and norms presented in this chapter
   - Description of the role of the nurses on this unit with regard to the development of the protocols and their implementation with women experiencing labor and birth complications
   - Description of emotional support measures provided to the women undergoing labor stimulation and their families
   - Identification of changes that you would propose regarding the care management of these clients; include the rationale for each of the proposed changes

2. *SEARCH* the nursing literature for articles related to the care management of women experiencing labor and birth complications discussed in the chapter. *CHOOSE* one article, and complete a bibliography card that includes the following:
   - Summary of the article's key points
   - Personal reaction to the ideas presented in the article
   - How the professional nurse can use the article's ideas to enhance and improve the quality of health care provided to women experiencing complications of labor and birth

3. *INTERVIEW* a woman who experienced an emergency cesarean birth as a result of one of the labor and birth complications discussed in this chapter to determine her perception of the event.
   - *PREPARE* a report that includes the woman's description of the following:
     - Her performance during childbirth
     - Stressors that she experienced
     - How she was prepared for the cesarean birth, including explanations given for the reasons for the cesarean and purposes of the preparatory measures performed
     - Support measures and persons she found to be helpful and those she found not to be helpful or lacking; how helpful these measures and persons were to her family or support persons
     - Additional support measures that she would have liked to have had available to her and her family
     - How this experience could affect future pregnancies and births
   - *DESCRIBE* how you would use this information when planning more sensitive care for laboring women who require an emergency cesarean birth.

# TOPICS FOR DISCUSSION

1. *Debate this issue:* Should a woman be forced to have a cesarean birth if she does not want this procedure even though it may be beneficial for the well-being of her fetus?

2. *Consider this question:* How does the American way of birth that emphasizes medical management contribute to the occurrence of dystocia?

3. *Support this statement:* Nursing care and support of the laboring woman play a major role in reducing the rate of cesarean birth.

# MERLIN PROJECT

1. Use MERLIN to assist you in searching the medical literature for research studies related to effective cervical ripening and labor stimulation techniques.
   - Create an annotated bibliography of at least five research studies.
   - Choose one study, and complete a bibliography card that includes the following:
     - Hypothesis; research question
     - Summary of the methodology used and key findings
     - Reliability of the study and its findings
     - Recommendations for further research
   - Describe how the findings of these studies could be used to develop a cervical ripening and labor stimulation protocol that is evidence-based.
2. Use MERLIN to access the CDC and the NCHS to gather statistical information regarding dystocia, cesarean birth, shoulder dystocia, prolapsed umbilical cord, uterine rupture, and amniotic fluid embolism. Create a chart that includes the following:
   - Incidence of each complication in your state and the nation as a whole
   - Characteristics of women who develop these complications
   - Impact of each complication on the woman and her fetus/newborn
   - Types of treatments used, such as cervical ripening, labor stimulation, forceps-assisted birth, and vacuum-assisted birth

Chapter

# 38 Postpartum Complications

## SUMMARY OF KEY CONCEPTS

Chapter 38 introduces students to major complications that can occur during the postpartum period. Hemorrhage and shock, coagulopathies, thromboembolic disease, and postpartum infections are explored.

Postpartum hemorrhage is described according to the timing of its occurrence, the most common causal factors, and typical medical and nursing management. Hemorrhagic shock and coagulopathies are highlighted in the description. A discussion of thromboembolic disease focuses on the incidence, etiology, manifestations, and management of superficial and deep venous thrombosis.

Endometritis, wound infections, urinary tract infections, and mastitis are included in a discussion of postpartum infection. Typical nursing diagnoses, expected outcomes, and interventions for women experiencing postpartum infection are identified. Boxes highlight predisposing factors for postpartum infection and instructions that a nurse can provide to postpartum women to prevent genital tract infections. A plan of care for postpartum infection develops the nursing diagnosis of infection of genital canal related to retained placental fragments. Several nursing interventions are included, along with rationales.

## LEARNING OBJECTIVES

Define the key terms.
Identify postpartum hemorrhage causes, signs and symptoms, possible complications, and medical and nursing management.
Describe hemorrhagic shock, including management and hazards of therapy.
Differentiate the causes of postpartum infection.
Apply the nursing process to care of women with postpartum infection.
Describe thromboembolic disorders including incidence, etiology, signs and symptoms, and management.
Summarize the role of the nurse in the home setting in assessing potential problems and managing care of women with postpartum complications.
Identify topics for nursing research related to postpartum complications.

# OUTLINE OF CHAPTER CONTENT WITH COURSE GUIDELINES

| CONTENT | GUIDELINE |
|---|:---:|
| Postpartum hemorrhage | A |
| – Definition and incidence | A |
| – Etiology and risk factors | A |
| – Uterine atony | A |
| – Lacerations of the genital tract | A |
| – Retained placenta | A |
| – Inversion of the uterus | B |
| – Subinvolution of the uterus | A |
| Care management | |
| – Assessment and nursing diagnoses | A |
| – Expected outcomes of care | A |
| – Plan of care and interventions | A |
| – Medical management | A |
| – Nursing interventions | A |
| – Evaluation | A |
| Hemorrhagic (hypovolemic) shock | B |
| – Medical management | B |
| – Nursing interventions | B |
| Coagulopathies | C |
| Thromboembolic disease | A |
| – Incidence and etiology | A |
| – Clinical manifestations | A |
| – Medical management | A |
| – Nursing interventions | A |
| Postpartum infections | A |
| – Endometritis | A |
| – Wound infection | A |
| – Urinary tract infection | A |
| – Mastitis | A |
| Care management | A |
| – Assessment and nursing diagnoses | A |
| – Expected outcomes of care | A |
| – Plan of care and interventions | A |
| – Evaluation | A |
| Plan of care | A |

# TEACHING STRATEGIES

1. Identify the risk factors for early postpartum hemorrhage, late postpartum hemorrhage, postpartum infection, and venous thrombosis. Encourage students to contribute risk factors from the case histories of the postpartum women for whom they cared during their clinical experiences.

2. Describe the nursing care management of hemorrhage, hypovolemic shock, puerperal infection, and venous thrombosis using case studies of postpartum women who experienced these complications associated with childbirth. Use case studies based on the client care experiences of the students if possible.

3. Discuss infection control practices that must be implemented when caring for women during childbirth and the postpartum period. Explain how these practices should be used by women after they are discharged to home.

4. Engage the students in a discussion of the essential role of the nurse in preventing the occurrence of postpartum complications. Emphasize the importance of discharge planning and teaching and postdischarge follow-up using telephone calls and home visits.

## SUGGESTED STUDENT LEARNING ACTIVITIES

1. *PREPARE* a discharge teaching plan for postpartum women that focuses on the prevention of the childbirth complications of hemorrhage and infection. Include visual aids to be used when implementing the plan and written materials to be given to the women and their families.

2. *EXAMINE* the care management approach used to prevent and treat postpartum hemorrhage and infection at the hospital where you have your clinical experience. Review protocols, and interview health care providers to gather the required information. *PREPARE* a report that includes the following:
   - Summary of the care management protocols
   - Comparison of the care management protocols of the hospital with professional standards and the recommendations in the textbook
   - Suggestions for changes in the protocols, including addition of other measures; explain the rationale for each proposed change

3. *INTERVIEW* a woman who experienced a postpartum hemorrhage or a postpartum infection.
   - *GATHER* information regarding the following:
     - The woman's description of the impact that the postpartum complication had on her postpartum recovery and her ability to care for her new baby and the impact that this complication had on her family
     - Coping mechanisms that the woman and her partner and family used to deal with the stressors encountered as a result of the complication and its treatment
     - The support measures, people, and services that she and her family found helpful, those that they found to be lacking or not helpful, and those that they would have liked to have been provided
     - Her impressions of the health care agency and health care providers who cared for her and the impact that they had on her well-being during treatment and after discharge
   - *DESCRIBE* how you would use this information to plan care that is effective in dealing not only with a woman's physical needs but also with a woman and her family's psychosocial and emotional needs when postpartum complications occur.

# TOPICS FOR DISCUSSION

1. *Support this statement:* The nurse plays a critical role in helping the postpartum woman prevent complications such as hemorrhage, venous thrombosis, and infection.

2. *Debate the issue:* Early postpartum discharge within 24 hours of birth does or does not increase a woman's risk for and severity of postpartum complications.

# MERLIN PROJECT

Use MERLIN to assist you in searching the medical literature for nursing journal articles related to the care management of postpartum complications of hemorrhage, infection, and venous thrombosis.
- Create an annotated bibliography of at least five nursing journal articles.
- Choose one article, and complete a bibliography card that includes the following:
  - Summary of the article's key points
  - Personal reaction to the ideas presented in the article
- Describe how you would use the information in these articles to develop a postpartum care management protocol that emphasizes prevention of postpartum complications and early detection and prompt treatment if they should occur.

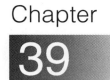

# Chapter

# 39

# Acquired Problems of the Newborn

## SUMMARY OF KEY CONCEPTS

Chapter 39 describes the impact that birth trauma, maternal diabetes, infection, and substance abuse can have on neonatal well-being, growth, and development. Each acquired problem is defined according to its incidence, typical clinical manifestations, and risk factors. The discussion of care management uses a nursing process framework with the identification of nursing diagnoses, expected outcomes, and effective care measures.

The student is informed about the risk factors associated with birth trauma, a significant source of neonatal morbidity, to identify those neonates most vulnerable to birth trauma and to prevent its occurrence. The most common birth injuries—soft tissue, skeletal, peripheral nervous system, and central nervous system—are described in terms of the typical clinical picture exhibited, the immediate and long-term effects, and the care management approaches found to be effective.

Infants of diabetic mothers are considered, with major emphasis on the assessment of the most common sequelae of ineffective maternal glucose control during pregnancy. A plan of care illustrates the use of the nursing process in the care management of an infant whose mother had gestational diabetes. The nursing diagnoses of anxiety and risks for injury, impaired gas exchange, and ineffective thermoregulation are developed.

A discussion of neonatal infection is presented in general terms, using a nursing process approach. Interventions are viewed as preventive, curative, and rehabilitative. A description of the clinical manifestations and typical care management of a variety of specific neonatal infections follows. TORCH, bacterial infections, and fungal infections are considered.

The student is made aware of the impact that maternal substance abuse can have on neonatal health and well-being immediately after birth and in the future. The magnitude of the problem is illustrated using statistical data. An overview of the care management of an infant and his or her family affected by substance abuse uses a nursing process framework. The impact and treatment related to specific substances including alcohol, heroin, methadone, marijuana, cocaine, phencyclidine, and tobacco are discussed. A plan of care describes the care management of an infant experiencing drug withdrawal. The nursing diagnoses of altered nutrition: less than body requirements, ineffective maternal coping, and risks for injury and fluid volume deficit are explored.

# LEARNING OBJECTIVES

Define the key terms.

Describe assessment of infants for birth trauma and for sequelae of a diabetic pregnancy.

Develop nursing care plans for complications typically seen in infants of diabetic mothers.

Summarize the care of the newborn with soft tissue, skeletal, and nervous system injuries.

Describe in detail the assessment of a newborn for infection.

Formulate nursing diagnoses for the infant and family for common bacterial and viral infections.

Review implementation and evaluation of care of infants with infections, including their families.

Assess the effects of maternal use of alcohol, heroin, methadone, marijuana, cocaine, and smoking on the fetus and newborn.

Describe the assessment of a newborn experiencing drug withdrawal.

Develop a care plan for the newborn experiencing drug withdrawal, including the infant's family.

Identify topics for nursing research related to acquired problems of the newborn.

# OUTLINE OF CHAPTER CONTENT WITH COURSE GUIDELINES

| CONTENT | GUIDELINE |
|---|:---:|
| Birth trauma—care management | A |
| – Assessment and nursing diagnoses | A |
| – Expected outcomes of care | A |
| – Plan of care and interventions | A |
| – Soft tissue injuries | A |
| – Skeletal injures | A |
| – Peripheral nervous system injuries | B |
| – Central nervous system injuries | B |
| – Evaluation | A |
| Infants of diabetic mothers | A |
| – Pathophysiology | A |
| – Congenital anomalies | A |
| – Macrosomia | A |
| – Birth trauma and perinatal hypoxia | A |
| – Respiratory distress syndrome | A |
| – Hypoglycemia | A |
| – Hypocalcemia and hypomagnesemia | B |
| – Cardiomyopathy | B |
| – Hyperbilirubinemia and polycythemia | A |
| – Nursing care | A |
| – Plan of care | A |
| Neonatal infections—care managment | A |
| – Sepsis | A |
| – Assessment and nursing diagnoses | A |
| – Expected outcomes or care | A |

| CONTENT | GUIDELINE |
|---|---|
| – Plan of care and interventions | A |
| – Preventive measures | A |
| – Curative measures | A |
| – Rehabilitative measures | A |
| – Evaluation | A |
| – TORCH infections | A |
| – Bacterial infections | A |
| – Fungal infections | A |
| Substance abuse | A |
| – Alcohol | A |
| – Heroin | A |
| – Methadone | A |
| – Marijuana | A |
| – Cocaine | A |
| – Phencyclidine | B |
| – Miscellaneous substances | B |
| – Tobacco | A |
| – Care management | A |
| Plan of care | A |

## TEACHING STRATEGIES

1. Describe the risk factors for and the clinical manifestations of common birth injuries. Identify measures that could be used to reduce the incidence and severity of birth trauma.

2. Identify the major problems encountered by infants of mothers who have pregestational and gestational diabetes. Specify the clinical manifestations for each problem identified. Discuss maternal factors that can influence the health and well-being of the fetus and newborn, including the occurrence and severity of the potential problems. Describe the care management of these problems using a case study of an infant born to a mother with pregestational diabetes and a case study of an infant born to a mother with gestational diabetes.

3. Describe the short-term and long-term impact of maternal infections during pregnancy on the growth and development of the fetus/newborn. Identify measures that can be used during the prenatal, natal, and postnatal periods to prevent infection or to accomplish early diagnosis and treatment if infection should occur. Discuss the nursing care management of the septic infant.

4. Describe the short-term and long-term impact of maternal substance abuse on the growth and development of the fetus/newborn. State the specific effects of the substances discussed in this chapter. Describe the care management of infants experiencing withdrawal and abstinence syndrome.

5. Discuss the ethical and legal responsibilities of the professional nurse when pregnant clients abuse substances that may be harmful to the fetus/newborn. Encourage students to share their feelings regarding substance abuse during pregnancy and the potentially harmful effects on the fetus and newborn.

6. Identify the treatment and support services available in your community to assist women who abuse drugs and alcohol and the infants who are affected by this abuse.

## SUGGESTED STUDENT LEARNING ACTIVITIES

1. *REVIEW* the protocols for acquired neonatal problems used in the hospital where you have your nursery experience. *DESCRIBE* the protocols used for each of the following newborn problems. *COMPARE* these protocols with the guidelines presented in this chapter. *INCLUDE* the manner in which the emotional needs of the newborns and their parents are met.
   - Newborns of pregestational and gestational diabetic mothers
   - Newborns born at risk for infection or already infected as a result of maternal TORCH, bacterial infections, or fungal infections
   - Newborns experiencing the effects of intrauterine exposure to such substances as cocaine, heroin, or methadone

2. *SURVEY* your community for the types of agencies available to support and care for newborns born to HIV-positive women or women addicted to illegal substances.
   - *PREPARE* a report that describes these agencies in terms of the following:
     - Type, eligibility requirements, accessibility, and services provided both for newborns who stay with their mothers and newborns whose mothers are unable to care for them
     - Degree to which these agencies are able to meet the community's need for these types of services—if they are inadequate, what would you propose as a solution?
   - *CREATE* a table that summarizes the information that you gathered so that it can be used by nurses who are caring for pregnant women.

3. *SEARCH* the nursing literature for articles related to care management of the acquired newborn problems described in this chapter. *CHOOSE* one article, and complete a bibliography card that includes the following:
   - Summary of the article's key points
   - Personal reaction to the ideas presented in the article
   - How the professional nurse could use the information to enhance and improve health care

## TOPICS FOR DISCUSSION

1. *Support these statements:*
   - Nurses can have a major impact on reducing the incidence of infection transmission to the fetus or newborn when caring for women before and after they are pregnant.
   - Nurses caring for women during labor and birth play a critical role in reducing the incidence of birth trauma.

2. *Debate these issues:*
   - Should routine HIV screening with counseling be mandated for all pregnant women?
   - Should all newborns be screened for the possibility that their mothers abused drugs during pregnancy?

3. *Address these questions:*
   - What can a woman with diabetes do to enhance the health and well-being of her fetus or newborn?
   - How can nurses use change theory to empower pregnant women to stop or at least reduce the use of tobacco?

## MERLIN PROJECT

Use MERLIN to contact the CDC and NCHS to gather statistical information regarding newborns affected by birth trauma, infection, and maternal substance abuse. Create a chart for each acquired problem of the newborn that includes the following:
   - Incidence in your state and in the nation as a whole
   - Characteristics of the mothers and infants who are likely to be affected by the problem
   - Impact of the problem on the newborn's health, well-being, and potential for growth and development
   - Types of approaches commonly used to care for the problem

# Chapter

## 40

# Hemolytic Disorders and Congenital Anomalies

## SUMMARY OF KEY CONCEPTS

Two major neonatal categories of health problems are the primary focus of Chapter 40—hemolytic disorders and congenital anomalies. The care management of each problem area is presented using the nursing process format.

A discussion of hyperbilirubinemia contrasts physiologic and pathologic jaundice. The major etiologic factor for pathologic jaundice is identified as hemolytic disorders associated with Rh or ABO incompatibility. A description of kernicterus is included in the discussion. Assessment focuses on the risk factors and findings present during the prenatal, perinatal, and postnatal periods. A variety of laboratory tests such as serum bilirubin levels and direct/indirect Coombs' tests are explained. Typical nursing diagnoses and expected outcomes of care for the neonate experiencing hyperbilirubinemia are identified. Treatment measures are categorized as preventive (emphasizing prophylaxis with $Rh_o$ [D] immune globulin [RhoGam]), curative (emphasizing phototherapy and exchange transfusion), and rehabilitative (emphasizing use of community resources to assist with the care of the child affected by kernicterus). A plan of care illustrates the use of the nursing process with a newborn affected by hyperbilirubinemia. The nursing diagnoses of risks for injury and knowledge deficit are developed.

The second part of the chapter discusses a variety of congenital anomalies. Prenatal, perinatal, and postnatal diagnoses of congenital disorders are explored. The student is introduced to the nature of parental responses and the care measures required when a diagnosis of an anomaly is made. Typical nursing diagnoses and expected outcomes are identified. Care management focuses on the neonate requiring surgery and the impact that this has on the family. An overview of common congenital disorders describes their etiology, clinical manifestations, and typical care management.

## LEARNING OBJECTIVES

Define the key terms.
Discuss assessment of the newborn for hyperbilirubinemia.
Develop a nursing plan of care for the prevention, identification, and management of
    hyperbilirubinemia in a newborn.
Compare Rh and ABO incompatibility.

Explain nursing management to prevent the pathologic consequences of hyperbilirubinemia.

Review prenatal diagnosis of neonatal disorders.

Present assessment strategies during the postnatal period to aid in diagnosis of congenital disorders.

Describe preoperative and postoperative nursing care of the newborn.

Develop a nursing plan of care for parents of a newborn with a defect or disorder.

Describe each congenital disorder presented in this chapter and identify the priority of nursing care for each.

Identify topics for nursing research related to developmental problems.

## OUTLINE OF CHAPTER CONTENT WITH COURSE GUIDELINES

| CONTENT | GUIDELINE |
|---|---|
| Hyperbilirubinemia | A |
| – Physiologic jaundice | A |
| – Pathologic jaundice | A |
| – Kernicterus | B |
| – Hemolytic disease of the newborn | A |
| – ABO incompatibility | A |
| – Rh incompatibility | A |
| Care management | A |
| – Assessment and nursing diagnoses | A |
| – Expected outcomes of care | A |
| – Plan of care and interventions | A |
| – Evaluation | A |
| Plan of care | A |
| Congenital anomalies | A |
| – Cardiovascular system anomalies | A |
| – Central nervous system anomalies | A |
| – Respiratory system anomalies | A |
| – Gastrointestinal system anomalies | A |
| – Musculoskeletal system anomalies | A |
| – Genitourinary system anomalies | A |
| – Teratoma | B |
| Care management | A |
| – Assessment and nursing diagnoses | A |
| – Prenatal diagnosis | A |
| – Perinatal diagnosis | A |
| – Postnatal diagnosis | A |
| – Expected outcomes of care | A |
| – Plan of care and interventions | A |
| – Newborn | A |
| – Parents and family | A |
| – Evaluation | A |

# TEACHING STRATEGIES

1. Compare and contrast physiologic and pathologic jaundice (hyperbilirubinemia).

2. Describe the care management of infants diagnosed with pathologic jaundice associated with hemolytic disease of the newborn. Compare the clinical manifestations and treatment approaches associated with Rh incompatibility and ABO incompatibility.

3. Use biostatistical data to describe the incidence of each of the congenital anomalies identified in this chapter and the impact that these problems have on infant morbidity and mortality. Compare the incidence of these problems in your community with the incidence in your state and in the nation as a whole. Point out regional differences with regard to incidence (i.e., urban or rural, north, south, east, or west). Identify factors that place a woman and her fetus or newborn at risk for the development of these problems.

4. Create a chart that identifies the presenting signs of major congenital anomalies that are apparent after birth. Use this chart to compare each anomaly and to point out similarities and differences.

5. Discuss the immediate care management of infants and their families when a congenital anomaly is diagnosed. (Select a major congenital anomaly from each of the body systems as the framework for the discussion.)

6. Identify the support services available in your community to assist children with developmental anomalies and their families.

# SUGGESTED STUDENT LEARNING ACTIVITIES

1. *REVIEW* the protocol used when treating newborns experiencing physiologic and pathologic jaundice at the hospital where you have your nursery experience. *PREPARE* a report that includes the following:
   - A description of each of the protocols used
   - A comparison of these protocols with the guidelines included in Chapters 27 and 40
   - A discussion of the support measures provided for parents during the treatment process of their newborn; include any changes that you would propose to enhance or improve the support measures provided

2. *SEARCH* the print media (newspapers or magazines) and electronic media (Internet or television) for information related to the influence of environmental factors on the incidence of congenital anomalies in a population group.
   - *COLLECT* two or three media resources related to one particular problem or group.
   - *SUMMARIZE* your findings.
   - *DESCRIBE* the influence that public awareness and actions had on the media presentations and initiation of interventions to rectify the problem and support those affected.
   - *DISCUSS* the role of the nurse in mobilizing public awareness and action.

3. *ASSESS* your community for the types of services that it offers to parents of infants born with congenital anomalies.
   - *DESCRIBE* the type and nature of the support services available, their cost, eligibility requirements, activities and services, and accessibility.
   - *PREPARE* a table that summarizes your findings so that they could be made accessible to families needing these services.
   - *DETERMINE* the adequacy of support services that are available.
   - *DISCUSS* approaches that nurses can take to improve the situation.

4. *VISIT* the March of Dimes chapter in your community. *PREPARE* a report that describes the types of services that it offers to prevent congenital anomalies, provide for early detection, and support the affected children and their parents.

## TOPICS FOR DISCUSSION

1. *Consider this question:* What is the role of the nurse when a child with a congenital disorder is born?

2. *Address this dilemma:* Early discharge can inhibit the ability of health care providers to detect physiologic alterations in the newborn early so that treatment can begin before permanent damage occurs. What can nurses do to facilitate timely detection of disorders within an early discharge system of health care delivery?

## MERLIN PROJECT

Use MERLIN to search the medical literature for nursing research studies related to the impact that a diagnosis of a congenital disorder can have on the infant's parents and the nursing measures that have been found to be most helpful in supporting the infant and the parents.
   - Create an annotated bibliography of at least four nursing studies.
   - Choose one study, and complete a bibliography card that includes the following:
     - Hypothesis; research question
     - Summary of methodology used and key findings
     - Reliability of the study and its findings
     - Recommendations for further research
   - Discuss how you would use the findings of these studies to develop an evidence-based support program for parents of infants diagnosed with a congenital disorder.

# Chapter

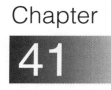

# Nursing Care of the High Risk Newborn

## SUMMARY OF KEY CONCEPTS

Chapter 41 focuses on the unique characteristics and complications faced by newborns as a result of their gestational age or their pattern of intrauterine growth. The nursing process provides the organizing framework for the care management of each deviation from expected gestation and intrauterine growth.

The discussion of the preterm infant begins with a description of physiologic assessment that focuses on identification of the most common potential problems of the preterm newborn related to respiratory, cardiovascular, central nervous system, and renal function; maintaining body temperature; adequate nutrition; hematologic status; and resisting infection. The manner in which parents respond to their preterm infant and the tasks that must be completed as parents adapt to the reality of a preterm infant are described and serve as the basis for nursing support measures directed toward meeting the needs of these parents. Typical nursing diagnoses and expected outcomes of care related to the preterm infant are listed. Implementation focuses on the prevention, early detection, and treatment of the common physiologic problems facing the preterm neonate with special emphasis on physical care, maintaining body temperature, providing oxygen therapy using several different methods, and using a variety of measures to ensure adequate nutrition and fluid balance. Mention is made of the use of surfactant to facilitate breathing. Respiratory distress syndrome (RDS) is described according to its pathophysiology, typical clinical manifestations, and required therapeutic measures. The possibility of oxygen-associated complications—retinopathy of prematurity, bronchopulmonary dysplasia, patent ductus arteriosus, and necrotizing enterocolitis—is explained. Students are informed about the critical need to assess and maintain nutritional, fluid, and electrolyte balance in the compromised newborn. Assessment focuses on weight and fluid measurement, criteria used to determine formula type and feeding schedule, and observation of elimination patterns. A description of methods for providing nourishment begins with oral feeding, the most natural and simple, and continues with gavage and gastrostomy feeding and parenteral fluids and nutrition (TPN). The benefits of nonnutritive sucking and guidelines for advancing infant feeding are included in the discussion.

The chapter continues with a description of the developmental and emotional aspects of care as related to preterm infants and their families. The impact of life in an intensive care nursery is illustrated with an emphasis on the sensory stimuli and environmental hazards facing these infants. Students are alerted to the need to consider the communication patterns of infants—their readiness for interaction, cues of overstimulation when appropriate infant stimulation is provided, and teaching parents about the meaning of their infant's behavior patterns. Kangaroo care is a suggested alternative to the "high tech" care emphasized in Western societies. A family's grief reaction as it applies to anticipated and actual loss is discussed.

A plan of care illustrates the use of the nursing process for the care management of the high risk newborn. Several nursing diagnoses are developed, including ineffective breathing pattern and thermoregulation, altered parenting, and risks for infection, altered nutrition: less than body requirements, fluid volume deficit or excess, impaired skin integrity, and injury.

Special attention is given to the infant's pain responses. Pain assessment, the ability of the infant to remember pain, and the consequences of untreated pain are described. Pain management focuses on both pharmacologic and nonpharmacologic approaches.

The problems faced by the postmature infant are described, including meconium aspiration syndrome and persistent pulmonary hypertension. Typical nursing diagnoses and expected outcomes of care as they relate to the postmature infant are identified. An overview of the care management approach required by the postmature infant is included.

The chapter includes a brief discussion of other problems related to gestation, including small for gestational age, intrauterine growth restriction, and large for gestational age. The physical findings exhibited by small for gestational age infants and the pathogenesis for their impeded growth and development are explained. Perinatal asphyxia, meconium aspiration, hypoglycemia, and heat loss are identified as the major problems faced by these newborns. A discussion of the characteristics and problems of the large for gestational age infant follows. The chapter concludes with a discussion of discharge planning that includes considerations related to transport to and from a regional center.

## LEARNING OBJECTIVES

Define the key terms.
Compare and contrast the characteristics of preterm, term, postterm, and postmature neonates.
Discuss respiratory distress syndrome and the approach to treatment.
Compare methods of oxygen therapy.
Describe nursing interventions for nutritional care of the preterm infant.
Discuss the pathophysiology of retinopathy of prematurity and bronchopulmonary dysplasia, and identify risk factors that predispose preterm infants to these problems.
List the signs and symptoms of perinatal asphyxia.
Describe meconium aspiration syndrome.
Plan developmentally appropriate care.
Examine the needs of parents of high risk infants.
Evaluate a neonatal transport plan.
Identify appropriate responses and interventions the nurse can use in caring for families experiencing anticipatory grief or loss and grief in the neonatal period.
Identify topics for nursing research related to high risk newborns.

# OUTLINE OF CHAPTER CONTENT WITH COURSE GUIDELINES

| CONTENT | GUIDELINE |
|---|:---:|
| Preterm infants—care management | |
|   – Assessment and nursing diagnoses | A |
|     – Physiologic assessment | A |
|     – Growth and development potential | A |
|     – Parental adaptation to preterm infant | A |
|   – Expected outcomes of care | A |
|   – Plan of care and interventions | A |
|     – Physical care | A |
|     – Maintaining body temperature | A |
|     – Oxygen therapy | A |
|       – Hood therapy; nasal cannula | A |
|       – Continuous positive airway pressure therapy | A |
|       – Mechanical ventilation | A |
|       – Surfactant administration | A |
|       – Extracorporeal membrane oxygenation therapy | C |
|       – High-frequency ventilation | C |
|       – Nitric oxide therapy | C |
|       – Weaning from respiratory assistance | A |
|     – Nutritional care | A |
|       – Types of nourishment | A |
|       – Weight and fluid loss or gain | A |
|       – Elimination patterns | A |
|       – Oral feeding | A |
|       – Gavage feeding | A |
|       – Gastrostomy feedings | B |
|       – Parenteral fluids | A |
|       – Advancing infant feedings | A |
|       – Nonnutritive sucking | A |
|       – Environmental concerns | A |
|     – Developmental care | A |
|       – Positioning | A |
|       – Reducing inappropriate stimuli | A |
|       – Infant communication | A |
|       – Infant stimulation | A |
|       – Kangaroo care | A |
|       – Parental support | A |
|       – Parent education | A |
|   – Evaluation | A |
| Plan of care | A |
| Complications in high risk infants | A |
|   – Respiratory distress syndrome | A |
|   – Complications associated with oxygen therapy | B |

| CONTENT | GUIDELINE |
|---|---|
| Infant pain responses | A |
|   – Pain assessment | A |
|   – Pain management | A |
| Postmature infants | A |
|   – Meconium aspiration syndrome | A |
|   – Persistent pulmonary hypertension | B |
|   – Care management | A |
| Other problems related to gestation | A |
|   – Small for gestational age and intrauterine growth restriction | A |
|     – Perinatal asphyxia | A |
|     – Hypoglycemia | A |
|     – Heat loss | A |
|     – Care management | A |
| Large for gestational age | A |
|   – Care management | A |
| Discharge planning | A |
| Transport to a regional center | B |
| Transport from a regional center | B |
| Anticipatory grief | A |
| Loss of an infant | A |

## TEACHING STRATEGIES

1. Contrast the physiologic function of a preterm infant with that of a full-term infant. Identify the physiologic and developmental problems that can arise as a result of the differences in function. Describe the nursing care management of preterm infants using a case study of a preterm infant born at 30 weeks and a case study of a preterm infant born at 36 weeks.

2. Compare the nursing care management of postmature infants and small for gestational age or IUGR infants. Point out the similarities with regard to potential problems and the care measures that these infants require.

3. Identify the factors that can compromise the health of a preterm newborn and place this newborn at risk. Indicate how these factors can interfere with the newborn's ability to breathe, maintain a stable body temperature, obtain sufficient nutrients, and meet growth and development standards.

4. Identify the sources of pain and discomfort encountered by infants in a neonatal intensive care unit (NICU). Describe the pain relief measures currently available and used.

5. Discuss the impact that a preterm newborn's compromised health status can have on parents and family.

6. Arrange for students to tour an NICU and shadow a nurse involved in the nursing care management of high risk newborns, including those that are preterm. Provide time for students to share their observations of the experience with the class.

Chapter 41: Nursing Care of the High Risk Newborn   183

7. Invite a nurse working in an NICU and parents of an infant who spent time in an NICU to participate in a panel discussion. The nurse should discuss the unique nursing care needs of the high risk newborn and his or her family. The parents should discuss the feelings, stressors, and fears that they experienced when their infant was hospitalized.

8. Identify the support groups available in your community to assist parents who have infants in NICUs.

## SUGGESTED STUDENT LEARNING ACTIVITIES

1. *VISIT* an intensive care nursery (ICN). Shadow one nurse as you observe the activities occurring in the nursery. *WRITE* a report about your experience that includes each of the following:
   - Description of your nursery observation according to the following:
     - Number of infants in the nursery and the types of health problems that they were facing
     - Technology and/or interventions used to meet the physical needs of the high risk infants for respiratory, thermoregulatory, nutritional, pain relief, and developmental support
     - Manner in which the emotional needs of the infants and their families were met
     - Discharge planning process—when it starts and what it entails
     - Cost of care and its impact on the family
     - Suggestions that you would make to improve the supportive care given to the families of the compromised infants
   - Description of the information collected during an interview of the nurse who you shadowed, including the following:
     - Educational background and experience of the nurse
     - The nurse's philosophy of nursing
     - The nurse's role in managing the care of high risk infants
     - The nurse's use and initiation of research
     - Rewards as well as frustrations or stressors encountered when caring for compromised infants and their families in an ICU environment
     - How the nurse copes with the day-to-day stressors of working in the ICN

2. *SURVEY* your community for the availability of support groups for parents whose infants are in an ICN. *ARRANGE* to attend a meeting of one group and to *INTERVIEW* one of the members of the group. *PREPARE* a report that includes the following:
   - Description of the formation of the group—who formed the group, when, and why?
   - Purpose and mission of the group
   - Process involved in publicizing the group and encouraging people to join
   - Services offered to the members of the group and their families to help them cope with the stressors of having an infant in the ICN
   - Perceptions of the ICN nurses and the degree of support that these nurses offer, including any suggestions that the parents would make to enhance the nursing support provided
   - Description of the meeting attended, including the group dynamics observed

3. *INTERVIEW* the parents of an infant who is preterm.
   - *GATHER* information concerning the following:
     - The psychosocial and economic impact that this birth has had on the parents and their family

- Their impressions and feelings with regard to their infant and the infant's environment (in the ICN)
- The type and effectiveness of nursing support measures provided *and* nursing support measures needed but not provided
- The learning needs that they identified with regard to their infant's status and care while hospitalized and their infant's care needs after discharge; the manner in which learning needs were met by the nurses involved in the care of their infant
- Resources that they have used to cope with the identified impact of this birth, including family, friends, support groups, and community resources and home care services
- *ASSESS* the manner in which these parents have reacted to the birth of their preterm infant and the degree to which they have met the psychologic tasks of parents with preterm infants. Use the information included in this chapter concerning parental adaptation to the preterm infant to facilitate your assessment.
- *DESCRIBE* how you would use the data gathered to help this family maximize its strengths and overcome its deficits to reach the goal of successful adaptation to and parenting of their preterm infant.

## TOPICS FOR DISCUSSION

1. *Address this question:* What can nurses do to help families adjust to the environment of an ICN and cope with the care management measures required by their infant?

2. *Support this statement:* The nurse plays an essential role in helping parents get ready for the discharge of their high risk infant to high-tech home care.

3. *Address these questions:*
   - How can nurses help parents of a preterm newborn cope with the care needs of their baby during hospitalization and after discharge?
   - What measures can a nurse working in the NICU use to help preterm infants meet their growth and developmental needs?

## MERLIN PROJECT

Use MERLIN to assist you in searching the medical literature for nursing journal articles related to the needs of infants requiring care in the NICU and their families and nursing measures found to be effective in meeting those needs. Focus your search on infants who are at risk as a result of problems related to gestational age and intrauterine growth.
- Create an annotated bibliography of at least five nursing journal articles.
- Choose one article, and complete a bibliography card that includes the following
  - Summary of the article's key points
  - Personal reaction to the ideas presented in the article
- Discuss how you would use the information in the articles to provide quality care to infants in the NICU that is also sensitive to the emotional and informational needs of the parents and families.

# Chapter

## 42

# Loss and Grief

## SUMMARY OF KEY CONCEPTS

In Chapter 42, the student is introduced to the concept of loss as a result of unexpected outcomes to pregnancy and the grief process as the family reacts to the loss.

Loss is viewed as failure to achieve what was hoped for, dreamed about, or planned, with the intensity and length of grief responses dependent upon an individual's characteristics and his or her perception of what was lost. The student is cautioned to avoid planning care based on stereotypical views about how an individual should perceive a loss. Rather, the student is encouraged to determine each person's views of the loss, the circumstances surrounding the loss, and his or her social support network as the basis for an appropriate, supportive plan of care.

The process of bereavement or mourning is contrasted with ineffective or complicated bereavement. Typical grief responses are described according to three phases—acute distress, intense grief, and reorganization. A box summarizes the signs and symptoms of each of the phases of the grief response. Swanson-Kauffman's caring framework is used to describe, in a concise manner, the nurse's role when working with bereaved parents and their families.

Care management with regard to loss and grief is further defined in terms of the nursing process. Assessment emphasizes the critical need for careful questioning and attentive listening to both the verbal and nonverbal responses. Typical nursing diagnoses and expected outcomes of care related to families experiencing loss are identified.

Communication and counseling techniques are the focal point of effective nursing support for grieving families. Two boxes, along with the text, provide helpful guidelines that alert students to the cultural and religious considerations regarding death and what to say or not say when working with grieving families. The student is informed about the need to not only meet the physical comfort needs of the bereaved mother but also to provide families with a variety of opportunities to create memories, such as viewing, holding, and caring for the baby who has died. Sample checklists are provided to facilitate meeting the needs of families experiencing an early or late pregnancy loss. Suggestions are made for the discharge of parents who experienced a loss and for follow-up after discharge, with phone calls at critical points in the mourning process.

The chapter includes a plan of care that illustrates the use of the nursing process when managing the care of a family experiencing a fetal death at 20 weeks' gestation. The nursing diagnoses of dysfunctional grieving and situational low self-esteem are explored. The final section of the chapter highlights special losses. Brief discussions are included regarding prenatal diagnoses with negative outcome, loss of one infant in a multiple birth, adolescent grief, and maternal death.

## LEARNING OBJECTIVES

Define the key terms.

Understand the personal and societal issues that may complicate responses to perinatal loss.

Describe emotional, behavioral, cognitive, and physical responses commonly experienced during the grieving process associated with perinatal loss.

Formulate appropriate nursing diagnoses for parents experiencing perinatal loss.

Identify specific nursing interventions to meet the special needs of parents and their families related to perinatal loss and grief.

Develop expected outcome criteria to evaluate nursing care for grieving families.

Differentiate among helpful and nonhelpful responses in caring for parents experiencing loss and grief.

Identify topics for nursing research related to perinatal loss and grief.

## OUTLINE OF CHAPTER CONTENT WITH COURSE GUIDELINES

| CONTENT | GUIDELINE |
|---|---|
| Grief responses | A |
| – Acute distress | A |
| – Intense grief | A |
| – Reorganization | A |
| – Grief of fathers | A |
| Care management | A |
| – Assessment and nursing diagnoses | A |
| – Expected outcomes of care | A |
| – Plan of care and interventions | A |
| – Help mother and father and other family members actualize loss | A |
| – Help parents with decision making | A |
| – Help the bereaved to acknowledge and express their feelings | A |
| – Normalize the grief process and facilitate positive coping | A |
| – Meet the physical needs of the postpartum bereaved mother | A |
| – Assist the bereaved in communicating with, supporting, and getting support from family | A |
| – Create memories for parents to take home | A |
| – Communicate using a caring framework | A |
| – Be concerned about cultural and spiritual needs of parents | A |
| – Provide sensitive care at discharge and after discharge | A |
| – Provide postmortem care | B |
| – Evaluation | A |

*continued*

| CONTENT | GUIDELINE |
|---|---|
| Plan of care | A |
| Special losses | B |
| – Prenatal diagnoses with negative outcomes | B |
| – Loss of one in a multiple birth | B |
| – Adolescent grief | B |
| – Maternal death | A |
| Complicated bereavement | B |

# TEACHING STRATEGIES

1. Describe the phases of the grief response and the tasks of mourners. Discuss the role of the nurse in helping parents and families cope with the death of their infant and/or of the mother.

2. Encourage students to share their feelings about death and dying, especially concerning the death of a newborn and/or the mother.

3. Invite a caregiver involved in pastoral care or grief counseling to discuss the approach that he or she uses when caring for families experiencing a pregnancy-related loss.

4. Identify support groups and services available in your community to assist families who have experienced a pregnancy-related loss.

# SUGGESTED STUDENT LEARNING ACTIVITIES

1. *ASSESS* the services provided by the hospital where you have your clinical experience for families who have experienced a loss related to pregnancy and its outcome (i.e., fetal, neonatal, or maternal death). *PREPARE* a report that includes each of the following:
   - Description of the types of support services offered and the role of the nurse in the development and provision of these services
   - Evaluation of the effectiveness of the services provided according to the principles presented in this chapter regarding loss and grief
   - Identification of any changes that you would propose to enhance or improve the services provided

2. *INTERVIEW* several labor and birth nurses related to their experiences with maternal, fetal, and neonatal death. *PREPARE* a report that describes the following:
   - Their feelings when the death occurred and then afterward
   - Measures that they used to deal with their feelings regarding the perinatal death
   - How they supported the family who experienced the loss
   - Measures that they used to help the families "make memories" when the fetus or newborn died
   - Services available in their agency or in the community that are designed to help families experiencing perinatal death
   - Measures that they used to support each other

3. *PREPARE* a packet of information, support materials, and resources that could be given at discharge to families who have experienced a loss related to pregnancy and its outcome. *USE* the information contained in this chapter as well as resources available in your community to guide your efforts.

4. *INTERVIEW* a family who experienced a loss related to pregnancy.
   - GATHER information regarding the following:
     - The family's description of the loss and the impact that it has had on their family and their ability to function
     - Coping mechanisms that the family used to deal with the loss they experienced
     - The support measures, persons, and services that the family found to be helpful, those that they found not to be helpful, and those that they found to be lacking
     - Types of support that they would have liked to have received but did not
   - *DESCRIBE* how you would use this information to plan care that is effective in helping families to grieve and cope effectively with a perinatal loss.

## Topics for Discussion

1. *Debate the issue:* Should parents be encouraged to view their dead fetus even if serious anomalies are present and visible?

2. *Support the statement:* Nurses have a responsibility in advocating for the development of bereavement support services in the hospitals where they work.

3. *Explore the questions:*
   - What are your beliefs and values regarding death and dying? What types of loss have you experienced in your life? How did you progress through the process of grieving and what coping mechanisms did you use? Who helped you deal with your loss? How did they help you?
   - How do different cultures view death and dying, including the nature of the grieving process?

## Merlin Project

Use MERLIN to assist you in searching the literature for research studies related to the responses of mothers and the responses of fathers to a pregnancy-related loss.
- Create an annotated bibliography that includes three research studies related to maternal grief responses and three studies related to paternal grief responses.
- Choose one study from each category, and complete two bibliography cards that include the following:
  - Hypothesis; research question
  - Summary of the methodology used and key findings
  - Reliability of the study and its findings
  - Recommendations for further research
- Use the results of the studies to compare and contrast maternal and paternal grief responses. Indicate how you would use this information to provide support for mothers and fathers that takes into consideration the characteristics of their grief response.

# Case Studies

Each of the case studies in this section reflects key concepts from one or more of the chapters in the text. The answer guidelines are included for each question in the case study, thereby providing a quick reference to use when helping students focus on the most important aspects of the required response.

## CASE STUDY 1: PREGNANT WOMAN DURING THE FIRST TRIMESTER

Teresa, 27 years old, calls the women's health clinic and tells her nurse-practitioner that her menstrual period, which usually occurs on a regular basis every 28 days, is 3 weeks late. She thinks that she may be pregnant since she and her husband of 2 years have been trying to have a baby for the last 6 months. An appointment is made to determine if Teresa is pregnant and to begin prenatal care if she is.

A. A pregnancy test confirms that Teresa is pregnant. She asks when to expect the baby's birth. Teresa reports that her last menstrual period began on August 11, 1999. What should the nurse explain to Teresa about her expected date of birth?

- **Use Nägele's rule: Subtract 3 months and add 7 days and 1 year; EDB = May 18, 2000.**
- **Caution Teresa that the EDB is not always accurate and that birth within 2 weeks before the date and 2 weeks after is considered acceptable. The fact that her menstrual cycles are regular and she keeps accurate dates increases the likelihood that she will give birth on or very near the date calculated.**

B. The nurse-practitioner prepares Teresa for her initial prenatal assessment. What components should be included as part of this assessment to ensure an adequate baseline database and to identify risk factors that may require immediate attention?

- **Components of a thorough assessment should include a health history interview, physical examination, and laboratory testing.**
- **Explain why each component is important and relevant and what should be included in each. A holistic and comprehensive approach is critical; risk factors should be determined.**
- **Since this is Teresa's first pregnancy, it is important to explain the purpose of each component, describe findings, and teach her about how her body will begin to change and what would indicate a developing problem.**

- Include a discussion of the approach that should be taken to enhance Teresa's comfort and security with prenatal care and establish a trusting rapport with the nurse-practitioner.

C. Since this is Teresa's first pregnancy, she expresses concern that she and her husband do not know exactly what to expect. State the nursing diagnosis reflective of Teresa's concern, one expected outcome, and appropriate nursing measures to use.

- **Nursing diagnosis: Anxiety related to lack of knowledge regarding adaptations to pregnancy.**
- **Expected outcome: Teresa will express knowledge regarding physical and psychosocial changes expected to occur during the first trimester.**
- **Nursing measures: Focus on teaching and planning out content over several visits; include expected changes, warning signs, and education for self-care; provide reading materials and suggest appropriate books, articles, and videos; give a reading assignment to complete before a visit and have Teresa indicate areas of questions and concern; provide a telephone number to call with questions. Consider that Teresa is in the first trimester and is working on the developmental task of "I am pregnant." Consider emotional and physical changes occurring during this time, including egocentricity, discomforts, and ambivalence; involve her husband in the teaching sessions.**

D. Teresa tells the nurse that she works full time and asks if it would be okay if she comes for prenatal care when she notices problems rather than coming on a regular basis according to a schedule. She assures the nurse that she will read a lot about pregnancy in her free time and consult with her friends for advice since many of them have already been pregnant. What should the nurse tell Teresa?

- **Fully discuss the importance of seeing and talking to a health care professional on a regular basis during pregnancy; caution against using only advice of friends and reading because misconceptions and misinterpretations can occur. Each woman's pregnancy is different, necessitating the care management of a health care professional to ensure an optimal outcome. Use biostatistics to emphasize importance of prenatal care for maternal and fetal well-being.**

E. Teresa calls the clinic 1 week after her first visit to tell the nurse that she has been feeling nauseous every morning and periodically during the day. She is especially concerned since her intake of food and fluids has decreased and she vomits about once and sometimes twice a day. What should the nurse do in response to Teresa's problem and concerns?

- **Use a similar approach with all discomforts: Never discount a woman's complaints, always fully assess, discuss the basis for discomfort, and offer appropriate suggestions for relief.**
- **Gather specific, exact information regarding the amount of vomiting and amount and type of food and fluid that is consumed and retained. Seek information regarding fluid balance— ask about urine characteristics and pattern, weight changes, thirst, and dryness of integument.**
- **Prenatal visit is warranted if signs of dehydration and weight loss are reported and/or Teresa's concerns remain despite advice given.**
- **Relief measures: Use natural measures first before any pharmacologic measures are suggested; many different measures can be cited, including timing and content of meals, use of fluids, types of foods to eat or to avoid, relaxation measures, acupressure, and environmental alterations.**

F. At the second prenatal visit, Teresa begins to ask questions about sexuality during pregnancy. She states that she and her husband enjoy each other sexually but now are afraid to do anything because it may hurt her or the baby. How should the nurse respond to Teresa's concern?

- **Approach: Obtain a sexual history; work with the couple together and alone, if needed; discuss how pregnancy can affect sexuality and suggest alternative means of sexual expression; encourage open communication of concerns and feelings.**
- **Use written materials and case histories of other couples and how they coped to illustrate measures that would be helpful.**

G. Teresa tells the nurse that even though she is usually happy about being pregnant, sometimes she feels that she should have waited a little longer to get pregnant so that she would have more time to get ready to be a mother. She also tells the nurse that she sometimes resents the baby for making her sick and that she gets moody and "cries at the drop of a hat." What approach should the nurse take in addressing Teresa's expressed emotions and feelings?

- **Discuss maternal emotional and psychosocial adaptation to pregnancy and impending parenthood; include basis for the adaptations discussed; emphasize the normalcy of her feelings and encourage her to continue to fully express them. Explain that she is experiencing ambivalence which is very typical of the first trimester and is part of the developmental task of accepting "I am pregnant."**
- **Discuss how her husband will undergo changes and adaptations as a result of the pregnancy.**
- **Include her husband in the discussion of emotional changes that each one can expect as they both adapt to pregnancy and parenthood.**

H. Teresa's body mass index (BMI) is 23. Based on this information, what should the nurse recommend to Teresa in terms of an overall weight gain and the specific weight gain pattern for each trimester?

- **BMI is a normal weight; weight gain amount and patterns should reflect this BMI.**
- **Discuss weight distribution regarding developing structures of pregnancy. Use graphs and illustrations; cite total recommended weight gain for pregnancy and the amount to be gained each week during the second and third trimesters.**

I. Describe the process that the nurse should use to help Teresa maintain an appropriate intake of foods and fluids during pregnancy.

- **Begin with an assessment of Teresa's current nutritional status and habits. Have Teresa complete a 24-hour or 3-day recall of what she eats, when she eats, where she eats, and how she prepares her food. Use this information to individualize interventions.**
- **Teach the importance of nutrition for herself and her developing baby; emphasize the hazards of not meeting the nutrient requirements for pregnancy.**
- **Plan a diet with Teresa that reflects her desires, lifestyle, and customs and requirements for calories, fluid, protein, vitamins, and minerals.**

# CASE STUDY 2: PREGNANT WOMAN DURING THE SECOND TRIMESTER

Anne, a multigravida, is pregnant again. She has two living children—twin daughters born at 36 weeks' gestation. Her first pregnancy ended with a spontaneous abortion at 10 weeks' gestation, and her third pregnancy ended with the stillbirth of a son at 38 weeks' gestation. She is currently 18 weeks pregnant and her health and well-being have been good, as determined during regular prenatal visits. Anne is married and works full time as a bank teller.

A. Explain the 5-digit system, and use this system to describe Anne's obstetric history.

- **In the 5-digit system, the first digit refers to gravida, or the number of times the woman has been pregnant.**
- **The next four digits refer to pregnancy outcomes. Use the acronym TPAL (term, preterm, abortion, living children) to determine the last four digits.**
- **Anne is pregnant now and has had three other pregnancies; the outcomes were as follows: one term birth (stillbirth), one preterm birth (twins), one abortion, and two living children (preterm twins); therefore she would be 4-1-1-1-2.**

B. During a prenatal visit, the nurse-practitioner assesses Anne's current health status. Outline the components for health assessment that should be used during regular prenatal visits to ensure a complete update of her progress during the second trimester of pregnancy.

- **Components of a thorough assessment during the second trimester should include an updated health history interview, physical examination, laboratory testing, and fetal assessment.**
- **Focus of assessment should be on updating the database in a holistic manner, including any changes since the last prenatal visit in the woman or her support system, including those that could indicate warning signs, risk factors, or the presence of discomforts; always compare findings obtained during the current visit with the findings obtained during previous visits.**

C. Anne expresses concern about a more irregular bowel elimination pattern over the last week or so. "I never had problems with my last pregnancy, and I certainly do not want to have any now." State the nursing diagnosis reflective of Anne's concern, one expected outcome, and appropriate nursing measures.

- **Nursing diagnosis: Risk for constipation related to alteration in intestinal motility associated with pregnancy; assessment measures should be used to determine the exact nature of the irregular bowel movements and characteristics of the stool and factors such as diet, stress, and activity that could be interfering with normal bowel elimination patterns.**
- **Expected outcome: Anne will achieve regular bowel elimination of soft, formed stool.**
- **Nursing measures: Use assessment findings to guide a discussion of the basis for the change in elimination patterns and the relief measures that would be appropriate, such as roughage, fluids, activity, and a regular schedule for elimination.**

D. Anne asks if she should continue to work, especially since she has two 4-year-old daughters to care for. How should the nurse reply?

- Consider Anne's employment as a full-time bank teller, and use anticipatory guidance regarding the discomforts that could occur from standing on her feet for long periods, such as varicosities, joint pain, backache, and ankle edema, and the relief measures that would be appropriate.
- Offer suggestions regarding clothing, posture, body mechanics, and physical activity.
- Discuss Anne's support system—who they are and how they can help her so that she can get the rest and relaxation she needs when she gets home from work.

E. Anne asks the nurse if she and her husband should prepare a birth plan, "so we could have more control over what is happening than the last time." What should the nurse tell Anne?

- The components and value of a birth plan should be discussed with the couple; plans should be realistic, developed with the couple's primary health care provider, and compatible with the policies of the setting that they will be using for their birth. Care plans can be valuable since they empower a couple to create a birth experience that is right for them.
- A birth plan should include the couple's wishes regarding birth setting, anesthesia and other interventions, persons who will be present, and prepared childbirth techniques that they will use.

F. Anne tells the nurse that her daughters are getting very excited about the new baby, especially since she has begun to "show." Anne states, "I have no idea how to prepare them for the reality of a newborn and how much care they require. I did not have to worry about this with my last pregnancy, when the girls were born." What suggestions could the nurse give to Anne?

- Offer suggestions for preparation for a new baby based on developmental status of the children, in this case, preschoolers.
- Offer to let the girls come in with Anne during prenatal visits to listen to the baby's heartbeat.
- Make referrals to sibling preparation classes.
- Prepare a list of appropriate children's storybooks, videos, and CD-ROMs that deal with the subject.
- Arrange for children to spend time with infants.

# CASE STUDY 3: PREGNANT WOMAN DURING THE THIRD TRIMESTER OF PREGNANCY

Sara is an unmarried, 20-year-old nulliparous woman beginning her third trimester. The father of the baby is actively involved in the pregnancy and plans to help Sara during labor and with the parenting of their child.

A. The nurse-practitioner assesses Sara's current health status. Outline the components for health assessment that should be used during regular prenatal visits to ensure a complete update of her progress during the third stage of pregnancy.

- Components of a thorough assessment during the third trimester should include an updated health history interview, physical examination, laboratory tests, and fetal assessment.
- Assessment should continue to be holistic in its approach and include warning signs of such potential problems as pregnancy-induced hypertension, placental disorders, and preterm labor.
- Begin to discuss changes indicating that labor is approaching; teach Sara signs of labor.
- Sara can begin daily fetal movement counts this trimester at about 27 weeks' gestation.

B. Sara asks the nurse if she and her partner should attend childbirth classes. "We have been watching videos and reading books about labor and what to do. We have even been practicing some of the techniques recommended." State the nursing diagnosis reflective of Sara's comment, one expected outcome, and appropriate nursing measures.

- Nursing diagnosis: Knowledge deficit regarding value of childbirth education classes related to lack of experience.
- Expected outcome: Sara and her partner will attend childbirth classes beginning in the seventh month of pregnancy.
- Nursing measures: Incorporate beneficial effects of childbirth classes into response to Sara's comment, including not only pain relief measures but also information regarding process of labor and birth, childbirth options, general health information about themselves as a couple and about the newborn, and interaction with other pregnant couples. Give them a list of classes, especially those designed for single parents; put them in touch with a teacher or a former student who found the classes to be helpful.

C. Why would it be helpful for Sara and her partner to begin to get things ready for the baby, including choosing a feeding method and finding a health care provider for the baby? How can the nurse assist in this process?

- Emphasize the importance of making decisions when conditions are less stressful. This is the time to consider the pros and cons of various options regarding their lifestyle, values, and beliefs; to visit or interview health care providers for their baby; and to get the best value and safety for items purchased to care for their baby.
- Encourage breastfeeding by discussing its benefits. This is a good time to learn basic information about breastfeeding, which can then be applied when the baby is born; refer to a prenatal breastfeeding class and/or lactation consultant.
- Help the couple to appreciate that onset of labor can be unpredictable and begin sooner than expected.

D. When Sara is at 32 weeks' gestation, she complains of having difficulty sleeping, even though she is tired. She asks for a prescription for a sleeping pill. How should the nurse respond to Sara's request?

- Assess Sara for physical problems, changes in status, and worries or concerns that could contribute to insomnia; have her describe what she is feeling at bedtime, what she thinks is keeping her awake, and measures that she has tried to help her sleep.
- Address issues raised in the assessment, for example, a worry or concern; suggest nonpharmacologic measures to help her relax and sleep, such as measures that she usually finds relaxing (music, warm milk, warm bath or shower).

- Involve her partner as appropriate in measures to help her relax and sleep, such as massage and assisting her into a supported, comfortable position for sleep.

# CASE STUDY 4: WOMAN IN FIRST STAGE OF LABOR

Tasha is a nulliparous woman at 39 weeks' gestation. She and her husband George attended childbirth education classes based on the Lamaze method. They also prepared a birth plan with their nurse-midwife. Tasha calls her nurse-midwife's office to report that she is in labor and asks if she should get her husband and leave for the birthing center right away.

A. How should the nurse approach this situation?

- Use a caring, respectful manner to gather information to determine if Tasha is experiencing true labor and to gain a sense of how far she has progressed. Outline questions that could be asked to determine Tasha's status.
- If in true labor, Tasha should be given guidance about when to come to the birthing center and what to do until it is time to leave home.

B. Tasha is in labor, and her husband brings her to the birthing center for admission. Outline the process of admission and assessment that the nurse who will care for Tasha and George should follow.

- Approach: Use a caring, respectful, confident manner to establish a trusting, therapeutic nurse-client relationship; involve George in the assessment process as appropriate; avoid questioning Tasha during contractions; discuss the birth plan.
- Components of assessment: Prenatal history, health history interview including status of this labor, physical examination including uterine contractions, condition of membranes and cervical changes, fetal assessment including FHR, station, presentation, position, and laboratory testing.

C. Tasha becomes tense and begins to cry when the nurse prepares to perform a vaginal examination as part of the admission process. What should this nurse do?

- It is important to put Tasha at ease and consider her comfort and feelings when the examination is performed, especially because several more will be required as labor progresses.
- Explain why the examination is done, consider her privacy and comfort needs during the examination, tell her what you are doing, and inform her about the results of the examination.
- Use infection control measures and Standard Precautions when performing the examination—perform perineal care before and after with clean gloves, use sterile gloves and lubricant for the examination, and limit the frequency of the examinations to times when they are indicated.

D. A priority nursing diagnosis for Tasha would be pain related to the increasing frequency, duration, and intensity of uterine contractions during the first stage of labor. State one expected outcome, and discuss the nonpharmacologic measures that the nurse could use to help reduce Tasha's pain and discomfort.

- Expected outcome: Tasha will participate in appropriate nonpharmacologic measures to reduce her pain and keep it within controllable limits.

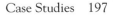

- Nonpharmacologic measures: Comfort and supportive measures, physical care and hygiene measures, pain management measures and relaxation techniques learned in childbirth education classes, and alternative measures including biofeedback, acupressure, TENS, water therapy, therapeutic touch, and birthing balls.
- Check the birth plan, and discuss proposed measures with Tasha and George to find out what would be acceptable and effective for them; take note of effectiveness of any measures implemented.

E. Tasha is very reluctant to change her semi-Fowler's position. She states that she feels just fine the way she is. What approach could the nurse take to help Tasha realize the importance of changing positions frequently throughout labor?

- Explain rationale for position change simply and in understandable terms, using diagrams and pelvic models as appropriate. Emphasize the beneficial effects for Tasha (increased comfort, shorter labor), her baby (enhanced circulation), and the progress of her labor (enhance progress).
- Give her a choice of positions, help her to change to the position, and stay with her to assess her response to the position in terms of her comfort and the well-being of the fetus.
- Teach her coach how to help in changing her position and why this is so important.

F. What measures could the nurse use to enhance and facilitate the progress of Tasha's labor?

- Identify stressors that can increase tension and impede labor; use this information to guide stress reduction measures.
- Ensure that energy and fluid needs are met to prevent dehydration and fatigue or energy depletion.
- Manage Tasha's pain and discomfort using nonpharmacologic and pharmacologic measures as appropriate.
- Keep bladder empty.
- Ambulate and change position frequently, thereby using gravity to enhance progress.
- Use support measures to reduce anxiety and fear.

G. Tasha is now in active labor. George appears more and more anxious as Tasha's labor progresses, especially when she has a contraction and her reaction to the pain becomes more evident. It is obvious that he is losing confidence in his ability to help Tasha as she becomes less responsive to his coaching efforts. What can the nurse do to help George regain his confidence and composure?

- Use supportive measures designed to help reduce the father or coach's anxiety; explain to him the normalcy of what Tasha is experiencing and how she is acting.
- Demonstrate and reinforce supportive measures that George can use to help Tasha now that her labor is more active.
- Give George a chance to talk about his feelings; provide time for him to meet his physical needs for rest and nutrition.

H. Since Tasha is in the active phase, ongoing assessment of her status, fetal well-being, and progress of labor becomes more critical. Outline the components of this ongoing assessment, the recommended frequency during the active phase, and the expected findings.

- Components include uterine contractions, cervical changes and vaginal show, maternal vital signs and behaviors, fetal descent and position, and FHR.
- Frequency of assessment and expected findings are based on the stage or phase of labor, condition of the maternal-fetal unit, and professional and agency standards/protocols.
- Include guidelines for using partograms and flow sheets to document findings.

I. Tasha and George included the option of epidural anesthesia in their birth plan. When Tasha reaches 5 cm, they request that the epidural anesthesia be administered if it would be safe for both Tasha and the baby.

1) What assessment data should be gathered before the induction of the anesthesia?
- Effects of epidural anesthesia should guide assessment measures—maternal vital signs and level of hydration, progress of labor, and FHR and pattern.
- Compare all findings with those obtained previously.

2) How should the nurse support Tasha and George just before and during the induction?
- Explain effects of the anesthesia, including assessment measures that will be used, what will be felt, how it will be administered, equipment that will be used, and measures that will be used to ensure safety.
- Help Tasha into position, and show George how to support Tasha.
- Keep Tasha and George informed as to what is happening during the induction.

3) What nursing measures should be implemented to ensure the safety of Tasha and the fetus after the epidural anesthesia is administered?
- Ongoing, more frequent assessment for maternal, fetal, and labor responses to the anesthetic—effects of the anesthetic should guide nursing measures and the assessment for problem development.
- Focus on blood pressure (hypotension), maternal breathing patterns (effect on diaphragm), FHR and pattern (alteration in placental perfusion), progress of labor (slowing), pain relief, loss of sensation to bladder (retention), and legs (injury).

# CASE STUDY 5: WOMAN IN THE SECOND AND THIRD STAGES OF LABOR

Barbara, a nulliparous woman, is in the transition stage of the first stage of labor and is nearing the second stage. She and her coach have been working together effectively for most of the labor, but Barbara lost control during transition. Barbara says that she is exhausted and cannot imagine how she will be able to go on and to push.

A. What criteria should be used to determine if Barbara has progressed to the second stage of labor?

- Cervix fully dilated and effaced is the definitive sign; other signs may also be observed at this time, including changes in behavior and physical signs and symptoms.

B. Barbara is confirmed to be in the second stage of labor. She is tired and does not want to push right now. Fetal station is 1+ and position is ROA. Barbara is not yet experiencing an urge to bear down. What would be an effective approach for the nurse to take at this time? Support your answer.

- **Recognize that Barbara is in the latent phase of the second stage of labor; a lull in the labor process occurs, therefore the nurse should let Barbara rest and get ready for the work of birth. Pushing is most effective when the urge to bear down is perceived as a result of Ferguson's reflex; changing positions, including upright positions, may facilitate progress as the fetus descends and applies pressure to the perineum.**
- **Use supportive measures to help Barbara relax until the urge to push begins.**
- **Be alert for signs that the descent phase is beginning, indicating that it is time for Barbara to start pushing.**

C. Barbara begins to feel the urge to bear down about 30 minutes after the second stage of labor begins. She is very anxious, stating that she cannot remember exactly what the childbirth teacher told her to do now. Her coach is unsure how to help her. What nursing action should be taken?

- **Redemonstrate the procedure of pushing by helping Barbara get into an appropriate position (e.g., lateral, sitting, squatting) and supporting her in this position.**
- **Remind her about what to do, not to hold her breath, and to follow what her body is telling her.**

D. Barbara's baby is born without the need for an episiotomy. Only a 1° perineal laceration occurred. What signs indicate that the expected events of the third stage of labor are occurring?

- **Separation and expulsion of the placenta are the expected events.**
- **Signs: Elevation of fundus, rounded shape of fundus, lengthening of umbilical cord, cessation of pulsation, and bleeding.**

E. At present, Barbara's flow is moderate to heavy with a few clots. What measures should be used to ensure fundal contraction?

- **Use massage when fundus is boggy, administer oxytocics as ordered to keep fundus firm, put baby to breast if breastfeeding, stimulate nipples, and keep bladder empty.**

F. Discuss the measures that the nurse should use to help Barbara and her husband bond with their new baby.

- **Measures to promote and support attachment include providing time to interact with their newborn, delaying eye prophylaxis, pointing out typical newborn behaviors and characteristics, and creating a celebratory atmosphere.**

# CASE STUDY 6: WOMAN DURING THE POSTPARTUM PERIOD

Rebecca, a primigravida, gave birth to a full-term, 8 pound, 2 ounce girl 30 minutes ago. Her placenta was intact and normal in appearance and size. Currently, her fundus is firm, at the umbilicus, and midline; her lochia is moderate rubra with no odor and a few small clots. A midline episiotomy was performed during the birth process. Rebecca has several large hemorrhoids that first developed late in the third trimester and increased in size as a result of Rebecca's bearing down efforts. Epidural anesthesia was used during labor and birth. Rebecca plans to breastfeed her baby.

A. Outline the assessment components that should be given priority when monitoring the progress of Rebecca's physiologic recovery during the fourth stage of labor.

- **Priorities for assessment: Focus on bleeding (fundus, lochia, episiotomy condition, vital signs, condition of bladder) and postanesthesia recovery (return of sensation to legs and bladder).**
- **Discuss rationale for the priorities given.**

B. During a postpartum assessment at 1½ hours after birth, Rebecca's fundus was no longer firm, and her lochial flow had increased in amount, saturating her pad in less than 1 hour. State in order of priority the actions that the nurse should take in response to these assessment findings.

- **Immediate response should be to massage the fundus until firm and then express clots that may be present.**
- **Check Rebecca's bladder for distension.**
- **Notify the primary health care provider to determine if oxytocics should be administered.**
- **Change Rebecca's pad, taking note of the time to aid in determining quantity of lochia.**
- **Increase frequency of postpartum assessments; document all findings, actions, and responses.**

C. Rebecca complains of perineal pain. She tells the nurse that she does not know which hurts worse, her episiotomy or her hemorrhoids. State the nursing diagnosis reflective of Rebecca's complaint, one expected outcome, and appropriate relief measures.

- **Nursing diagnosis: Pain related to presence of a midline episiotomy and hemorrhoids.**
- **Expected outcome: Rebecca will experience a reduction in pain after implementation of perineal relief measures.**
- **Always fully assess the client's pain experience (character, location, severity) before taking action.**
- **Consider nonpharmacologic and local measures for pain relief since the pain is of perineal origin—ice packs (first 12 to 24 hours to limit swelling and to numb), sitz bath (after first 12 to 24 hours to soothe, cleanse, and enhance healing), perineal cleansing, maternal positioning, and topicals.**
- **Consider pharmacologic relief measures if the pain is severe and/or the other measures are ineffective; be sure to determine the safety of any medication for the lactating woman.**
- **Pain relief is important so that the woman can rest and care for her baby.**

D. Rebecca is very concerned about having her first bowel movement. "I have hemorrhoids and stitches— it is going to be awful until I heal. Maybe I should hold back from having a bowel movement for a few days until I feel a little less sore." How should the nurse respond?

- **Emphasize that delaying bowel elimination will only dry the stool, making it harder to pass; discuss measures to enhance bowel elimination, such as roughage, fluids, activity, and the use of stool softener with or without a laxative.**

- Discuss measures to reduce discomfort after the bowel movement, such as perineal cleansing, a sitz bath, and topicals.

E. Rebecca and her husband Andy are worried about how they will manage when they go home with their new baby at 48 hours after birth. "We never even baby sat when we were kids or helped take care of younger siblings." What can the nurse do to help Rebecca and Andy take care of their new baby effectively?

- Use strategies such as promotion of parenting skills, coping mechanisms, and discharge planning and teaching; demonstrate skills and encourage parents to redemonstrate; recommend videos and provide reading materials; encourage "rooming-in."
- Discuss with the primary health care provider the possibility of referral to a home care agency for a postpartum home visit.
- Consider referral to parenting support groups, telephone follow-up, and a warm line.

F. During a home health care visit 4 days after birth, Rebecca and Andy ask the nurse about postpartum blues. They relate to the nurse that Rebecca has been "feeling down" since coming home from the hospital 2 days ago. What approach should the nurse take in responding to this couple's concern?

- Determine what Rebecca and Andy mean by "feeling down."
- Review the phases of maternal postpartum adjustment with Rebecca and Andy; describe the postpartum blues in terms of what they are and why they happen.
- Assess Rebecca for risk factors associated with postpartum depression.
- Discuss strategies to help Rebecca cope with postpartum blues in an effective manner; include Andy in the discussion since he is affected by Rebecca's emotions and is important in helping her cope; emphasize that Rebecca needs rest and sleep, adequate nutrition, and time to meet her own needs.

# CASE STUDY 7: FULL-TERM NEWBORN

Baby girl Melissa was born 1 hour ago. She is a full-term newborn weighing 7 pounds, 12 ounces. Her Apgar scores were seven at 1 minute and nine at 5 minutes. The parents of Melissa are participating in the mother-baby care program at the hospital where she was born.

A. Outline the components of a newborn assessment during the first 2 hours after birth.

- Assessment needs to emphasize the newborn's adequate adjustment to extrauterine life with major focus on breathing, circulation, thermoregulation, and glucose regulation.
- Be sure to include the parents in the assessment process as a teaching-learning methodology, especially because they are participating in the mother-baby care program.

B. Describe the measures that a nurse should use to facilitate newborn respiration and adequate oxygenation during the first 2 hours after birth.

- Information related to how infants breathe and normal characteristics of breathing and how infants lose and generate heat and the impact of cold stress on breathing should be applied when formulating the answer.

- Maintain airway patency with appropriate suctioning to prevent blockage of airway, and position to facilitate chest expansion.
- Measures to stabilize and maintain a normal body temperature and prevent chilling include application of the methods of heat loss (conduction, convection, radiation, evaporation), assessment of temperature, and use of radiant heat shield/warmer.
- Parents should be instructed regarding measures used to facilitate breathing and maintaining body temperature so that they can use these measures in the home after discharge.

C. Since Melissa is staying with her mother in the same room, the nurse assesses and cares for Melissa while her parents are present. The same nurse also cares for Melissa's mother. What are the advantages of this approach to health care during the postpartum period?

- This approach facilitates teaching-learning process.
- Parents get to know their baby and practice care measures with supervision.
- Care is not fragmented; it avoids duplication of efforts and streamlines care, including health teaching.
- The nurse is able to observe progress of attachment and development of parenting skills; the need for referrals becomes more apparent.

D. Identify the most critical newborn assessment measures that Melissa's parents should learn before discharge. Give rationale for measures included.

- Emphasize breathing and airway patency, temperature/thermoregulation, skin color, feeding and elimination patterns, signs of fluid and nutritional adequacy, healing of cord including signs of infection, and symmetry and strength of movement.
- Parents should have demonstrations and a chance to redemonstrate newborn care skills such as bathing, diapering, cord care, and feeding.
- Parents should learn signs of common problems and who they should call to discuss concerns and report findings.

E. Melissa's parents ask the nurse what they should do to make sure that their home is a safe place for Melissa. What should the nurse tell them?

- Use principles of a safe environment for a newborn/infant to adapt home environment and care measures appropriately.
- Discuss developmental changes to expect and when and how to alter the environment to accommodate the new capabilities of their infant.
- Provide parents with safety-related literature and emergency phone numbers.
- Refer them to a first aid and CPR course for infants and children.

F. When Melissa is 26 hours old, signs of jaundice begin to appear. As the bilirubin level rises, the jaundice becomes more noticeable. Melissa's parents become more concerned when phototherapy (light) is initiated. They state that their friend recently died from liver cancer and his skin was very yellow toward the end of his life.

1) What is the basis for the jaundice exhibited by Melissa?
- Normal RBC destruction, immature liver function, and limited oral intake resulting in limited bowel elimination are the factors involved in physiologic jaundice, which occurs after the first 24 hours.

- **Be sure to emphasize the characteristics that distinguish physiologic from pathologic jaundice.**

2) What nursing measures are required for Melissa and her parents related to the phototherapy being administered?
   - **Care measures related to physiologic jaundice and phototherapy include skin exposure and care, temperature assessment and maintenance, protection of eyes, frequent feeding to stimulate bowel and maintain hydration, checking level of bilirubin, and providing time for parents to interact with their baby.**
   - **Care measures for parents include teaching about jaundice and phototherapy and supporting and keeping them informed about Melissa's progress.**

G. Melissa's parents ask the nurse if they should have their baby receive the hepatitis B vaccine before going home. How should the nurse respond?

   - **Immunizing newborns for hepatitis B is becoming increasingly popular and is safe; explain the impact of hepatitis B and the advantages of immunizations; discuss any side effects that could occur and how they will be handled; emphasize the need for two more injections to complete the series and ensure immunity.**
   - **This would be a good time to discuss other important immunizations, when they should be given, and where parents can go for this type of health care.**

H. Melissa is being breastfed. This is her mother's first experience with breastfeeding. She tells the nurse that she has read several books, watched some videos, and even attended a prenatal class about breastfeeding. Yet she appears anxious and tells the nurse, "Why am I so awkward and nervous now when I try to breastfeed Melissa? I worked so hard during pregnancy to get ready. Maybe this is not for me."

1) How should the nurse reply to this mother's comments?
   - **Even though she did a great job with the theoretic (cognitive) portion of learning, breastfeeding is a psychomotor skill that must be practiced in order for her to become proficient. Provide her with positive reinforcement and encourage her husband to do the same; be available to offer assistance as she breastfeeds.**

2) Melissa's mother has contacted a lactation consultant who will make a home visit within 2 days of discharge. What should the nurse emphasize during health teaching before discharge, considering that another nurse will follow-up in the home?
   - **Focus on the information required to ensure adequate hydration and safety of Melissa and to preserve nipple integrity of the mother.**
   - **Topics should include feeding readiness cues, basic process of latch-on, removal, maternal-infant positions, signs of adequate nutrition and feeding patterns, let-down reflex, nutrition and fluid intake, timing and frequency of feeding, waking a sleepy baby, and position after feeding.**

# CASE STUDY 8: WOMAN DIAGNOSED WITH PREECLAMPSIA

Beth is 36 years old and a recently divorced primigravida at 30 weeks' gestation. She is an active career woman who experiences a moderate to sometimes severe level of stress with her job. Her diet consists of a lot of fast foods to "save time," especially when she has to eat on the run or while working. Beth was diagnosed with mild preeclampsia. When the diagnosis is explained, she states that her mother and one of her sisters had a blood pressure problem when they were pregnant.

A. What is preeclampsia, and what are the expected clinical manifestations of this disorder?

- **Preeclampsia is a pregnancy-related, multisystem disorder associated with varying degrees of such clinical manifestations as hypertension, proteinuria, edema, CNS irritability, and hepatic involvement.**
- **Clinical manifestations—which occur and to what degree—are dependent upon the severity of the disorder in the individual woman.**

B. What risk factors for this disorder does Beth present?

- **Risk factors: Age > 35, unmarried (recently divorced), poor diet, stressful career, first pregnancy, and family history.**

C. Since her preeclampsia is mild at this point, Beth's health problem will be managed on an outpatient–home care basis. She is instructed to record her daily health status in a log or diary. What should the nurse tell Beth to include in her diary?

- **Items to include in the diary: BP, weight, protein in urine, daily fetal movement count, presence of any warning signs, and general feeling related to well-being and being able to cope with and implement the treatment regimen.**
- **The nurse must teach Beth each aspect of the health assessment, how to perform the assessment accurately, and how to interpret findings in terms of being expected or a sign of worsening preeclampsia.**
- **Beth must be informed about the importance of attending her prenatal appointments and who to call if signs of worsening preeclampsia are noted.**

D. Describe the major components of Beth's care management at home.

- **Components of home care: Daily self-assessment of health status, activity restriction, nutrition, and stress management.**
- **Beth will need strategies to cope with the sudden change in her lifestyle now that her career is on hold; members of her support group need to be identified and enlisted to help her; home care services may be required.**

E. State three priority nursing diagnoses related to Beth's health problem and its impact on her pregnancy and her lifestyle/career.

- **Nursing diagnoses should consider circulatory changes leading to altered tissue perfusion, anxiety level, interference with role performance, risk for maternal and fetal injury, and safety issues resulting from CNS irritability.**

F. Beth's condition advances to severe preeclampsia, and she is admitted to the hospital. A magnesium sulfate intravenous infusion is initiated.

1) State the expected outcome associated with this medication.
   - **Seizures do not occur or are controlled because magnesium sulfate acts as a central nervous system depressant and anticonvulsant.**

2) What is the recommended infusion rate?
   - **Loading dose of 4 to 6 g in 100 ml over 20 to 30 minutes then a maintenance infusion of 2 to 4 g/hour.**
   - **Keep in mind that protocols may vary from agency to agency and from physician to physician.**

3) What are the priority nursing assessments and frequency of assessments for Beth while she is receiving magnesium sulfate therapy?
   - **Components of assessment: CNS and respiratory function, renal function, maternal vital signs, intake and output, and FHR and pattern.**
   - **Expected effects and potential toxic effects should be the foundation for the assessment findings gathered and documented.**

4) Identify the signs that Beth would exhibit related to magnesium toxicity.
   - **CNS depression is the basis for the major toxic effects that occur as a result of magnesium therapy.**
   - **These effects include hyporeflexia (diminished or absent of DTRs), respiratory depression, and decreased LOC.**

5) What emergency measures should be implemented related to Beth's current health status?
   - **Seizure prevention and precaution measures, including padded side rails, decreased environmental stimuli, and immediate availability of emergency equipment such as oxygen and suctioning.**
   - **Bedside availability of calcium gluconate, which is the antidote for magnesium toxicity, will be administered IV.**

G. Beth begins to exhibit signs of the HELLP syndrome. What are the major dangers for which the nurse must be alert? State the basis for each danger.

   - **Dangers of the HELLP syndrome: Hemolysis (anemia), liver involvement (dysfunction, hematoma formation and rupture), low platelets/coagulopathy (excessive bleeding), abruptio placentae, fetal compromise, renal failure, pulmonary edema, and seizures.**

# CASE STUDY 9: WOMAN DIAGNOSED WITH RUPTURED ECTOPIC PREGNANCY, ENDOMETRIOSIS

Hillary, a 30-year-old woman with a history of endometriosis, is admitted to the emergency room, complaining of severe unilateral lower abdominal pain referred to her shoulder. She is accompanied by her husband John. Hillary is restless and apprehensive and states that she feels lightheaded. Her pulse is rapid, and she is slightly hypotensive. A small amount of vaginal bleeding is noted. To assist with diagnosis, a vaginal ultrasound and a pregnancy test are performed. A diagnosis of ruptured (tubal) ectopic pregnancy is made.

A. What factors may have placed Hillary at risk for ectopic pregnancy?

- **The incidence of ectopic pregnancy has been increasing as a result of a number of risk factors, especially reproductive tract infection; other risk factors include endometriosis, tubal/pelvic surgery, history of infertility, and use of IUD.**

B. Identify the major care management concern related to Hillary's diagnosis.

- **Major concern is hemorrhage—Hillary is exhibiting early signs of hemorrhagic/hypovolemic shock.**

C. State two priority nursing diagnoses for Hillary.

- **Nursing diagnoses: Consider fluid deficit, pain, risk for infection, and anticipatory grieving.**

D. Hillary is scheduled for surgery to remove the affected tube. Describe the preoperative and postoperative nursing care measures that Hillary will require.

- **Typical perioperative care measures including comprehensive, holistic assessment, physical care regarding preparation for surgery (e.g., catheter, IV, skin preparation) and care after surgery (e.g., pain control, prevention of complications, hydration and nutritional support, elimination, infection control) and emotional support should be discussed.**

E. Hillary and John are devastated by the diagnosis. They tell the nurse that they had been trying to have a baby for 2 years now and thought that they had succeeded, despite Hillary's problem with endometriosis. How could the nurse help this couple deal with their loss?

- **Apply the theory of the grief/bereavement process and the principles of effective nursing management to facilitate the process of grieving; keep in mind that this couple has already experienced difficulty achieving pregnancy and is likely to continue to have difficulty in the future.**
- **Make referrals to counseling and infertility care as appropriate.**

F. Before discharge, Hillary asks the nurse if her endometriosis had anything to do with her ectopic pregnancy. What should the nurse tell Hillary about endometriosis and its effect on fertility and pregnancy?

- **Explain to Hillary how the endometrial tissue implants in the pelvis and on pelvic organs, bleeds cyclically, and results in an inflammatory response; the implants and scarring/adhesions can pull, twist, and block the tubes.**

G. After Hillary's recovery, her primary health care provider places her on Synarel. This is the first time Hillary will be taking this medication. What should the nurse teach Hillary about this medication?

- **Synarel is a gonadotropin-releasing hormone (GnRH) agonist that is sprayed into the nostrils BID.**
- **Tell Hillary the actions of the drug (how it works), how to administer the medication for maximum effectiveness, when and who she should call if she has any concerns or notes side effects, and approximately how long she will need to continue this therapy.**

# CASE STUDY 10: PREGNANT WOMAN WITH PREGESTATIONAL DIABETES

Dana, a 23-year-old newly married woman, was diagnosed with diabetes when she was 16 years old. Her diabetes has been fairly stable for several years, although she occasionally experiences glucose control problems requiring reevaluation of her insulin dosage and diet. Dana and her husband are planning to become pregnant in about a year.

A. Explain why Dana and her husband Sam should seek preconception care as soon as possible.

- **Purpose of preconception are: Because optimal outcome of pregnancy hinges on maternal glycemic control, it is important that Dana's health be assessed and her diabetes be regulated in preparation for pregnancy; maternal and fetal/newborn risks and complications including congenital anomalies and worsening of maternal diabetic condition can be significantly reduced.**
- **Components of preconception care: This care addresses many issues regarding a healthy lifestyle and becoming physically, emotionally, and psychosocially ready for pregnancy and parenting. Males and females should participate in this care; the care includes holistic, comprehensive assessment and counseling and guidance to alter lifestyle and care for health problems, which, in this case, is diabetes.**

B. Identify the maternal and fetal/newborn risks and complications associated with pregestational diabetes, especially if glucose control is not maintained within an acceptable range. Discuss the basis for each risk and complication identified.

- **Maternal risks and complications: PIH, hydramnios, ketoacidosis, infection, hypoglycemia, and preterm labor and birth.**
- **Fetal/newborn risks and complications: Congenital anomalies, macrosomia, IUGR, RDS, hypoglycemia/hypocalcemia, and polycythemia/hyperbilirubinemia.**

C. One year later, Dana does become pregnant. She is now 4 weeks pregnant. Describe what Dana can expect regarding her insulin needs during pregnancy.

- **Emphasize that they are expected to change as a result of adaptations to pregnancy, usually decreasing during the first half of pregnancy and increasing during the second half of pregnancy.**
- **Inform her that she may be more prone to hypoglycemia (first half) and ketoacidosis (second half); review signs of each, measures to prevent, and actions to take if they occur.**
- **Emphasize importance of monitoring blood glucose levels and urine for ketones several times a day as instructed (e.g., ensure that insulin dosage and nutritional intake are appropriate).**

D. At her second prenatal visit, Dana's glycosylated hemoglobin was 5%. Explain what this finding indicates.

- **Reflects glucose control over time, with this finding indicating good control.**

E.  How should Dana's diet be modified to meet the requirements of pregnancy?

- **Nutritional requirements are increased using her prepregnancy diet as a foundation; increases should maintain acceptable blood glucose levels, achieve recommended weight gain, and prevent ketoacidosis; importance of a bedtime snack should be emphasized; a careful distribution of nutrients throughout the day should be planned; diet should reflect a balance of all nutrients.**

F.  Dana may experience increased stress as a result of the change in her diabetes associated with pregnancy. What measures could a nurse use to help prevent or reduce Dana's level of stress?

- **Full explanations of changes to expect and why they occur can reduce Dana's worry that something is wrong or that her diabetes is getting worse.**
- **Plan for more frequent prenatal visits, and provide a telephone contact to facilitate discussion of concerns.**
- **Encourage healthy lifestyle measures such as exercise, infection prevention, and relaxation measures to prevent complications from occurring that would further increase stress; involve Sam in helping her cope in a healthy manner and decrease her stress.**

G.  During the third trimester, Dana asks the nurse if she will be able to breastfeed her baby. What should the nurse tell Dana?

- **Breastfeeding is safe and could even facilitate glucose control during the postpartum period; care must be taken to carefully monitor blood glucose level and adjust caloric intake accordingly.**
- **Maintain integrity of the nipples because a woman with diabetes is more prone to infection.**

H.  After a successful, uncomplicated vaginal birth, Dana's primary health care provider advises her to avoid another pregnancy for at least 2 years. Dana plans to resume the use of a diaphragm as her method of contraception. What should the nurse emphasize regarding the use of this method?

- **Emphasize the need to have the diaphragm refitted when healing is complete at 6 weeks after birth.**
- **Review principles for effective use with special emphasis on measures to prevent infection.**
- **Discuss alternative methods, such as condoms with spermicide for contraception until the diaphragm can be refitted; encourage Dana and Sam to wait until Dana is healed because infection is a real concern with persons who have diabetes. Spermicide may be useful as a vaginal lubricant if Dana is breastfeeding because prolactin suppresses estrogen secretion and thereby decreases vaginal secretions.**

# CASE STUDY 11: PREGNANT WOMAN WITH A CLASS III CARDIAC DISORDER

Betsy is a 30-year-old pregnant woman at 4 weeks' gestation. She has been diagnosed with a Class III cardiac disorder for several years. Her cardiac condition has remained stable. Both she and her husband Jeff desperately want to have one child and are "willing to take a chance." They state that they will work together with each other and with the health care team to do all they can to ensure Betsy's safety and their baby's safety. Both Betsy and Jeff come from large, supportive families who are all available to "pitch in and help whenever they are needed."

A. What complications do Betsy and her fetus face as a result of her cardiac status?

- **Cardiac disease is a major cause of nonobstetric maternal mortality with cardiac decompensation and MI major concerns; spontaneous abortion, preterm labor and birth, and IUGR are also possible.**

B. Describe the factors that should be emphasized while assessing Betsy during each prenatal visit.

- **Holistic approach should be used to identify factors that can place stress on the heart, including those related to lifestyle and emotions.**
- **Physical examination emphasizes in-depth cardiopulmonary assessment. The couple should be fully informed of findings and taught about what to observe for when at home, including the effect that stress can have on cardiac function; include warning signs in teaching.**

C. Betsy is at high risk for cardiac decompensation. Identify the signs and symptoms that Betsy would exhibit and experience if cardiac decompensation was occurring.

- **Signs of cardiac decompensation: Increasing pulmonary edema with fatigue, dyspnea, crackles, and productive cough.**

D. What are the specific prenatal care management recommendations related to Betsy's Class III cardiac status?

- **Care management includes an emphasis on activity restriction, primarily bed rest, measures to reduce stress on the heart, infection prevention, and balanced nutrition for appropriate weight gain and prevention of anemia and constipation; ensure appropriate use of medications such as cardiac medications and anticoagulants.**
- **Mobilize family members and home care as needed; make referrals as appropriate.**

E. Describe the intrapartal care management recommendations related to Betsy's Class III cardiac status.

- **Care management during labor and birth should emphasize assessment for and prevention of cardiac decompensation by reducing stress on the heart—decrease anxiety and fear, recommend effective pain control with epidural anesthesia, position on her side to enhance cardiac output, facilitate birth with controlled open glottis pushing and appropriate use of forceps or vacuum extraction and episiotomy, and administer antibiotic prophylaxis.**

F. Betsy successfully gave birth to a baby girl at 36 weeks' gestation. She is at high risk for cardiac decompensation during the first 24 to 48 hours after birth. What prevention measures should be implemented?

- **Care management: Emphasize balance of rest and activity, stress reduction, appropriate nutrition, and supervised interaction with and care of the newborn; assist as needed with ADLs; avoid urinary retention and constipation; advise not to breastfeed and to consider sterilization, especially if cardiac decompensation occurred with this pregnancy.**
- **Organize home care and mobilize family; make needed referrals.**

210   Case Studies

# CASE STUDY 12: PREGNANT WOMAN AT RISK FOR PRETERM LABOR

Jane is a 24-year-old unmarried African-American multigravida (4-0-1-2-1). She is 15 weeks pregnant and has finally come to the women's health clinic for her first prenatal visit because she is afraid that she will have another premature baby. Her first two pregnancies resulted in spontaneous abortions at 13 and 14 weeks. Her third pregnancy resulted in the birth of her 4-year-old daughter at 30 weeks' gestation. Jane smokes one pack of cigarettes every 1 to 2 days. Her health history reveals that she has been hypertensive since age 20 and often experiences bladder infections. Her stress level has increased since her boyfriend, the father of the baby, has started to "pick fights with her and hit her." She cannot understand why he is doing this because he never hit her before when he would get angry.

A. What risk factors associated with preterm labor and birth does Jane's history reveal?

- **Risk factors for preterm labor and birth in this situation: Violence and stress in the partner relationship, race, unmarried status, history of two spontaneous second trimester abortions, preterm labor and birth with third pregnancy, hypertension, UTIs, limited prenatal care, and habit of smoking.**

B. The nurse managing Jane's care recognizes that violence has become part of Jane's relationship with her boyfriend.

1) Why can pregnancy precipitate violence in a relationship?
- **Battery during pregnancy can increase as a result of stress of the pregnancy and impending responsibility of parenting, jealousy of fetus, anger against the woman or the child, or a need to end the pregnancy; this violence increases the risk for LBW, poor maternal weight gain, infections, anemia, smoking, alcohol and drug use; inadequate prenatal care may occur.**

2) What does the nurse need to do to regarding the abuse described by Jane?
- **Consider legal and ethical issues regarding what to do with the knowledge of the abuse.**
- **Use appropriate communication techniques to further assess extent of abuse and the relationship between Jane and her boyfriend; use the ABCDES tool to help Jane deal with the situation effectively; consider community and health care services that may be helpful for Jane and also for her partner.**
- **Help Jane to develop a plan that she can follow if she and her daughter should face a dangerous situation with her boyfriend and need to "escape" for their safety.**

C. Jane elects to stay in her relationship for now because her boyfriend has agreed to try counseling to help him deal with his anger. What care management measures must be instituted to prevent preterm labor if possible or to detect it early if it should occur?

- **Use risk factors identified above to formulate a plan.**
- **Continue to monitor Jane's relationship with her partner, making sure that Jane knows about the cycle of violence, has a plan of action to provide for her and her daughter's safety if the battery continues, and has access to hotlines, shelters, and other support if she should be in need.**
- **Encourage her regular participation in prenatal care so that her condition can be monitored.**

- Use appropriate genital hygiene measures to prevent genitourinary tract infections.
- Empower Jane to stop smoking or at least reduce the amount to less than 10 each day.
- Encourage good nutrition to facilitate appropriate weight gain, maintain fluid balance, avoid dehydration, and balance rest and moderate activity.
- Teach about signs of preterm labor and what to do.

D. Jane asks the nurse about what signs to look for when preterm labor is occurring. "With my daughter, everything seemed to happen so fast without any warning." What should the nurse teach Jane about the signs of preterm labor and what to do if she detects them?

- Signs of labor are vague, necessitating knowledge of exactly what to observe for and how subtle the changes could be; teach Jane how to palpate her uterus for contractions, assess for fetal activity, and weigh herself accurately every day.
- If signs of labor appear, Jane should empty her bladder, drink 3 to 4 glasses of water, rest in bed on her side, and palpate for uterine contractions; if they continue, she should call for further instructions.

E. Jane goes into labor at 24 weeks' gestation. Conservative measures fail to suppress labor, necessitating admission to the hospital. Tocolytic therapy with magnesium sulfate is successful, and Jane is discharged to home care. A terbutaline pump is being used to keep labor suppressed, and home uterine monitoring has been arranged. How should the nurse prepare Jane for discharge?

- Health teaching should include terbutaline, its effects, care of the pump, and the site care and observation.
- Discuss and demonstrate the use of a home uterine monitor.
- Explain guidelines and rationale for bed rest, diet, and fluid intake, avoiding orgasm and nipple stimulation.
- Make referrals for home care and mobilize Jane's support system to help her and her daughter.

F. Identify the side effects of terbutaline.

- Side effects of terbutaline should be discussed with Jane, and the home care nurse should observe for them at every visit.

# CASE STUDY 13: PRETERM NEWBORN

Baby girl Laura is born at 32 weeks' gestation after attempts to suppress her mother's preterm labor fail. She is admitted to the neonatal intensive care unit (NICU) because of concern by health care providers for Laura's compromised respiratory function. Her parents are distraught, wondering what they could have done to cause this to happen to their baby. They become highly anxious when they see Laura and all the equipment surrounding her.

A. What clinical manifestations would indicate that Laura is experiencing respiratory distress?

- Effect of respiratory distress on rate, effort, pattern, and sound of respirations and on color of integument should be identified, including tachypnea, cyanosis, nasal flaring, sternal retractions, chin tugs, and grunting.

B. Since Laura is exhibiting some of the signs of respiratory distress, oxygen is administered via an oxygen hood. What guidelines should the nurse follow to ensure the safety and effectiveness of the oxygen administration?

- **Guidelines identified should include careful monitoring of oxygen administration equipment, infant's respiratory status, including characteristic of respirations, oxygen saturation, $PaO_2$, process of weaning, and parental support measures.**

C. Laura received artificial surfactant. State the rationale for this treatment approach.

- **Rationale relates to easing respiratory effort at the alveolar level; surfactant facilitates expansion of alveoli and prevents their collapse.**

D. What supportive measures should the nurse use to enhance Laura's respiratory effort?

- **Supportive measures: Maintain airway patency, prevent cold stress, position to enhance chest expansion, maintain nutritional intake because requirements are increased with stress, and use measures to calm infant and decrease the activity level.**

E. Because cold stress can lead to respiratory distress or make it worse if it is already present, nurses must implement measures to prevent or minimize temperature instability. Identify what these measures should include.

- **Prevention of cold stress: Use concepts of heat loss mechanisms—radiation, conduction, convection, and evaporation—to guide preventive measures implemented, and create a neutral thermal environment.**
- **Observe for signs of cold stress, and instruct parents about these signs and how measures being used will prevent cold stress from occurring.**

F. Laura's sucking is too weak to complete an oral feeding. The neonatologist orders intermittent gavage feedings. What guidelines should the nurse administering this type of feeding follow to ensure safety and maximum effectiveness?

- **Major steps in procedure: Process of insertion, checking placement and amount of residual gastric contents, flow rate of feeding, and removal.**
- **Assess effectiveness of feeding: Monitoring weight, fluid loss and gain, and elimination patterns.**
- **Assess for overfeeding: Measure amount of residual gastric contents before beginning a gavage feeding.**
- **Use nonnutritive sucking to enhance effectiveness.**

G. How could Laura's nurse help her parents cope with Laura's health status and her care requirements?

- **Be aware of what typical parents feel, how they respond and adjust, and the tasks that they must accomplish in order to cope with a preterm newborn.**
- **Supportive measures: Reassure them that preterm labor and birth often occurs with no definitive cause and that it is difficult in many cases to suppress preterm labor; orient them to Laura's environment, and explain all the procedures that are done and why. Help them to participate in her care and offer her comfort and appropriate stimulation. Keep them fully informed of Laura's progress; refer them to a support group if available or to parents of infants who have successfully "graduated from the NICU."**

# CASE STUDY 14: INFANT OF WOMAN WITH GESTATIONAL DIABETES

Baby girl Judy was born 1 hour ago. Her gestational age is confirmed to be 38 weeks, indicating that Judy's weight of 11 pounds reflects macrosomia and LGA status (large for gestational age). Judy's mother was diagnosed with gestational diabetes at 28 weeks' gestation. She had difficulty maintaining a stable blood glucose level.

A.  What health problems must the nurse be alert for when assessing Judy's physiologic status? Indicate the clinical manifestations of each health problem identified and its pathophysiologic basis.

- **Signs of birth trauma that can occur as a result of macrosomia, signs of RDS, hypoglycemia, hypocalcemia, and hyperbilirubinemia/polycythemia.**

B.  State three priority nursing diagnoses that reflect the most common health problems associated with infants of diabetic mothers.

- **Nursing diagnoses should reflect the health problems that can occur if an infant has a mother with gestational diabetes. Consider the risk for injury, altered nutrition: less than body requirements for glucose, impaired gas exchange, altered parenting, and parental anxiety.**

C.  Describe the recommended care measures to prevent and treat hypoglycemia when caring for Judy.

- **Measures related to hypoglycemia: Promote feeding, prevent chilling (cold stress), minimize stress, facilitate and support respiration, monitor blood glucose levels, and observe for signs of hypoglycemia.**

# Test Bank

## CHAPTER 1

### Contemporary Issues in Maternity and Women's Health Care

1-1 A woman has just learned that she is pregnant for the first time. She would like to have a midwife deliver her baby, but she is concerned about the safety of birth with a midwife as attendant. The nurse knows that her teaching is effective when the woman makes which of the following comments?
a. "I am glad to hear that research has found that midwifery care has as good an outcome as that of physicians."
b. "I am grateful to learn that I'd better go to an obstetrician if I want pain relief in labor."
c. "I did not know that midwives could only deliver women who are on Medicaid."
d. "I want a midwife because my husband can be with me during birth."

1-2 Managed care is gaining popularity. This rise in popularity is most often guided by which of the following considerations?
a. Concern for the quality of care
b. Means of controlling costs of care
c. Greater access to physicians
d. Allowance for early discharge

1-3 The role of the professional nurse has evolved to emphasize:
a. Providing direct care to clients at the bedside
b. Planning client care to cover longer hospital stays
c. Leading the activities of a team of interdisciplinary health care providers
d. Managing care to cure health problems once they have occurred

1-4 To assess for the risk of having a low-birth-weight (LBW) infant, which of the following factors is the most important for the nurse to consider?
a. African-American race
b. Cigarette smoking
c. Poor nutritional status
d. Limited maternal education

1-5 A 23-year-old African-American woman is pregnant with her first child. Based on the statistics related to infant mortality, which of the following plans is most important for the nurse to implement?
   a. Perform a nutrition assessment.
   b. Refer the woman to a social worker.
   c. Advise the woman to see an obstetrician and not a midwife.
   d. Explain to the woman the importance of keeping her prenatal care appointments.

1-6 The nurse will know that teaching to increase self-care is effective when the client makes which of the following comments?
   a. "I'll do whatever you say; you're the nurse."
   b. "I don't think I can quit smoking."
   c. "I exercise for 30 minutes 3 days a week."
   d. "What do you think I should do?"

1-7 A pregnant woman at 29 weeks' gestation has been diagnosed with preterm labor. Her labor is being controlled with tocolytic medications. She asks when she might be able to go home. Which of the following responses by the nurse is most accurate?
   a. "After the baby is born."
   b. "When we can arrange for a nurse to visit you at home."
   c. "Whenever the doctor says that it is okay."
   d. "It depends on what kind of insurance coverage you have."

1-8 When managing health care for pregnant women at a prenatal clinic, the nurse should recognize that the most significant barrier to access to care is the pregnant woman's:
   a. Age
   b. Minority status
   c. Educational level
   d. Inability to pay

1-9 What is the primary role of practicing nurses in the research process?
   a. Designing research studies
   b. Collecting data for other researchers
   c. Identifying researchable problems
   d. Seeking funding to support research studies

1-10 A pregnant couple's fetus has been diagnosed with anencephaly. They have learned that this condition is incompatible with life. They asked the nurse for advice on what they should do. Which of the following nursing plans is likely to be most therapeutic?
   a. Refer the couple to a genetic counselor
   b. Refer the couple to a minister
   c. Refer the couple to an ethics committee
   d. Refer the couple to their physician

1-11 When the nurse is unsure about how to perform a client care procedure, the nurse's best action would be to:
   a. Ask another nurse
   b. Discuss the procedure with the client's physician
   c. Look up the procedure in a nursing textbook
   d. Consult the agency procedure manual and follow the guidelines for the procedure

# CHAPTER 2

## The Family and Culture

2-1  A married couple lives in a single-family house with their newborn son and the husband's daughter from a previous marriage. Based on the information given, which of the following family forms best describes this family?
   a. Blended family
   b. Extended family
   c. Nuclear family
   d. Same-sex family

2-2  In which of the following family forms do families tend to be most socially vulnerable?
   a. Blended family
   b. Extended family
   c. Nuclear family
   d. Single-parent family

2-3  Health care functions that are carried out by families to meet its members' needs include:
   a. Developing family budgets
   b. Socialization of children
   c. Meeting nutritional requirements
   d. Teaching family members about birth control

2-4  Using family development theory as a base, which of the following family development tasks would you expect to see in a family where the husband and his wife have two young children and a newborn?
   a. Concentrating on their relationship with their best friends
   b. Making decisions on how they will help each other with household chores
   c. Actively assisting with the care of the wife's elderly mother
   d. Getting to know each other again as their young children start school

2-5  The criteria used for making decisions and problem solving within families is primarily based on family:
   a. Rituals and customs
   b. Values and attitudes
   c. Boundaries and channels
   d. Socialization processes

2-6  During your prenatal assessment of a family, you notice that a 22-year-old pregnant woman is accompanied by her mother. Using a systems perspective for assessment, you determine that this is a family with relatively closed boundaries. Based on this, you realize that the pregnant daughter will most readily accept prenatal advice from:
   a. Her mother
   b. Her friends
   c. The nurse
   d. The media

2-7 Using family stress theory as an intervention approach for working with families experiencing parenting, the nurse can help the family change internal context factors. These include:
a. Biologic and genetic makeup
b. Maturation of family members
c. The family's perception of the event
d. The prevailing cultural beliefs of society

2-8 While working in the prenatal clinic, you care for a very diverse group of clients. When planning interventions for these families, you realize that the acceptance of the interventions will be most influenced by the:
a. Educational achievement
b. Income level
c. Subcultural group
d. Individual beliefs

2-9 The nurse's care of a Hispanic family includes teaching about infant care. When developing a plan of care, the nurse bases interventions on the knowledge that in traditional Hispanic families:
a. Breastfeeding is encouraged immediately after birth
b. Circumcision is typically performed on male infants
c. The maternal grandmother will participate in the care of the mother and her infant
d. Special herbs mixed in water are used to stimulate the passage of meconium

2-10 You are working in the prenatal clinic of a large urban center where the clients represent a variety of cultural backgrounds. You note that clients are frequently late for their appointments. You learn that this may be a factor of culture. Which of the following time orientations best describes these individuals?
a. Future
b. Present
c. Past
d. Transition

# CHAPTER 3

## Community and Home Care

3-1 The perinatal continuum of care begins with:
a. Diagnosis of pregnancy
b. The period of time just before birth
c. Identification of a pregnant woman as high risk
d. Family planning and preconception care

3-2 A statistic widely used to compare the health status of different populations would be:
a. Incidence of specific infections such as AIDS and TB
b. Infant mortality rate
c. Maternal mortality rate
d. Incidence of low-birth-weight infants

3-3 Which of the following health care services represents the primary level of prevention?
   a. Immunizations
   b. Breast self-examination
   c. Home care for high risk pregnancies
   d. Blood pressure screening

3-4 What is the primary difference between hospital care and home health care?
   a. Home care is routinely delivered continuously by professional staff.
   b. Home care is delivered on an intermittent basis by professional staff.
   c. Home care is delivered for emergency conditions.
   d. Home care is not available 24 hours a day.

3-5 Which of the following statements is inaccurate regarding effective teaching plans?
   a. Verbal instructions can be reinforced with written materials.
   b. Plans are coordinated with hospital and home care providers to avoid duplication.
   c. Plans are based on the nurse's perceptions of what constitutes essential information.
   d. Plans can prevent the woman from getting conflicting information from different care providers.

3-6 Which of the following situations would be considered safe when encountered by the nurse who is making a home visit?
   a. A group of teens are sitting on the stairs in front of the client's apartment.
   b. Parking is three blocks away from the client's house because there is no space in front of the house.
   c. The family dog is on a chain in the front yard.
   d. The door of the home is open when the nurse arrives.

3-7 The woman's family members are present when the nurse arrives for a postpartum and newborn visit. What should the nurse do?
   a. Observe interactions of family members with the newborn and each other.
   b. Ask the woman to meet with her and the baby alone.
   c. Do a brief assessment on all family members present.
   d. Reschedule the visit for another time so that the mother and infant can be assessed privately.

3-8 Which of the following is a limitation of a home postpartum visit?
   a. Ability to teach is limited by the presence of many distractions.
   b. Identified problems cannot be resolved in the home setting.
   c. Necessary items for infant care are not available.
   d. Visits between families may require traveling a great distance.

3-9 A breastfeeding mother who is concerned that her baby is not getting enough to eat would find which of the following resources most helpful and most cost-effective on the day after discharge?
   a. Visiting a pediatric screening clinic at the hospital
   b. Placing a call to the hospital nursery "warm line"
   c. Calling the pediatrician for a lactation consult referral
   d. Requesting a home visit

3-10 Which of the following areas within the home environment would be appropriate to include in a physical assessment of the home?
    a. Stove, refrigerator, sink, countertops, inside china cabinet drawers
    b. Baby's bed, changing table, baby's clothes, inside diaper bag, inside keepsake box
    c. Bedroom closets, inside jewelry boxes, under beds
    d. Electrical wall outlets, telephones, bathroom sink and faucets, inside the bathtub

3-11 Which of the following personal safety precautions should guide the nurse working in home care?
    a. Do not carry personal items such as extra car keys or a cellular phone.
    b. Avoid making a visit with another nurse.
    c. Schedule visits during daylight hours.
    d. Never wear a name tag.

# CHAPTER 4

## Alternative and Complementary Therapies

4-1 Alternative and complementary therapies:
    a. Replace standard or allopathic medicine
    b. Involve interaction of body within the environment
    c. Are especially beneficial in the care of clients with chronic illnesses
    d. Are more expensive than standard medicine, especially if used for health maintenance

4-2 Many alternative and complementary therapies share which of the following concepts?
    a. The use of herbs is a cornerstone of good health.
    b. Clients are capable of decision making and should be a part of the health care team.
    c. Touch should be used to relieve pain and reduce anxiety.
    d. Clients should place the responsibility for their health and healing in the hands of alternative healers.

4-3 A client is learning to relax and consciously control his breathing to improve his asthma. Specially designed electronic equipment is monitoring his progress. This alternative therapy is called:
    a. Guided imagery
    b. Energetic healing
    c. Reflection
    d. Biofeedback

4-4 A woman experiences dysmenorrhea. The nurse could recommend which of the following as an effective alternative to nonsteroidal antiinflammatory agents?
    a. Increasing intake of milk and dairy products
    b. Taking vitamins A and D daily
    c. Using guided imagery
    d. Taking feverfew supplements

4-5 St.-John's-wort can be used to reduce:
a. Migraine headaches
b. Hot flashes
c. Anxiety
d. Heavy menstrual flow

# CHAPTER 5

## Health Promotion and Prevention

5-1 The abuse of which of the following substances is the leading cause of mental retardation in the United States?
a. Alcohol
b. Tobacco
c. Marijuana
d. Heroin

5-2 _____ is a powerful central nervous system stimulant that can lead to spontaneous abortion, preterm labor, premature separation of the placenta, and stillbirth.
a. Heroin
b. Alcohol
c. PCP
d. Cocaine

5-3 _____ abuse during pregnancy causes vasoconstriction and decreased placental perfusion resulting in maternal and neonatal complications.
a. Alcohol
b. Caffeine
c. Tobacco
d. Chocolate

5-4 During her annual gynecologic check-up, a 17-year-old woman states that recently she has been experiencing cramping and pain during her menstrual periods. The nurse would document this complaint as:
a. Amenorrhea
b. Dysmenorrhea
c. Dyspareunia
d. Premenstrual syndrome

5-5 One purpose of preconception care is to:
a. Make sure pregnancy complications do not occur
b. Identify women who should not get pregnant
c. Encourage healthy lifestyles
d. Make sure women know about prenatal care

5-6 A woman with insulin-dependent diabetes plans to try to get pregnant in approximately 6 months. She sought the advice of her nurse-midwife on how to improve her chances of having a healthy baby and uneventful pregnancy. Which of the following plans by the midwife is most effective?

a. "Just keep taking your insulin as your doctor prescribed."

b. "Maintain your blood sugar at a constant range within normal limits."

c. "There is really nothing you can do to change the outcome of pregnancy when you are a diabetic who uses insulin."

d. "Maintain a daily caloric intake of 2000 kcal or less per day, and increase your insulin by 5 units."

5-7 A woman who has come to the clinic for preconception counseling because she wants to start trying to get pregnant in 3 months can expect the following advice:

a. "Discontinue all contraception now."

b. "Lose weight so that you can gain more during pregnancy."

c. "You may take any medications that you have been taking regularly."

d. "Make sure you include adequate folic acid in your diet."

# CHAPTER 6

## Assessment of Women

6-1 The two primary functions of the ovary are:

a. Normal female development and sex hormone release

b. Ovulation and internal pelvic support

c. Sexual response and ovulation

d. Ovulation and hormone production

6-2 The uterus is a muscular, pear-shaped organ that is responsible for:

a. Cyclic menstruation

b. Sex hormone production

c. Fertilization

d. Sexual arousal

6-3 The unique pattern of muscle fibers makes the uterine myometrium ideally suited for:

a. Menstruation

b. Labor

c. Hemostasis

d. Fertilization

6-4 The hormone responsible for the maturation of mammary gland tissue is:

a. Estrogen

b. Testosterone

c. Prolactin

d. Progesterone

6-5 Because of the effect of cyclic ovarian changes on the breast, the best time for breast self-examination is:
   a. 6 to 7 days after menses cease
   b. Day 1 of the endometrial cycle
   c. Mid-menstrual cycle
   d. Any time

6-6 Menstruation is periodic uterine bleeding:
   a. That occurs every 28 days
   b. In which the entire uterine lining is shed
   c. That is regulated by ovarian hormones
   d. That leads to fertilization

6-7 Individual irregularities in the menstrual cycle are most often caused by:
   a. Variations in the follicular (preovulatory) phase
   b. An intact hypothalamic-pituitary feedback mechanism
   c. A functioning corpus luteum
   d. A prolonged ischemic phase

6-8 Prostaglandins are produced in most organs of the body but are found in the highest concentration in the:
   a. Ovaries
   b. Fallopian tubes
   c. Endometrium
   d. Vagina

6-9 Physiologically, sexual response can be characterized by:
   a. Coitus, masturbation, and fantasy
   b. Myotonia and vasocongestion
   c. Erection and orgasm
   d. Excitement, plateau, and orgasm

6-10 Passive immunity can occur when:
   a. Infants receive immunizations
   b. Antibodies are transferred from the mother to the newborn through colostrum
   c. A person has the infectious disease itself, for example, rubella
   d. A person receives a booster vaccination

6-11 Before beginning the health history interview, the nurse should:
   a. Smile and ask the client if she has any special concerns
   b. Speak in a relaxed manner, with an even, nonjudgmental tone
   c. Make the client comfortable
   d. Tell the client that the information she provides is considered confidential

6-12 The nurse guides a woman to the examination room and asks her to remove her clothes and put on an examination gown with the front open. The woman states, "I have special undergarments that I do not remove for religious reasons." The most appropriate response from the nurse would be:

a. "You cannot have an examination without removing all your clothes."
b. "I will ask the doctor to modify the examination."
c. "Tell me about your undergarments. I will explain the examination procedure, and then we can discuss how you can have your examination comfortably."
d. "What? I have never heard of such a thing! That sounds unbelievable."

6-13 A 62-year-old woman has not been to the clinic for an annual examination for 5 years. The recent death of her husband has reminded her that she should come for a visit. Her family doctor has retired, and she is going to see the woman's health nurse-practitioner for her visit. To facilitate a positive health care experience, the nurse should:

a. Remind the woman that she is long overdue for her examination and that she should come in annually
b. Listen carefully and allow for extra time for this woman's health history interview
c. Reassure this woman that a nurse-practitioner is just as good as her old doctor
d. Encourage the woman to talk about the death of her husband and her fears surrounding her own death

6-14 A blind woman has arrived for an examination. Her guide dog assists her to the examination room. She appears nervous and says, "I have never had a pelvic examination." The nurse's most appropriate response would be:

a. "Do not worry. It will be over before you know it."
b. "Try to relax. I will be very gentle and will not hurt you."
c. "Your anxiety is common. I was anxious when I first had a pelvic examination."
d. "I will let you touch each item that I will use during the examination as I tell you how it will be used."

6-15 During a health history interview, a woman tells the nurse that her husband physically abuses her. The nurse's first response should be to:

a. Advise the woman of state reporting laws pertaining to abuse and confidentiality
b. Reassure the woman that the abuse is not her fault
c. Give the woman referrals to local agencies and shelters where she can obtain help
d. Formulate an escape plan for the woman that she can use the next time her husband abuses her

6-16 During a health history interview, a woman states that she thinks that she has "bumps" on her labia. She also states that she is not sure how to check herself. The correct response would be to:

a. Reassure the woman that the examination will reveal any problems
b. Explain to the woman the process of vulvar self-examination and reassure her that she should become familiar with normal and abnormal findings during the examination
c. Reassure the woman that "bumps" can be treated
d. Reassure her that most women have "bumps" on their labia

6-17 A woman arrives at the clinic for her annual examination. She tells the nurse that she thinks that she has a vaginal infection and she has been using an over-the-counter cream for the past 2 days to treat the infection. The nurse's initial response should be to:

a. Inform the woman that vaginal cream may interfere with the Pap test for which she is scheduled

b. Reassure the woman that using vaginal cream is not a problem for the examination

c. Ask the woman to describe the symptoms that indicate to her that she has a vaginal infection

d. Ask the woman to reschedule the appointment for the examination

6-18 At a routine annual examination, a woman states, "I never check my breasts. I feel so anxious about doing it correctly." The nurse's most appropriate response would be:

a. "There is no need for you to be anxious. Of course you are doing it correctly."

b. "Let me remind you how to examine your breasts, and then you can practice while I observe how you do."

c. "Tell me about your anxiety; maybe I can help."

d. "You should check your breasts once a month, just after your menses begins."

# CHAPTER 7

## Common Reproductive Concerns

7-1 Hypogonadotropic amenorrhea is least likely to be caused by:

a. Oral contraceptives

b. Rapid weight loss

c. Strenuous exercise

d. Stress

7-2 When counseling a woman for primary dysmenorrhea, which of the following nonpharmacologic interventions would be used?

a. Increasing intake of red meat and simple carbohydrates

b. Reducing intake of diuretic foods such as peaches and asparagus

c. Temporarily substituting sedentary activity for physical activity, including exercise

d. Using a heating pad on the abdomen to relieve cramping

7-3 Which of the following symptoms described by a woman is characteristic of premenstrual syndrome (PMS)?

a. "I feel irritable and moody a week before my period is supposed to start."

b. "I have lower abdominal pain beginning the third day of my menstrual period."

c. "I have nausea and headaches after my period starts, and they last 2 to 3 days."

d. "I experience abdominal bloating and breast pain at the onset of my period."

7-4 A woman complains of severe abdominal and pelvic pain around the time of menstruation that has gotten worse over the last 5 years. She also complains of pain during intercourse and has tried unsuccessfully to get pregnant for the past 18 months. These symptoms are most likely related to:
a. Endometriosis
b. PMS
c. Primary dysmenorrhea
d. Secondary dysmenorrhea

7-5 Nafarelin is currently used as a treatment for mild to severe endometriosis. The nurse should tell the woman being treated that this medication:
a. Stimulates the secretion of gonadotrophic-releasing hormone, therefore stimulating ovarian activity
b. Should be sprayed into one nostril every other day
c. Should be injected into her subcutaneous tissue BID
d. Can cause her to experience some hot flashes and vaginal dryness

7-6 While interviewing a 31-year-old woman before her routine gynecologic examination, the nurse collects data about her recent menstrual cycles. The nurse should collect additional information about which of these areas?
a. Her menstrual flow lasts 5 to 6 days.
b. She describes her flow as heavy.
c. She reports a small amount of spotting midway between her periods.
d. The length of her menstrual cycle varies from 26 to 29 days.

7-7 Nurses who provide health care for women should recognize that the most commonly reported gynecologic problem for women of any age group is:
a. Dysmenorrhea
b. Menorrhagia
c. Dyspareunia
d. Endometriosis

7-8 Amenorrhea is most commonly a result of:
a. Stress
b. Excessive exercise
c. Pregnancy
d. Eating disorders

7-9 A 36-year-old woman has been diagnosed as having uterine fibroids. When planning care for this client the nurse should know that:
a. Fibroids are malignant tumors of the uterus requiring radiation or chemotherapy
b. Fibroids will increase in size during the perimenopausal period
c. Menorrhagia is a common finding, necessitating assessment for signs of anemia
d. The woman is unlikely to become pregnant as long as the fibroids are in her uterus

7-10 When assessing a woman for menopausal discomforts, the nurse would expect the woman to describe the most frequently reported discomforts, which would be:
a. Headaches
b. Hot flashes
c. Mood swings
d. Vaginal dryness with dyspareunia

7-11 Which of the following is a risk factor for osteoporosis?
a. African-American race
b. Low protein intake
c. Obesity
d. Cigarette smoking

7-12 When teaching perimenopausal women about estrogen replacement therapy, the nurse would include the risks of:
a. Cervical cancer
b. Endometrial cancer
c. Osteoporosis
d. Atherosclerosis

# CHAPTER 8

## Sexually Transmitted Diseases and Other Infections

8-1 The two primary areas of risk for sexually transmitted diseases are:
a. Sexual orientation and socioeconomic status
b. Age and educational level
c. Large numbers of sexual partners and race
d. Sexual behaviors and inadequate preventive health behaviors

8-2 The most common perinatal complications associated with bacterial sexually transmitted diseases are:
a. Preterm labor and low birth weight
b. Newborn eye infections and low Apgar scores
c. Nausea, vomiting, and frequent urinary tract infections
d. Congenital anomalies and infertility

8-3 The most common bacterial sexually transmitted infection is:
a. Gonorrhea
b. Syphilis
c. Chlamydia
d. Candidiasis

8-4 The viral sexually transmitted disease affecting the most people in the United States today is:
a. Herpes simplex virus-2 (HSV-2)
b. Human papillomavirus (HPV)
c. Human immunodeficiency virus (HIV)
d. Cytomegalovirus (CMV)

8-5 The CDC recommends that human papillomavirus be treated with:
   a. Miconazole ointment
   b. Topical application of podofilox 0.5% solution or gel
   c. Penicillin intramuscularly for two doses
   d. Metronidazole by mouth

8-6 A woman exhibits a thick, white, lumpy, cottage cheese–like discharge with patches on her labia and in her vagina. She complains of intense pruritus. The nurse-practitioner could order which of the following preparations for treatment?
   a. Fluconazole
   b. Tetracycline
   c. Metronidazole
   d. Acyclovir

8-7 Once HIV enters the body, seroconversion to HIV positivity usually occurs within:
   a. 6 to 10 days
   b. 2 to 4 weeks
   c. 6 to 12 weeks
   d. 6 months

8-8 Human immunodeficiency virus (HIV) may be perinatally transmitted:
   a. Only in the third trimester from the maternal circulation
   b. By a needlestick injury at birth with contaminated instruments
   c. Only through the ingestion of amniotic fluid
   d. Through the ingestion of breast milk from an infected mother

8-9 Health care workers are at greatest risk of being infected with:
   a. Hepatitis A virus
   b. Human immunodeficiency virus
   c. Hepatitis B virus
   d. Cytomegalovirus

8-10 Care management of a woman diagnosed with acute pelvic inflammatory disease would most likely include which of the following?
   a. Oral antibiotic therapy
   b. Bed rest in a semi-Fowler's position
   c. Antibiotic regimen continued until symptoms subside
   d. Frequent pelvic examination to monitor progress of healing

8-11 Upon vaginal examination of a 30-year-old woman, the nurse documents the following findings: profuse, thin grayish-white vaginal discharge with a "fishy" odor; complains of pruritus. Based on these findings, the nurse suspects that this woman has:
   a. Bacterial vaginosis
   b. Candidiasis
   c. Trichomoniasis
   d. Gonorrhea

8-12 The recommended treatment for the prevention of HIV transmission to the fetus during pregnancy is:
   a. Acyclovir
   b. Ofloxacin
   c. Podophyllin
   d. Zidovudine

# CHAPTER 9

## Contraception and Abortion

9-1 A woman has chosen the calendar method of conception control. During the assessment process, it is most important that the nurse:
   a. Obtain a history of menstrual cycle lengths for the last 6 to 12 months
   b. Determine her weight loss and gain pattern for the previous year
   c. Examine skin pigmentation and hair texture for hormonal changes
   d. Explore her previous experiences with conception control

9-2 A woman is using the basal body temperature method of contraception. She calls the clinic and tells the nurse, "My period is due in a few days and my temperature has not gone up." The nurse's most appropriate response would be:
   a. "This probably means you are pregnant."
   b. "Don't worry; it is probably nothing."
   c. "Have you been sick this month?"
   d. "You probably did not ovulate during this cycle."

9-3 A married couple is discussing alternatives for pregnancy prevention and has asked about the fertility awareness method. The nurse's most appropriate reply is:
   a. "It is not very effective, and it is very likely that you will get pregnant."
   b. "It can be effective for many couples, but it requires motivation."
   c. "There are few advantages to this method and several health risks."
   d. "You would be much safer going on the pill and not having to worry."

9-4 A woman has been using a vaginal foam spermicide for pregnancy prevention since she gave birth 3 months ago. She tells you that lately her partner "feels less down there during sex." You are concerned that this may be:
   a. Evidence of a postpartum marital problem
   b. Related to her alterations in body image
   c. Associated with the use of a vaginal spermicide
   d. Indicative of the need for STD evaluation

9-5 A male client asks the nurse why it is better to purchase condoms that are lubricated with nonoxynol-9. The nurse's most appropriate response is:
   a. "The lubricant prevents vaginal irritation."
   b. "Nonoxynol-9 provides some protection against STDs."
   c. "The additional lubrication improves sex."
   d. "Nonoxynol-9 improves penile sensitivity."

9-6  A woman who has a seizure disorder and takes barbiturates and phenytoin sodium daily asks the nurse about the pill as a contraceptive choice. The nurse's most appropriate response would be:
  a. "This is a highly effective method, but it has some side effects."
  b. "Your current medications will decrease the effectiveness of the pill."
  c. "The pill will decrease the effectiveness of your seizure medication."
  d. "This is a good choice for your age and personal history."

9-7  A woman who has just undergone a first trimester abortion will be using oral contraceptives. To be protected from pregnancy, she should be advised to:
  a. Avoid sexual contact for at least 10 days after starting the pill
  b. Use condoms and foam for the first few weeks as backup
  c. Use another method of contraception for one full cycle on the pill
  d. Begin sexual relations once vaginal bleeding has ended

9-8  Injectable progestins (DMPA, Depo-Provera) are a good contraceptive choice for women who:
  a. Desire menstrual regularity and predictability
  b. Have a history of thrombotic problems or breast cancer
  c. Have difficulty remembering to take oral contraceptives daily
  d. Are homeless or mobile and rarely receive health care

9-9  A woman currently uses a diaphragm and spermicide for contraception. She asks the nurse what the major differences are between the cervical cap and diaphragm. The nurse's most appropriate response would be:
  a. "No spermicide is used with the cervical cap, so it is less messy."
  b. "The diaphragm can be left in place longer after intercourse."
  c. "Repeated intercourse with the diaphragm is more convenient."
  d. "The cervical cap can safely be inserted several hours before intercourse without adding more spermicide later."

9-10  A woman was recently treated for toxic shock syndrome. She has intercourse occasionally and uses over-the-counter protection. Based on her history, what contraceptive method should she and her partner avoid?
  a. Cervical cap
  b. Condom
  c. Vaginal film
  d. Vaginal sheath

9-11  Postcoital contraception with Ovral:
  a. Requires that the first dose be taken within 72 hours of unprotected intercourse
  b. Requires that the woman take a second and third dose at 24 and 36 hours after the first dose
  c. Has an effectiveness rate in preventing pregnancy of approximately 50%
  d. Is commonly associated with the side effect of menorrhagia

9-12 An unmarried young woman describes her sex life as "active" with "many" partners. She wants a contraceptive method that is reliable and does not interfere with sex. She requests an intrauterine device (IUD). The nurse's most appropriate response would be:
a. "The IUD does not interfere with sex."
b. "The risk of pelvic inflammatory disease (PID) is higher for you."
c. "The IUD will protect you from STDs."
d. "Pregnancy rates are high with the IUD."

9-13 A married couple is discussing male and female sterilization with the nurse. Which of the following statements is most appropriate for the nurse to make?
a. "Male and female sterilization methods are 100% effective."
b. "A vasectomy may have a slight effect on sexual performance."
c. "Tubal ligation can be easily reversed if you change your mind in the future."
d. "Major complications after sterilization are rare."

9-14 A 26-year-old woman is scheduled for a first trimester abortion in the morning. A Laminaria tent is inserted as part of the vacuum aspiration procedure. The nurse explains to the woman that Laminaria is used to:
a. Stimulate the uterus to contract
b. Prevent postabortion infection
c. Reduce pain by numbing the cervix
d. Dilate the cervix for easier insertion of the aspirator

9-15 A woman is 16 weeks pregnant and has elected to terminate her pregnancy. The nurse knows that the most common technique used for the medical termination of a pregnancy in the second trimester would be:
a. Administration of prostaglandins
b. Instillation of hypertonic saline into the uterine cavity
c. Intravenous administration of Pitocin
d. Vacuum aspiration

# CHAPTER 10

## Infertility

10-1 Which of the following tests used to diagnose the basis of infertility is done during the luteal or secretory phase of the menstrual cycle?
a. Hysterosalpingogram
b. Endometrial biopsy
c. Laparoscopy
d. FSH level

10-2 A physician prescribes clomiphene citrate (Clomid, Serophene) for a woman experiencing infertility. She is very concerned about the risk for multiple births. The nurse's most appropriate response is:

a. "This is a legitimate concern. Would you like to discuss this further before your treatment begins?"

b. "No one has ever had more than triplets with Clomid."

c. "Ovulation will be monitored with ultrasound so that this will not happen."

d. "Ten percent is a very low risk, so you do not need to worry too much."

10-3 A man smokes two packs of cigarettes a day. He wants to know if smoking is contributing to the difficulty that he and his wife are having with getting pregnant. The nurse's most appropriate response is:

a. "Your sperm count seems to be okay in the first semen analysis."

b. "Only marijuana cigarettes affect sperm count."

c. "Smoking can give you lung cancer, even though it has no effect on sperm."

d. "Smoking can decrease the quality of your sperm."

10-4 A couple is present for an infertility work-up, having attempted to get pregnant for 2 years. The woman, age 37, has always had irregular menstrual cycles but is otherwise healthy. The man has fathered two children from a previous marriage and had a vasectomy reversal 2 years ago. The man has had two normal semen analyses, but the sperm seem to be clumped together. What additional test is needed?

a. Testicular biopsy

b. Anti-sperm antibodies

c. FSH level

d. Examination for testicular infection

10-5 A couple is trying to cope with an infertility problem and wants to know what they can do to preserve their emotional equilibrium. The nurse's most appropriate response is:

a. "Tell your friends and family so that they can help you."

b. "Talk only to other friends who are infertile since only they can help."

c. "Get involved with a support group. I will give you some names."

d. "Start adoption proceedings immediately, since obtaining an infant is very difficult."

10-6 Bromocriptine (Parlodel) may be prescribed for an infertile woman if she has:

a. Thyroid dysfunction

b. Elevated levels of prolactin

c. Inadequate levels of follicle-stimulating hormone

d. Acidic cervical mucus

10-7 An infertile woman will begin pharmacologic treatment. As part of the regimen, she will be taking purified FSH (Metrodin). The nurse will instruct her that this medication is administered in the form of a(n):

a. Intranasal spray

b. Vaginal suppository

c. Intramuscular injection

d. Tablet

# CHAPTER 11

## Violence Against Women

11-1 The justification for the victimization of women very early in history was that:
   a. Women were regarded as possessions
   b. Women were the "weaker sex"
   c. Control of women was necessary for protection
   d. Women were created subordinate to men

11-2 The primary theme of the feminist perspective on violence against women recognizes the:
   a. Role of testosterone as the underlying cause of men's violent behavior
   b. Basic human instinctual drive toward aggression
   c. Dominance and coercive control over women by men
   d. Cultural norm of violence in Western society

11-3 The nurse suspects that a client who comes to the maternity clinic for a pregnancy test is in an abusive relationship. The nurse includes the abuse assessment screen as part of the assessment. Although the woman was very emotional and hesitant in responding to the questions, verbally she denied abuse as being a problem. While waiting for the results of the pregnancy test, the nurse decides to teach the client about partner abuse anyway. Rationale for the nurse's decision is that all women should be informed about:
   a. The nurse's ethical responsibility to protect clients
   b. The cycle of violence, indicating that it continues and escalates over time once it begins
   c. Women's legal rights not to be controlled by men
   d. The masochistic nature of women who stay in abusive relationships

11-4 In assessing a woman for potential abuse, the nurse directly asks the woman if someone is harming her. Since denial is often a defense for women in abusive relationships, which of the following information communicated by the nurse would be conducive to the woman's disclosure?
   a. The woman's situation is not unique, and the bruises and injuries that she has are very common in women who have been abused.
   b. X-rays show an old fracture of her upper arm, which is atypical in women.
   c. The nurse is aware of the build and size of the woman's husband, against whom she would not have a chance in a physical battle.
   d. The nurse is aware that the woman seems very unhappy about news of her pregnancy.

11-5 The primary responsibility of the nurse who suspects or confirms any type of violence against a woman is to:
   a. Report the incident to legal authorities
   b. Provide information to social services
   c. Call a client advocate who can assist in the client's decision making about what action to take
   d. Document the incident (or findings) accurately and concisely in the client's record

11-6 The nurse's best measure when evaluating the care of a woman in an abusive situation is based on the:
- a. Woman's decision to leave her partner
- b. Woman's declaration of a safety plan
- c. Couple's follow-through on a referral for counseling
- d. Woman's gratitude to the nurse for the helpful information

11-7 Intervention for the sexual abuse survivor is often not attempted by maternity and women's health nurses because of the concern about increasing the distress of the woman and the lack of expertise in counseling. Which of the following initial interventions is appropriate and most important in facilitating the woman's care?
- a. Initiating a referral to an expert counselor
- b. Setting limits on what the client discloses
- c. Listening and encouraging therapeutic communication skills
- d. Acknowledging the nurse's discomfort to the client as an expression of empathy

11-8 Sexual assault is:
- a. Limited to rape
- b. An act of force in which unwanted and uncomfortable sexual acts occur
- c. A legal term for sexual violence
- d. An act of violence in which the partner is unknown

11-9 A young woman arrives at the emergency department and states that she "thinks" she has been raped. She is sobbing extensively and expresses disbelief that this could happen because the man was her "best friend." In an effort to calm the client to do a thorough assessment and physical examination, the nurse acknowledges her fear and anxiety and tells the woman:
- a. "Rape is not limited to strangers and frequently occurs by someone who is known to the victim."
- b. "I would be very upset if my best friend did that to me; that is very unusual."
- c. "You must feel very betrayed. In what way do you think you might have been seductive?"
- d. "Some friend! I hope you will report this incident to the police."

11-10 The nurse's best measure of evaluating care of a rape victim is that:
- a. All legal evidence is preserved during the physical examination
- b. The victim appreciates the legal information but decides not to pursue legal proceedings
- c. The victim states that she is going to advocate against sexual violence
- d. The victim leaves the health care facility without feeling revictimized

# CHAPTER 12

## Problems of the Breast

12-1 Fibrocystic change in breasts is:
- a. A disease of the milk ducts and glands in the breasts
- b. A premalignant disorder characterized by lumps found in the breast tissue
- c. Lumpiness found in varying degrees in breast tissue of healthy women during menstrual cycles
- d. Lumpiness accompanied by tenderness after menses

12-2 The nurse who is teaching a group of women about breast cancer would tell the women that:
   a. Risk factors identify more than 50% of women who will develop breast cancer
   b. Nearly 90% of lumps found by women are malignant
   c. One in ten women in the United States will develop breast cancer in her lifetime
   d. The exact cause of breast cancer is unknown

12-3 Which of the following diagnostic tests is used to confirm a suspected diagnosis of breast cancer?
   a. Mammogram
   b. Ultrasound
   c. Fine-needle aspiration (FNA)
   d. CA 15-3

12-4 A healthy 60-year-old African-American woman regularly receives her health care at the clinic in her neighborhood. She is due for a mammogram. At her first clinic visit, her physician, concerned about the 3-week wait at the neighborhood clinic, made an appointment for her to have a mammogram at a teaching hospital across town. She did not go to the appointment and returned to the clinic today to have the nurse check her blood pressure. What would be the most appropriate thing for the nurse to say to this client?
   a. "Do you have transportation to the teaching hospital so that you can get your mammogram?"
   b. "I am concerned that you missed your appointment; let me make you another one."
   c. "It is very dangerous to skip your mammograms; your breasts need to be checked."
   d. "Would you like for me to make an appointment for you to have your mammogram here?"

12-5 A client's oncologist has just finished explaining the diagnostic work-up results to her, and she still has questions. The woman states, "The doctor says I have a slow-growing cancer. Very few cells are dividing. How does she know this?" What is the name of the test that gave the physician this information?
   a. Tumor ploidy
   b. S-phase index
   c. Nuclear grade
   d. Estrogen receptor assay

12-6 What are the common complications that the nurse must watch for in the client who has undergone saline implant placement?
   a. Swelling in the axilla and leakage of the implant
   b. Delayed wound healing and muscle contractions
   c. Delayed wound healing and swelling in the axilla
   d. Delayed wound healing and hematoma

12-7 A client has had adjuvant tamoxifen therapy prescribed for her. Which of the following is a list of the common side effects that she should look for?
   a. Nausea, hot flashes, and vaginal bleeding
   b. Vomiting, weight loss, and hair loss
   c. Nausea, vomiting, and diarrhea
   d. Hot flashes, weight gain, and headaches

12-8 After a mastectomy, a woman should be instructed to:
   a. Empty surgical drains twice a day and as needed
   b. Avoid lifting more than 4.5 kg (10 lb) or reaching above her head until given permission by her surgeon
   c. Wear clothing with snug sleeves to support the tissue of the arm on the operative side
   d. Report immediately any decrease in sensation or tingling at the incision site or the affected arm during the first few weeks postoperatively

# CHAPTER 13

## Structural Disorders and Neoplasms of the Reproductive System

13-1 A pessary would be most effective in the treatment of which of the following disorders?
   a. Cystocele
   b. Uterine prolapse
   c. Rectocele
   d. Stress urinary incontinence

13-2 A postmenopausal woman at age 54 has been diagnosed with two leiomyomas. Which of the following assessment findings is most commonly associated with the presence of leiomyomas?
   a. Abnormal uterine bleeding
   b. Diarrhea
   c. Weight loss
   d. Acute abdominal pain

13-3 Which of the following women is at high risk for psychologic complications after hysterectomy?
   a. A 55-year-old woman who has been having abnormal bleeding and pain for 3 years
   b. A 46-year-old woman who has three children and has just been promoted at work
   c. A 62-year-old widow who has three friends who have had uncomplicated hysterectomies
   d. A 36-year-old woman who had a ruptured uterus after giving birth to her first child

13-4 What information will the nurse include in planning for the care of a woman who has had a vaginal hysterectomy?
   a. The woman should expect to be fully recovered in 4 to 6 weeks.
   b. The woman should expect no changes in her hormone levels.
   c. The woman should expect surgical menopause.
   d. The woman should take tub baths to aid in healing.

13-5 A 48-year-old woman has just had a hysterectomy for endometrial cancer. Which statement alerts the nurse that further teaching is needed?
   a. "I can't wait to go on the cruise that I have planned for this summer."
   b. "I know that the surgery saved my life, but I will miss having sexual intercourse with my husband."
   c. "I have asked my daughter to come and stay with me next week after I am discharged from the hospital."
   d. "Well, I don't have to worry about getting pregnant anymore."

13-6 A woman has preinvasive cancer of the cervix. In discussing available treatments, the nurse would include which of the following?
   a. Cryosurgery
   b. Colporrhaphy
   c. Hysterectomy
   d. Internal radiation

13-7 The nurse knows that teaching about external radiation therapy is effective when the woman:
   a. Uses her special moisturizer to keep her skin from drying out
   b. Washes the irradiated area with deodorant soap
   c. Eats a diet high in protein and drinks at least 2000 ml fluid a day
   d. Washes off the markings for the radiation site after each treatment

13-8 In planning for treatment of a pregnant woman who has cancer, which of the following statements about timing or type of treatment is correct?
   a. The fetus is most at risk during the first trimester.
   b. The fetus is most at risk during the second trimester.
   c. The fetus is most at risk during the third trimester.
   d. Surgery is more risky than chemotherapy in the first trimester.

13-9 During internal radiation therapy for cervical cancer, the woman should:
   a. Maintain a diet high in roughage
   b. Urinate in the bedpan or bathroom every 2 hours
   c. Avoid moving her legs
   d. Deep breathe every 2 hours

# CHAPTER 14

## Conception, Fetal Development, and Genetics

14-1 A father and mother are carriers of phenylketonuria (PKU). Their 2-year-old daughter has PKU. The couple told the nurse that they were planning to have a second baby. Since their daughter has PKU, they believe that their next baby is sure not to be affected. Which of the following responses by the nurse is most accurate?
   a. "Good idea; you need to take advantage of the odds in your favor."
   b. "I think you'd better check with your doctor first."
   c. "You are both carriers, so each baby has a 25% chance of being affected."
   d. "Just hope for a boy; he's sure to be okay."

14-2 A newly married couple plans to use natural family planning. It is important for them to know how long an ovum can live after ovulation. The nurse knows that teaching is effective when the couple responds that an ovum is considered fertile for:
   a. 6 to 8 hours
   b. 24 hours
   c. 2 to 3 days
   d. 1 week

14-3 A woman's cousin gave birth to an infant with a congenital heart anomaly. The woman asked the nurse when such anomalies occur. Which of the following responses by the nurse is most accurate?
a. "We don't really know when such defects occur."
b. "It depends on what caused the defect."
c. "They occur between the third and fifth week of development."
d. "They usually occur in the first 2 weeks of development."

14-4 The volume of amniotic fluid is an important factor in assessing fetal well-being. Oligohydramnios (having less than 300 ml of amniotic fluid) is associated with which kind of fetal anomalies?
a. Renal
b. Cardiac
c. Gastrointestinal
d. Neurologic

14-5 A woman is 8 months pregnant. She told the nurse that she knows her baby listens to her, but her husband thinks she is imagining things. Which of the following responses by the nurse is most appropriate?
a. "Many women imagine what their baby is like."
b. "Babies in utero do respond to their mother's voice."
c. "You'll need to ask the doctor if the baby can hear yet."
d. "Thinking that your baby hears will help you bond to the baby."

14-6 A pregnant woman at 25 weeks' gestation told the nurse that she dropped a pan last week and her baby jumped at the noise. Which of the following responses by the nurse is most accurate?
a. "That must have been a coincidence; babies cannot respond like that."
b. "The fetus is demonstrating the aural reflex."
c. "Babies respond to sound starting at about 24 weeks' gestation."
d. "Let me know if it happens again; we need to report that to your midwife."

14-7 A woman is 5 months pregnant. On routine ultrasound, the physician discovered that the fetus has a diaphragmatic hernia. The woman became distraught and asked the nurse what she should do. Which of the following actions by the nurse is the most appropriate?
a. Talking to the woman and referring her to a genetic counselor
b. Suggesting that the woman travel to a fetal treatment center and have intrauterine surgery
c. Doing nothing
d. Suggesting that the woman terminate the pregnancy

14-8 Meconium is produced by:
a. Fetal intestines
b. Fetal kidneys
c. Amniotic fluid
d. Placenta

14-9 The placenta:
a. Produces nutrients for fetal nutrition
b. Secretes both estrogen and progesterone
c. Forms a protective impenetrable barrier to microorganisms such as bacteria and viruses
d. Excretes prolactin and insulin

14-10 A pregnant couple at 14 weeks' gestation has just been told that they both are carriers of an autosomal-recessive disorder. The nurse who is providing genetic counseling should:
a. Tell the couple that they need to have an abortion within 2 to 3 weeks
b. Explain that there is a 50% chance that their baby will have the disorder
c. Discuss options with the couple, including amniocentesis to determine if their fetus is affected
d. Refer them to a psychologist for emotional support

# CHAPTER 15

## Anatomy and Physiology of Pregnancy

15-1 A woman's obstetric history indicates that she has had three children, all of whom are living. One was born at 39 weeks' gestation, another at 34 weeks' gestation, and another at 35 weeks' gestation. What is her gravity and parity using the GTPAL system?
a. 4-1-1-1-3
b. 3-1-2-0-3
c. 3-0-3-0-3
d. 4-2-1-0-3

15-2 A woman is 6 weeks pregnant. She has had a previous spontaneous abortion at 14 weeks' gestation and a pregnancy that ended at 38 weeks with the birth of a stillborn girl. What is her gravity and parity using the GTPAL system?
a. 2-0-0-1-1
b. 2-1-0-1-0
c. 3-1-0-1-0
d. 3-0-1-1-0

15-3 Over-the-counter (OTC) pregnancy tests usually rely on which of the following technologies to test for the presence of hCG?
a. Radioimmunoassay
b. Radioreceptorassay
c. Latex agglutination test
d. Enzyme-linked immunosorbent assay

15-4 A woman at 10 weeks' gestation who is seen in the prenatal clinic with presumptive signs and symptoms of pregnancy will likely have which of the following?
a. Amenorrhea
b. A positive pregnancy test
c. Chadwick's sign
d. Hegar's sign

15-5 The nurse teaches a pregnant woman about the presumptive, probable, and positive signs of pregnancy. The woman demonstrates understanding of the nurse's instructions if she states that a positive sign of pregnancy is:
a. A positive pregnancy test
b. Fetal movement palpated by the nurse-midwife
c. Braxton Hicks contractions
d. Quickening

15-6 A woman is at 14 weeks' gestation. The nurse would expect to palpate the fundus at which of the following levels?
a. Not palpable above the symphysis at this time
b. Slightly above the symphysis pubis
c. At the level of the umbilicus
d. Slightly above the umbilicus

15-7 On physical examination, the nurse notes that the lower uterine segment is soft upon palpation. The nurse would document this finding as:
a. Hegar's sign
b. McDonald's sign
c. Chadwick's sign
d. Goodell's sign

15-8 Cardiovascular system changes occur during pregnancy. Which of the following findings would be considered normal for a woman in her second trimester?
a. Heart sounds ($S_1$, $S_2$) less audible
b. Increase in pulse rate
c. Increase in blood pressure
d. Decrease in red blood cell production

15-9 A number of changes in the integumentary system occur during pregnancy. Which of the following changes will remain after recovery from pregnancy has been achieved?
a. Epulis
b. Chloasma
c. Telangiectasia
d. Striae gravidarum

15-10 The musculoskeletal system adapts to the changes that occur during pregnancy. A woman can expect to experience which of the following changes?
a. Her center of gravity will shift backward.
b. She will experience an increased lumbosacral curve.
c. She will have increased abdominal muscle tone.
d. She will notice decreased mobility of her pelvic joints.

# CHAPTER 16

## Maternal and Fetal Nutrition

16-1 A 22-year-old pregnant woman with a single fetus was at normal weight (BMI 24) before pregnancy. When she was seen in the clinic at 14 weeks' gestation, she had gained 1.8 kg (4 lb) since conception. How would the nurse interpret this?
a. This large weight gain indicates possible pregnancy-induced hypertension (PIH).
b. This small weight gain indicates that her infant is at risk for intrauterine growth restriction.
c. It is impossible to evaluate this weight gain until the woman has been followed for several more weeks.
d. The woman's weight gain is appropriate for this stage of pregnancy.

16-2 Which meal would provide the most absorbable iron?
   a. Toasted cheese sandwich, celery sticks, tomato slices, and a grape drink
   b. Oatmeal, whole wheat toast, jelly, and low-fat milk
   c. Black bean soup, wheat crackers, ambrosia (orange sections, coconut, and pecans), and lemonade
   d. Red beans and rice, cornbread, mixed greens, and decaffeinated tea

16-3 What nutrient's recommended dietary allowance (RDA) is higher during lactation than during pregnancy?
   a. Energy (kcal)
   b. Iron
   c. Calcium
   d. Folic acid

16-4 A pregnant woman's diet consists almost entirely of whole grain breads and cereals, fruits, and vegetables. The nurse would be least concerned about this woman's intake of:
   a. Calcium
   b. Protein
   c. Vitamin $B_{12}$
   d. Folic acid

16-5 A pregnant woman experiencing nausea and vomiting should:
   a. Drink a glass of water with a fat-free carbohydrate before getting out of bed in the morning
   b. Eat small, frequent meals (every 2 to 3 hours)
   c. Increase the intake of high-fat foods to keep the stomach full and coated
   d. Limit fluid intake throughout the day

16-6 A pregnant woman reports that she is still playing tennis competitively at 32 weeks' gestation. The nurse would be most concerned whether this woman consumes which of the following during and after tennis matches?
   a. Several glasses of fluid
   b. Extra protein sources such as peanut butter
   c. Salty foods to replace lost sodium
   d. Easily digested sources of carbohydrate

16-7 Which statement made by a lactating woman would lead the nurse to believe that the woman might have lactose intolerance?
   a. "I always have heartburn after I drink milk."
   b. "If I drink more than a cup of milk, I usually have abdominal cramps and bloating."
   c. "Drinking milk usually makes me break out in hives."
   d. "Sometimes I notice that I have bad breath after I drink a cup of milk."

16-8 A pregnant woman's diet history indicates that she likes the foods listed below. Which food would the nurse encourage this woman to consume more of to increase her calcium intake?
   a. Fresh apricots
   b. Canned clams
   c. Spaghetti with meat sauce
   d. Canned sardines

16-9 A 27-year-old pregnant woman was underweight (18.0 BMI) before pregnancy. The nurse would be aware that this woman's total recommended weight gain during pregnancy should be at least:
   a. 20 kg (44 lb)
   b. 16 kg (35 lb)
   c. 12.5 kg (27.5 lb)
   d. 10 kg (22 lb)

16-10 A pregnant woman in her 34th week of pregnancy reports that she is very uncomfortable because of heartburn. The nurse would suggest that the woman:
   a. Substitute other calcium sources for milk in her diet
   b. Lie down after each meal
   c. Decrease the amount of fiber that she consumes
   d. Eat five small meals daily

# CHAPTER 17

## Nursing Care During Pregnancy

17-1 Prenatal care should ideally begin:
   a. Before the first missed menstrual period
   b. After the first missed menstrual period
   c. After the second missed menstrual period
   d. After the third missed menstrual period

17-2 A woman arrives at the clinic for a pregnancy test. Her last menstrual period (LMP) was February 14, 2000. Her expected date of birth (EDB) would be:
   a. September 17, 2000
   b. November 7, 2000
   c. November 21, 2000
   d. December 17, 2000

17-3 Women who wish to breastfeed should:
   a. Wash nipples with soap and water each day
   b. Understand that no special preparation is required
   c. Roll the nipples each day
   d. Rub the nipples with a towel each day

17-4 HIV prenatal testing is recommended for which of the following women?
   a. All women, regardless of risk factors
   b. A woman who has had more than one sexual partner
   c. A woman who has had an STD
   d. A woman who is monogamous with her partner

17-5 Which of the following symptoms would be considered a first trimester warning sign and should be reported immediately by the pregnant woman to her health care provider?
a. Nausea with occasional vomiting
b. Fatigue
c. Urinary frequency
d. Vaginal bleeding

17-6 A pregnant woman at 10 weeks' gestation jogs 3 to 4 times per week. She is concerned about the effect of exercise on the fetus. The nurse would inform her that:
a. "You do not need to modify your exercising any time during your pregnancy."
b. "Stop exercising because it will harm the fetus."
c. "You may find that you need to modify your exercising to walking later in your pregnancy around the seventh month."
d. "Jogging is too hard on your body; switch to walking now."

17-7 Condoms should be used in pregnancy by:
a. Unmarried pregnant women
b. Women at risk for acquiring or transmitting STDs
c. All pregnant women
d. Women at risk for candidiasis

17-8 Which of the following blood pressure (B/P) assessment findings during the second trimester indicate a risk for pregnancy-induced hypertension?
a. Baseline B/P 120/80, current B/P 126/85
b. Baseline B/P 100/70, current B/P 130/85
c. Baseline B/P 140/85, current B/P 130/80
d. Baseline B/P 110/60, current B/P 110/60

17-9 The triple marker test is used to assess the fetus for which condition?
a. Down syndrome
b. Spina bifida
c. Congenital cardiac abnormality
d. Anencephaly

17-10 A pregnant woman who is 32 weeks pregnant is informed by the nurse that a warning sign of pregnancy could be:
a. Constipation
b. Alteration in the pattern of fetal movement
c. Heart palpitations
d. Edema in ankles and feet at the end of the day

17-11 A pregnant woman is 23 weeks pregnant. She calls to tell the nurse that she thinks she is leaking fluid from her vagina. The nurse would tell her:
a. "As long as the baby is still moving around, there is nothing to worry about."
b. "Come into the office right away so that we can check the fluid."
c. "Call me back in 2 hours and tell me if there is any change in the leakage."
d. "You are probably leaking urine. We can wait until your next appointment to check you."

17-12 A woman who is 14 weeks pregnant tells the nurse that she always had a glass of wine with dinner before she became pregnant. She has abstained during her first trimester and would like to know if it is safe for her to have a drink with dinner now. You would tell her:
  a. "As you are in your second trimester, there is no problem with having one drink with dinner."
  b. "One drink every night is too much. One drink three times a week should be fine."
  c. "As you are in your second trimester, you can drink as much as you'd like."
  d. "Because no one knows how much or how little alcohol it takes to cause fetal problems, it is recommended that you abstain throughout your pregnancy."

17-13 A pregnant woman at 18 weeks' gestation calls the clinic to report that she has been experiencing occasional backaches of mild to moderate intensity. The nurse would recommend that she:
  a. Do Kegel exercises
  b. Do pelvic rock exercises
  c. Use a softer mattress
  d. Stay in bed for 24 hours

17-14 For which of the following reasons would breastfeeding be contraindicated?
  a. Hepatitis B
  b. Everted nipples
  c. History of breast cancer 3 years ago
  d. Hepatitis C

7-15 A pregnant woman is in her third trimester. She asks the nurse to explain how she can tell true labor from false labor. The nurse would tell her that true labor contractions:
  a. Increase with activity such as ambulation
  b. Decrease with activity
  c. Are infrequent and mild
  d. Continue to follow an irregular pattern

17-16 A woman who is 39 weeks pregnant expresses fear about her impending labor and how she will manage. The nurse's best response would be:
  a. "Don't worry about it; you'll do fine."
  b. "It's normal to be anxious about labor. Let us discuss what makes you afraid."
  c. "Labor is scary to think about, but the actual experience isn't."
  d. "You can have an epidural. You won't feel anything."

17-17 A woman is 3 months pregnant. At her prenatal visit, she told the nurse that she doesn't know what is happening; one minute she is happy that she is pregnant, and the next minute she cries for no reason. Which of the following responses by the nurse is most appropriate?
  a. "Don't worry about it; you'll feel better in a month or so."
  b. "Have you talked to your husband about this?"
  c. "Perhaps you really don't want to be pregnant."
  d. "Hormone changes during pregnancy commonly result in mood swings."

17-18 Which of the following roles is the partner's main role in pregnancy?
  a. Provide financial support
  b. Protect the pregnant woman from "old wives' tales"
  c. Support and nurture the pregnant woman
  d. Ensure that the pregnant woman keeps prenatal appointments

17-19 During the first trimester of pregnancy, a woman can expect which of the following changes in her sexual desire?
    a. An increase because of enlarging breasts
    b. A decrease because of nausea and fatigue
    c. No change in the first trimester
    d. An increase because there are no changes

17-20 Which of the following behaviors indicates that a woman is "seeking safe passage" for herself and her infant?
    a. She keeps all prenatal appointments.
    b. She "eats for two."
    c. She drives her car slowly.
    d. She wears only low-heeled shoes.

17-21 A 3-year-old girl's mother is 6 months pregnant. Which of the following concerns is this girl likely to experience?
    a. How the baby will "get out"
    b. What the baby eats
    c. Whether her mother will die
    d. What color eyes the baby has

17-22 In her work with pregnant women of various cultures, a nurse-practitioner has observed various practices that seemed strange or unusual. She has learned that cultural rituals and practices during pregnancy seem to have one purpose in common. Which of the following statements best describes that purpose?
    a. To promote family unity
    b. To ward off the "evil eye"
    c. To appease the gods of fertility
    d. To protect the mother and fetus during pregnancy

# CHAPTER 18

## Childbirth Education

18-1 Conscious relaxation is associated with which method of childbirth preparation?
    a. Grantly Dick-Read
    b. Lamaze
    c. Bradley
    d. Psychoprophylactic

18-2 Active relaxation and control are associated with which method of childbirth preparation?
    a. Grantly Dick-Read
    b. Lamaze
    c. Bradley
    d. Natural childbirth

18-3 The childbirth preparation method associated with a quiet environment and working in harmony with the body is known as the:
   a. Grantly Dick-Read
   b. Lamaze
   c. Bradley
   d. Psychoprophylactic

18-4 The nurse advises the woman who wishes to have a nurse-midwife provide obstetric care that:
   a. She will have to give birth at home
   b. She must see an obstetrician as well as the midwife during pregnancy
   c. She will not be able to have an epidural analgesia for labor pain
   d. She must be experiencing a low risk pregnancy

18-5 Which of the following birth setting choices allows only for laboring and giving birth in the same place?
   a. LDR
   b. LDRP
   c. Free-standing birth center
   d. Alternative birth center

18-6 A woman and her partner want to give birth at home. Birth at home and at the hospital have some similar advantages. Which of the following is an advantage of home birth only?
   a. The family can be in control of the experience.
   b. Attachment among the parents, the newborn, and siblings can occur immediately.
   c. Birth is less expensive.
   d. The family can assist and be part of the birth experience.

18-7 Which of the following situations could adversely affect the safety of a home birth?
   a. The woman lives 15 minutes away from the hospital.
   b. Only the woman and her midwife will be present.
   c. Medical backup is not arranged because the pregnancy is considered low risk.
   d. The woman's family does not wish her to give birth at home.

18-8 During labor, a doula would be expected to:
   a. Help the woman to do Lamaze breathing techniques
   b. Check the fetal monitor tracing for effect of labor process on FHR
   c. Take the place of the baby's father as a coach and for support
   d. Administer pain medications as needed by the woman

# CHAPTER 19

## Labor and Birth Processes

19-1 A new mother asks the nurse when the "soft spot" on her son's head will go away. The nurse's answer is based on the knowledge that the anterior fontanel closes after birth by:
   a. 2 months
   b. 8 months
   c. 12 months
   d. 18 months

19-2 The relationship of the fetal body parts to each other is called fetal:
  a. Lie
  b. Presentation
  c. Attitude
  d. Position

19-3 When assessing the fetus using Leopold's maneuvers, the nurse feels a round, firm, movable fetal part in the fundal portion of the uterus and a long, smooth surface in the mother's right side close to midline. What is the likely position of the fetus?
  a. ROA
  b. LSP
  c. RSA
  d. LOA

19-4 The nurse has received a report about a woman in labor. The woman's last vaginal examination was recorded as 3 cm, 30%, and −2. The nurse's interpretation of this assessment is that:
  a. The cervix is effaced 3 cm, dilated 30%, and the presenting part is 2 cm above the ischial spines
  b. The cervix is 3 cm dilated, effaced 30%, and the presenting part is 2 cm above the ischial spines
  c. The cervix is effaced 3 cm, dilated 30%, and the presenting part is 2 cm below the ischial spines
  d. The cervix is dilated 3 cm, effaced 30%, and the presenting part is 2 cm below the ischial spines

19-5 Which of the following positions would be least effective when gravity is desired to assist in fetal descent?
  a. Lithotomy
  b. Kneeling
  c. Sitting
  d. Walking

19-6 Which position would the nurse suggest for second stage labor if the pelvic outlet needs to be increased?
  a. Semi-recumbent
  b. Sitting
  c. Squatting
  d. Side-lying

19-7 A pregnant woman is at 38 weeks' gestation. She wants to know if there are signs that indicate "labor is getting closer to starting." The nurse informs the woman that which of the following is a sign that labor will begin soon?
  a. Weight gain of 1.5 to 2 kg (3 to 4 lb)
  b. Increase in fundal height
  c. Urinary retention
  d. Surge of energy

19-8 Which stage of labor varies the most in length?
   a. First
   b. Second
   c. Third
   d. Fourth

19-9 Which of the following fetal heart rate findings would be a concern to the nurse during labor?
   a. Accelerations with fetal movement
   b. Early decelerations
   c. Average FHR of 126 beats per minute
   d. Late decelerations

19-10 Which of the following maternal cardiovascular findings is expected during labor?
   a. Increased cardiac output
   b. Decreased pulse rate
   c. Decreased white blood cell count
   d. Decreased blood pressure

# CHAPTER 20

## Management of Discomfort

20-1 An 18-year-old pregnant woman, gravida 1 para 0, is admitted to the labor and birth unit with moderate contractions every 5 minutes, lasting 40 seconds. The woman states, "My contractions are so strong, and I do not know what to do." The nurses should:
   a. Assess for fetal well-being
   b. Encourage the woman to lie on her side
   c. Disturb the woman as little as possible
   d. Recognize that pain is personalized for each individual

20-2 A woman who is pregnant for the first time is dilated 3 cm with contractions every 5 minutes. She is groaning with excessive perspiration and states that she did not attend childbirth classes. The most important nursing action is to:
   a. Notify the woman's health care provider
   b. Administer the prescribed narcotic analgesic
   c. Assure her that her labor will be over soon
   d. Give simple breathing and relaxation instructions

20-3 The following are nursing care measures commonly offered to women in labor. Which nursing measure reflects application of the gate control theory?
   a. Massage the woman's back.
   b. Change the woman's position.
   c. Give the prescribed medication.
   d. Encourage the woman to rest between contractions.

20-4 The following breathing patterns are taught to laboring women. Which breathing pattern would the nurse support for the woman and her coach during the latent phase of the first stage of labor if they attended Lamaze classes?
a. Slow-paced breathing
b. Deep abdominal breathing
c. Modified-paced breathing
d. Patterned-paced breathing

20-5 If a narcotic antagonist is administered to a laboring woman, she should be told that:
a. Her pain will return
b. Her pain will decrease
c. She will feel less anxious
d. She will no longer feel the urge to push

20-6 A laboring woman received meperidine (Demerol) IV 90 minutes before she gave birth. Which of the following medications should be available to decrease the postnatal effects of Demerol on the neonate?
a. Fentanyl (Sublimaze)
b. Promethazine (Phenergan)
c. Naloxone (Narcan)
d. Nalbuphine (Nubain)

20-7 A woman in labor has just received an epidural block. The most important nursing intervention is to:
a. Limit oral fluids
b. Monitor the fetus for possible tachycardia
c. Monitor blood pressure for possible hypotension
d. Monitor maternal pulse for possible bradycardia

20-8 A woman experienced shivering and her blood pressure dropped from 120/80 mm Hg to 102/68 mm Hg shortly after giving birth. The nurse immediately removed the wet drapes and applied a warm blanket. The woman's fundus was firm, and there was no excessive bleeding. The woman asked, "Why was I unable to stop shivering?" The nurse's most appropriate response would be:
a. "You were shivering because of the pain that you experienced. The shivering will stop soon now that the pain is gone."
b. "You were shivering because your body cooled. This is a normal response, and the shivering will stop shortly."
c. "Your doctor will be here shortly to talk about your shivering."
d. "Don't worry. Your doctor will give you a pain medication that will cause your shivering to stop."

20-9 An effective plan to achieve adequate pain relief without maternal risk is most effective if:
a. The mother has the baby without any analgesic or anesthetic
b. The mother and the family priorities and preferences are incorporated into the plan
c. The primary health care provider decides the best pain relief for the mother and family
d. The nurse informs the family of all alternative methods of pain relief available in the hospital setting

20-10 A woman in the active phase of the first stage of labor is using a shallow pattern of breathing, which is about twice the normal adult breathing rate. She starts to complain about feeling lightheaded and dizzy and states that her fingers are tingling. The nurse should:
   a. Notify the woman's physician
   b. Tell the woman to slow the pace of her breathing
   c. Administer oxygen via mask or nasal cannula
   d. Help her to breathe into a paper bag

20-11 A woman is experiencing back labor and complains of intense pain in her lower back. An effective relief measure would be to use:
   a. Counter pressure against the sacrum
   b. Pant-blow (breaths and puffs) breathing techniques
   c. Effleurage
   d. Conscious relaxation or guided imagery

# CHAPTER 21

## Fetal Assessment

21-1 Fetal tachycardia is most common during:
   a. Maternal fever
   b. Umbilical cord prolapse
   c. Regional anesthesia
   d. MgSO$_4$ administration

21-2 Fetal bradycardia is most common during:
   a. Intraamniotic infection
   b. Fetal anemia
   c. Prolonged umbilical cord compression
   d. Tocolytic treatment using ritodrine

21-3 The most common cause of decreased variability of the fetal heart rate (FHR) is:
   a. Altered cerebral blood flow
   b. Fetal hypoxemia
   c. Umbilical cord compression
   d. Fetal sleep cycles

21-4 Early decelerations are caused by:
   a. Altered fetal cerebral blood flow
   b. Umbilical cord compression
   c. Uteroplacental insufficiency
   d. Spontaneous rupture of membranes

21-5 Accelerations with fetal movement:
   a. Are reassuring
   b. Are caused by umbilical cord compression
   c. Warrant close observation
   d. Are caused by uteroplacental insufficiency

21-6 Variable FHR decelerations are caused by:
a. Altered fetal cerebral blood flow
b. Umbilical cord compression
c. Uteroplacental insufficiency
d. Fetal hypoxemia

21-7 Late FHR decelerations are caused by:
a. Altered cerebral blood flow
b. Umbilical cord compression
c. Uteroplacental insufficiency
d. Meconium fluid

21-8 Amnioinfusion is used to treat:
a. Variable decelerations
b. Late decelerations
c. Fetal bradycardia
d. Fetal tachycardia

21-9 Maternal hypotension can result in:
a. Early decelerations
b. Fetal dysrhythmias
c. Uteroplacental insufficiency
d. Spontaneous rupture of membranes

21-10 Maternal cardiac output can be increased by:
a. Position change
b. Oxytocin administration
c. Regional anesthesia
d. Intravenous analgesic

21-11 When evaluating an external monitor tracing of a woman in active labor whose labor is being induced, the nurse notes that the FHR begins to decelerate at the onset of several contractions and returns to baseline before each contraction ends. The nurse should:
a. Change the woman's position
b. Discontinue the oxytocin infusion
c. Insert an internal monitor
d. Document the finding in the client's record

# CHAPTER 22

## Nursing Care During Labor

22-1 The nurse recognizes that a woman is in true labor when she states:
a. "I passed some thick, pink mucus when I urinated this morning."
b. "My bag of waters just broke."
c. "The contractions in my uterus are getting stronger and closer together."
d. "My baby dropped and I have to urinate more frequently now."

22-2 The nurse teaches a pregnant woman about the characteristics of true labor contractions. The nurse evaluates understanding of the instructions when the woman states:
a. "True labor contractions will subside when I walk around."
b. "True labor contractions will cause discomfort over the top of my uterus."
c. "True labor contractions will continue and get stronger even if I relax and take a shower."
d. "True labor contractions will remain irregular but become stronger."

22-3 When a nulliparous woman telephones the hospital to report that she is in labor, the nurse should initially:
a. Tell the woman to stay home until her membranes rupture
b. Emphasize that food and fluid intake should stop
c. Arrange for the woman to come to the hospital for labor evaluation
d. Ask the woman to describe why she believes that she is in labor

22-4 Which of the following is an expected characteristic of amniotic fluid?
a. Deep yellow color
b. Clear, with small white particles
c. Nitrazine test: acidic result
d. Absence of ferning

22-5 When planning care for a laboring woman whose membranes have ruptured, the nurse recognizes that the woman's risk for _____ has increased.
a. Intrauterine infection
b. Hemorrhage
c. Precipitous labor
d. Supine hypotension

22-6 The uterine contractions of a woman early in the active phase of labor are assessed by an internal uterine pressure catheter (IUPC). The nurse notes that the intrauterine pressure at the peak of the contraction ranges from 65 to 70 mm Hg and the resting tone range is 6 to 10 mm Hg. The uterine contractions occur every 3 to 4 minutes and last an average of 55 to 60 seconds. Based on this information, the nurse should:
a. Notify the woman's primary health care provider immediately
b. Prepare to administer an oxytocic to stimulate uterine activity
c. Document the findings since they reflect the expected contraction pattern for the active phase of labor
d. Prepare the woman for the onset of the second stage of labor

22-7 Which of the following actions is correct when using palpation to assess the characteristics and pattern of uterine contractions?
a. Place hand on abdomen below the umbilicus, and palpate uterine tone with fingertips.
b. Determine frequency by timing the end of one contraction until the end of the next contraction.
c. Evaluate intensity by pressing fingertips into the uterine fundus.
d. Assess uterine contractions every 30 minutes throughout the first stage of labor.

22-8 When assessing a woman in the first stage of labor, the nurse recognizes that the most conclusive sign that uterine contractions are effective would be:
a. Dilation of cervix
b. Descent of fetus
c. Rupture of amniotic membranes
d. Increase in bloody show

22-9 The nurse who performs vaginal examinations to assess a woman's progress in labor should:
a. Perform an examination at least once every hour during the active phase of labor
b. Perform the examination more frequently if vaginal bleeding is present
c. Wear two clean gloves for each examination
d. Discuss findings with the woman and her partner

22-10 A multiparous woman has been in labor for 8 hours. Her membranes have just ruptured. The nurse's initial response would be to:
a. Prepare the woman for imminent birth
b. Notify the woman's primary health care provider
c. Document the characteristics of the fluid
d. Assess the fetal heart rate and pattern

22-11 The nurse would assist the laboring woman into a hands-and-knees position when the:
a. Occiput of the fetus is in a posterior position
b. Fetus is at or above the ischial spines
c. Fetus is in a vertex presentation
d. Membranes rupture

22-12 A nulliparous woman is in the transition phase of the first stage of labor. She becomes very irritable and tells her partner to stop touching her and to leave her alone. The nurse should:
a. Tell the partner that this is a good time to leave the room and take a break
b. Explain to the partner that the woman's behavior is normal and help him to continue to coach her
c. Inform the partner that a nurse would be a more effective coach at this time
d. Reassure the partner that the woman does not mean what she is saying and he should ignore it

22-13 A nulliparous woman who has just begun the second stage of her labor would most likely:
a. Experience a strong urge to bear down
b. Exhibit perineal bulging
c. Feel tired yet relieved that the worst is over
d. Exhibit an increase in bright-red bloody show

22-14 The nurse knows that the second stage of labor has begun when the:
a. Amniotic membranes rupture
b. Cervix cannot be felt during a vaginal examination
c. Woman experiences a strong urge to bear down
d. Presenting part is below the ischial spines

22-15 When managing the care of a woman in the second stage of labor, the nurse uses a variety of measures to enhance the progress of fetal descent. These measures include:
a. Encouraging the woman to try a variety of upright positions, including squatting and standing
b. Telling the woman to start pushing as soon as her cervix is fully dilated
c. Continuing an epidural anesthetic so that pain is reduced and the woman can relax
d. Coaching the woman to use sustained, 10- to 15-second, closed glottis bearing down efforts with each contraction

22-16 The nurse evaluates that expected outcomes of the second and third stages of labor for nulliparous women have been met if:
a. Both the mothers and fathers participated in the birth of their child
b. The women eagerly breastfed their newborns immediately after birth
c. The second stage of labor did not exceed 1 hour
d. The women expressed satisfaction with the childbirth companions that they chose to be present

22-17 The most critical nursing action when caring for the newborn immediately after birth is:
a. Keeping the newborn's airway clear
b. Fostering parent-newborn attachment
c. Drying the newborn and wrapping him or her in a blanket
d. Administering eye drops and vitamin K

22-18 When assessing a multiparous woman who has just given birth to an 8-pound boy, the nurse notes that the woman's fundus is firm and has become globular in shape. A gush of dark red blood comes from her vagina. The nurse concludes that:
a. The placenta has separated
b. A cervical tear occurred during birth
c. The woman is beginning to hemorrhage
d. Clots have formed in the upper uterine segment

22-19 The nurse expects to administer an oxytocic (e.g., Pitocin, Methergine) to a woman after an expulsion of her placenta to:
a. Relieve pain
b. Stimulate uterine contraction
c. Prevent infection
d. Facilitate rest and relaxation

22-20 A nulliparous woman has just given birth to a baby girl after 20 hours of labor that included 1 hour of pushing. She refuses to breastfeed her baby at this time, stating, "I am exhausted and just want to sleep. I will breastfeed her later when I feel better." The nurse recognizes this reaction as:
a. Typical of a woman who has experienced a long labor
b. A warning sign of maternal-newborn conflict
c. Disappointment over the sex of the baby
d. A cultural belief not to breastfeed until the milk comes in

22-21 After an emergency birth, the nurse encourages the woman to breastfeed her newborn. The primary purpose for this action is to:
a. Facilitate maternal-newborn interaction
b. Stimulate the uterus to contract
c. Prevent neonatal hypoglycemia
d. Initiate the lactation cycle

# CHAPTER 23

## Postpartum Physiology

23-1 A woman gave birth to a baby boy 12 hours ago. Where would the nurse expect to locate the fundus of this woman's uterus?
a. One centimeter above the umbilicus
b. Two centimeters below the umbilicus
c. Midway between the umbilicus and the symphysis pubis
d. Nonpalpable abdominally

23-2 The most common causes of subinvolution are:
a. Postpartum hemorrhage and infection
b. Multiple gestation and postpartum hemorrhage
c. Uterine tetany and overproduction of oxytocin
d. Retained placental fragments and infection

23-3 Which of the following clients is most likely to experience strong afterpains?
a. A woman who exhibited oligohydramnios
b. A woman who is a gravida 4, para 4 0 0 4
c. A woman who is bottle feeding her baby
d. A woman whose baby weighed 5 pounds, 3 ounces

23-4 A woman gave birth to a healthy baby boy 5 days ago. What type of lochia would the nurse expect to find when assessing this woman?
a. Lochia rubra
b. Lochia sangra
c. Lochia alba
d. Lochia serosa

23-5 Which of the following hormones remain elevated in the immediate postpartum period of the breastfeeding woman?
a. Estrogen
b. Progesterone
c. Prolactin
d. Human placental lactogen

23-6 Two days ago, a woman gave birth to a full-term infant. Last night, she awakened several times to urinate and noted that her gown and bedding were wet from profuse diaphoresis. One mechanism for the diaphoresis and diuresis that this woman is experiencing during the early postpartum period is:
a. Increased temperature caused by postpartum infection
b. Increased basal metabolic rate after giving birth
c. Loss of increased blood volume associated with pregnancy
d. Increased venous pressure in the lower extremities

23-7 A woman gave birth to a 7-pound, 3-ounce baby boy 2 hours ago. The nurse determines that the woman's bladder is distended because her fundus is now 3 cm above the umbilicus and to the right of the midline. In the immediate postpartum period, the most serious consequence likely to occur from bladder distension is:
a. A urinary tract infection
b. Excessive uterine bleeding
c. A ruptured bladder
d. Bladder wall atony

23-8 Yesterday, a woman gave birth to a full-term baby girl. Which of the following laboratory results indicates a deviation from normal at this time?
a. Hematocrit of 34%
b. White blood cell count of 15,000
c. Prolonged PT and PTT
d. +1 proteinuria

23-9 Breast engorgement is caused by:
a. Overproduction of colostrum
b. Accumulation of milk in the lactiferous ducts
c. Hyperplasia of mammary tissue
d. Congestion of veins and lymphatics

23-10 A woman gave birth to a 7-pound, 6-ounce baby girl 1 hour ago. The birth was vaginal, and the estimated blood loss was less than 500 ml. When assessing vital signs, the nurse would expect to see:
a. Temperature 37.9°, heart rate 88, respirations 20, blood pressure 110/60
b. Temperature 37.4°, heart rate 100, respirations 36, blood pressure 100/50
c. Temperature 38.5°, heart rate 80, respirations 16, blood pressure 110/80
d. Temperature 36.8°, heart rate 60, respirations 28, blood pressure 140/90

# CHAPTER 24

## Assessment and Care During the Postpartum Period

24-1 A 25-year-old gravida 2, para 2 0 0 2 gave birth 4 hours ago to a 9-pound, 7-ounce boy after augmentation of labor with Pitocin. She puts on her call light and asks for her nurse right away, stating, "I'm bleeding a lot." The most likely cause of postpartum hemorrhage in this woman would be:
   a. Retained placental fragments
   b. Unrepaired vaginal lacerations
   c. Uterine atony
   d. Puerperal infection

24-2 On examining a woman who gave birth 5 hours ago, the nurse finds that the woman has completely saturated a perineal pad within 15 minutes. The nurse's first action is to:
   a. Begin an IV infusion of Ringer's lactate solution
   b. Assess the woman's vital signs
   c. Call the woman's primary health care provider
   d. Palpate the woman's fundus

24-3 A woman gave birth vaginally to a 9-pound, 12-ounce girl yesterday. Her primary health care provider has written orders for perineal ice packs, use of a sitz bath tid, and a stool softener. Which of the following information is most closely correlated with these orders?
   a. The woman is a gravida 2, para 2.
   b. The woman had a vacuum-assisted birth.
   c. The woman received epidural anesthesia.
   d. The woman has an episiotomy.

24-4 The laboratory results of a postpartum woman are as follows: blood type, A; Rh status, positive; Rubella titer, 1:4 (EIA 0.70); hematocrit, 30%. How would the nurse best interpret this data?
   a. Rubella vaccine should be given.
   b. A blood transfusion is necessary.
   c. Rh immune globulin is necessary within 72 hours of birth.
   d. A Kleihauer-Betke test should be performed.

24-5 A woman gave birth 48 hours ago to a healthy baby girl. She has decided to bottle feed. During your assessment, you notice that both breasts are swollen, warm, and tender upon palpation. The woman should be advised that this condition can best be treated by:
   a. Running warm water on her breasts during a shower
   b. Applying ice to the breasts for comfort
   c. Expressing small amounts of milk from the breasts to relieve pressure
   d. Wearing a loose-fitting bra to prevent nipple irritation

24-6 A new breastfeeding mother becomes agitated when her baby cries. The baby is rooming with her mother. The nurse should:

a. Leave the crying baby with her mother so that they can get acquainted
b. Tell the mother that the baby is hungry and that she should breastfeed her immediately
c. Refer the mother to a lactation consultant for assistance
d. Demonstrate ways that the mother can comfort her baby

24-7 Mrs. Kim is a 25-year-old multiparous woman who gave birth to a baby boy 1 day ago. Today her husband brings a large container of brown seaweed soup to the hospital. When the nurse enters the room, Mr. Kim asks the nurse for help with warming the soup so that his wife can eat it. The nurse's most appropriate response would be:

a. "Mrs. Kim, didn't you like your lunch?"
b. "Does your doctor know that you are planning to eat that?"
c. "What is that anyway?"
d. "I will warm the soup in the microwave for you."

24-8 A primiparous woman is to be discharged from the hospital tomorrow with her baby girl. Which behavior indicates a need for further intervention by the nurse before she can be discharged? The woman:

a. Leaves the baby on her bed while she takes a shower
b. Continues to hold and cuddle her baby after she has fed her
c. Reads a magazine while her baby sleeps
d. Changes her baby's diaper then shows the nurse the contents of the diaper

24-9 Which of the following would prevent early discharge of a postpartum woman?

a. Hgb < 10 g
b. Birth was at 38 weeks' gestation
c. Voids about 200 to 300 ml per void
d. Episiotomy exhibits slight redness and edema and is dry and approximated

24-10 Which of the following findings could prevent early discharge of the newborn who is now 12 hours old?

a. Birth weight of 3000 g
b. One meconium stool since birth
c. Voided clear pale urine three times since birth
d. Breastfed once with some difficulty latching on and sucking and once with some success for about 5 minutes on each breast

24-11 The Newborns and Mothers Health Protection Act of 1996 requires that all health care plans allow for a minimum length of stay after a normal vaginal birth of:

a. 24 hours
b. 36 hours
c. 48 hours
d. 96 hours

24-12 Decreasing length of postpartum hospital stay primarily is the result of the influence of:

a. HMO and private insurers
b. Consumer demand
c. Hospitals
d. The federal government

# CHAPTER 25

## Transition to Parenthood

25-1 After giving birth to a healthy baby boy, a primiparous woman, age 16, is admitted to the post-partum unit. An appropriate nursing diagnosis for her at this time is "risk for altered parenting, related to knowledge deficit of newborn care." In planning for the woman's discharge, the nurse should be certain to include which of the following in the plan of care?
   a. Tell the woman how to feed and bathe her baby.
   b. Give the woman written information on bathing her baby.
   c. Advise the woman that all mothers instinctively know how to care for their babies.
   d. Provide time for the woman to bathe her baby after she views a baby bath demonstration.

25-2 A 30-year-old multiparous woman has a boy who is 2½ years old and now a baby girl. She tells the nurse, "I don't know how I'll ever manage both children when I get home." Which suggestion would best help this woman decrease sibling rivalry?
   a. Tell the older child that he is a big boy now and should love his new sister.
   b. Let the older child stay with his grandparents for the first 6 weeks to allow him to adjust to the new baby.
   c. Ask friends and relatives not to bring gifts to the older sibling because you do not want to spoil him.
   d. Realize that the babyish behavior in the older child is a typical reaction and that he needs extra love and attention at this time.

25-3 The nurse observes several interactions between a postpartum woman and her new son. Which of the following behaviors, if exhibited by this woman, would the nurse identify as a possible maladaptive behavior regarding parent-infant attachment?
   a. Talks and coos to her son
   b. Seldom makes eye contact with her son
   c. Cuddles her son close to her
   d. Tells visitors how well her son is feeding

25-4 The nurse observes that a 15-year-old mother seems to ignore her newborn. A strategy that the nurse can use to facilitate mother-infant attachment in this mother is to:
   a. Tell the mother that she must pay attention to her baby
   b. Show the mother how the baby initiates interaction and attends to her
   c. Demonstrate for the mother different positions for holding her baby while feeding
   d. Arrange for the mother to watch a video on parent-infant interaction

25-5 The nurse hears a primiparous woman talking to her son and telling him that his chin is just like his dad's chin. This woman's statement reflects:
   a. Mutuality
   b. Synchrony
   c. Claiming
   d. Reciprocity

25-6 New parents express concern that, because of the mother's emergency cesarean birth under general anesthesia, they did not have the opportunity to hold and "bond" with their daughter immediately after her birth. The nurse's response should convey to the parents that:
a. Attachment or bonding is a process that occurs over time and does not require early contact
b. The time immediately after birth is a critical period for humans
c. Early contact is essential for optimum parent-infant relationships
d. They should just be happy that the baby is healthy

25-7 By the second postpartum day, the nurse would expect a new mother who had an uncomplicated vaginal birth to:
a. Request help with ambulation and perineal care
b. Be interested in learning more about infant care
c. Sleep most of the time when the baby is not present
d. Be very excited and talkative about the birth experience

25-8 During a phone follow-up conversation with a woman who is 4 days postpartum, the woman tells the nurse, "I don't know what is wrong. I love my son, but I feel so let down. I seem to cry for no reason!" The nurse would recognize that the woman is experiencing:
a. Taking-in
b. Postpartum depression
c. Postpartum blues
d. Attachment difficulty

25-9 The nurse can help a father in his transition to parenthood by:
a. Pointing out that the infant turned at the sound of his voice
b. Encouraging him to go home to get some sleep
c. Telling him to tape the baby's diaper a different way
d. Suggesting that he let the baby sleep in the bassinet

25-10 Common symptoms of postpartum blues are:
a. Anxiety, panic attacks, insomnia, and disinterest in the infant
b. Delusions, hallucinations, disorganized speech, and catatonic behavior
c. Flight of ideas, distractibility, psychomotor agitation, and a decreased need for sleep
d. Mood swings, anxiety, tears, and fatigue

25-11 The nurse notes that Mrs. Nguyen does not cuddle or interact with her newborn other than to feed him, change his diapers or soiled clothes, or put him to bed. In evaluating Mrs. Nguyen's behavior with her infant, the nurse realizes that:
a. What appears to be a "lack of interest" in the newborn is, in fact, the Vietnamese way of demonstrating intense love by attempting to ward off evil spirits
b. Mrs. Nguyen is inexperienced in caring for newborns
c. Mrs. Nguyen needs a referral to a social worker for further evaluation of her parenting behaviors once she goes home with the baby
d. Extra time needs to be planned for assisting Mrs. Nguyen in bonding with her newborn

# CHAPTER 26

## Physiology and Physical Adaptations of the Newborn

26-1 A woman gave birth to a healthy 7-pound, 13-ounce baby girl. The nurse suggests that the woman place the infant to her breasts within 15 minutes after birth. The nurse knows that breastfeeding would be effective during the first 30 minutes after birth because this is the:
a. Transitional period
b. First period of reactivity
c. Organizational stage
d. Second period of reactivity

26-2 Part of the health assessment of a newborn includes observing the newborn's breathing pattern. A full-term newborn's breathing pattern is predominantly:
a. Abdominal with synchronous chest movements
b. Chest breathing with nasal flaring
c. Diaphragmatic with chest retraction
d. Deep with a regular rhythm

26-3 The average expected apical pulse range of a full-term, quiet alert newborn would be:
a. 80 to 100 beats per minute
b. 100 to 120 beats per minute
c. 120 to 140 beats per minute
d. 150 to 180 beats per minute

26-4 A newborn is placed under a radiant heat warmer. The nurse knows that thermoregulation presents a problem for newborns because:
a. Their renal function is not fully developed and heat is lost in the urine
b. Their small body surface area favors heat loss more rapidly than an adult's body surface area
c. They have a relatively thin layer of subcutaneous fat that provides poor insulation
d. Their normal flexed posture favors heat loss through perspiration

26-5 A newborn is placed under a radiant heat warmer, and the nurse evaluates the baby's body temperature every hour. It is important to maintain the baby's body temperature to prevent:
a. Respiratory depression
b. Cold stress
c. Tachycardia
d. Vasoconstriction

26-6 An African-American woman noticed some bruises on her newborn baby girl's buttocks. She asks the nurse who spanked her daughter. The nurse explains to the woman that these marks are called:
a. Lanugo
b. Vascular nevi
c. Nevus flammeus
d. Mongolian spots

26-7 When examining a newborn, the nurse notes uneven skin folds of the buttocks and a click when performing Ortolani's maneuver. The nurse recognizes these findings as a sign that the baby probably has:
a. Polydactyly
b. Clubfoot
c. Hip dysplasia
d. Webbing

26-8 A new mother states that her baby must be cold because the hands and feet are blue. The nurse explains that this is a common and temporary condition called:
a. Acrocyanosis
b. Erythema neonatorum
c. Harlequin color
d. Vernix caseosa

26-9 The nurse assessing a newborn knows that the most critical physiologic change required of the newborn is:
a. Closure of fetal shunts in its circulatory system
b. Full function of the immune defense system at birth
c. Maintenance of a stable temperature
d. Initiation and maintenance of respirations

26-10 A primiparous woman is watching her newborn sleep. She wants him to wake up and respond to her. The mother asks the nurse how much he will sleep every day. The nurse's response to her is:
a. "He will only wake up to be fed, and you should not bother him between feedings."
b. "The newborn sleeps about 17 hours a day with periods of wakefulness gradually increasing."
c. "He will probably follow your same sleep and wake patterns, and you can expect him to be awake soon."
d. "He is being stubborn by not waking up when you want him to. You should try to keep him awake during the daytime so that he will sleep through the night."

26-11 Parents of a newborn ask the nurse how much the baby can see. The parents specifically want to know what type of visual stimuli they should provide for their newborn. The nurse responds to the parents by telling them:
a. "Babies can see very little until about 3 months of age."
b. "Infants at 2 weeks of age can distinguish patterns and seem to like medium-colored or black and white geometric shapes and patterns."
c. "The infant's eyes must be protected, and the infant enjoys looking at brightly colored stripes."
d. "It is important to shield the newborn's eyes. You should ask your physician what the infant should look at."

26-12 When evaluating the reflexes of a newborn, the nurse notes that with a loud noise the new-born symmetrically abducts and extends his arms, the fingers fan out and form a "C" with the thumb and forefinger, and he has a slight tremor. The nurse would document this finding as a positive:
a. Tonic neck reflex
b. Glabellar (Myerson's) reflex
c. Babinski's reflex
d. Moro's reflex

26-13 When assessing the integument of a 24-hour-old newborn, the nurse notes a pink papular rash with vesicles superimposed on the thorax, back, and abdomen. The nurse should:
a. Notify the physician immediately
b. Move the newborn to an isolation nursery
c. Document the finding as erythema toxicum
d. Take the newborn's temperature and obtain a culture of one of the vesicles

# CHAPTER 27

## Assessment and Care of the Newborn

27-1 A baby boy was born just a few minutes ago. The nurse is conducting the initial assessment. Part of the assessment includes the Apgar score. The Apgar assessment is performed:
a. Only if the newborn is in obvious distress
b. Once, just after the birth by the obstetrician
c. At least twice, 1 minute and 5 minutes after birth
d. Every 15 minutes during the newborn's first hour after birth

27-2 A new father wants to know what medication was put into his baby's eyes and why it was need-ed. The nurse explains to the father that the purpose of the Ilotycin ophthalmic ointment is to:
a. Destroy an infectious exudate caused by staphylococcus that could make the baby blind
b. Prevent gonorrheal and chlamydial infection of the baby's eyes potentially acquired from the birth canal
c. Prevent potentially harmful exudate from invading the tear ducts of the baby's eyes, leading to dry eyes
d. Prevent the baby's eyelids from sticking together and help the baby see

27-3 The nurse is assessing a newborn girl who is 2 hours old. Which of the following findings would warrant a call to the pediatrician?
a. Blood glucose of 45 mg/dl using a Dextrostix
b. Heart rate of 160 beats per minute after crying vigorously
c. A crepitant-like feeling when assessing the clavicles
d. Passage of a dark black-green substance from the intestines

27-4 The nurse administers vitamin K to the newborn for which of the following reasons?
   a. Most mothers have a diet deficient in vitamin K, which results in the infant being deficient.
   b. Vitamin K prevents the synthesis of prothrombin in the liver and must be given by injection.
   c. Bacteria that synthesize vitamin K are not present in the newborn's intestinal tract.
   d. The supply of vitamin K is inadequate for at least 3 to 4 months, and the newborn must be supplemented.

27-5 The nurse is using the new Ballard scale to determine the gestational age of a newborn. Which assessment finding is consistent with a gestational age of 40 weeks?
   a. Flexed posture
   b. Abundant lanugo
   c. Smooth pink skin with visible veins
   d. Faint red marks on the soles of the feet

27-6 Before a newborn is discharged, the nurse places a warm diaper on the newborn's foot so that a heel stick can be performed to obtain blood for the PKU test. The newborn's mother wants to know why this test needs to be performed. The nurse tells the mother that the test will determine if her newborn will need:
   a. Lifelong dietary management
   b. Blood transfusions
   c. Medications to prevent infection
   d. Iron-enriched formula

27-7 A newborn is jaundiced and is receiving phototherapy. An appropriate nursing intervention when caring for an infant with hyperbilirubinemia and receiving phototherapy would be to:
   a. Apply an oil-based lotion to the newborn's skin to prevent dying and cracking
   b. Limit the newborn's intake of milk to prevent nausea, vomiting, and diarrhea
   c. Place eye shields over the newborn's closed eyes
   d. Change the newborn's position every 4 hours

27-8 Early this morning, a baby boy was circumcised using the Plastibell method. The nurse tells the mother that she and the baby can be discharged after:
   a. The bleeding stops completely
   b. Yellow exudate forms over the glans
   c. The Plastibell rim falls off
   d. The infant voids

27-9 A mother expresses fear about changing her infant's diaper after he is circumcised. What does the woman need to be taught to take care of the baby when she gets home?
   a. Cleanse the penis with prepackaged diaper wipes every 3 to 4 hours.
   b. Apply constant, firm pressure by squeezing the penis with the fingers for at least 5 minutes if bleeding occurs.
   c. Cleanse the penis gently with water, and put petroleum jelly around the glans after each diaper change.
   d. Wash off the yellow exudate that forms on the glans at least once every day to prevent infection.

27-10 A nurse is responsible for teaching new parents about the hygienic care of their newborn. The nurse should tell the parents to:
    a. Avoid washing the head for at least 1 week to prevent heat loss
    b. Begin tub baths when the cord is dried and the clamp is removed
    c. Cleanse the ears and nose with cotton-tipped swabs such as Q-tips
    d. Create a draft-free environment of at least 75° F when bathing their baby

27-11 When preparing to administer a hepatitis B vaccine to a newborn, the nurse should:
    a. Obtain a syringe with a 25-gauge, $\frac{5}{8}$-inch needle
    b. Confirm that the newborn's mother has been infected with the hepatitis B virus
    c. Assess the dorsogluteal muscle as the preferred site for injection
    d. Confirm that the newborn is at least 24 hours old

# CHAPTER 28

## Newborn Nutrition and Feeding

28-1 A new mother recalls from prenatal class that she should try to feed her newborn daughter when she exhibits feeding readiness cues rather than waiting until her baby is crying frantically. Based on this recollection, this woman should feed her baby about every 2½ to 3 hours when she:
    a. Waves her arms in the air
    b. Makes sucking motions
    c. Has hiccups
    d. Stretches her legs out straight

28-2 A new father is ready to take his wife and newborn son home. He proudly tells the nurse who is discharging them that within the next week he plans to start feeding the baby cereal in between breastfeeding sessions. The nurse can explain to him that beginning solid foods before 4 to 6 months may:
    a. Decrease the infant's intake of sufficient calories
    b. Lead to early cessation of breastfeeding
    c. Help the baby sleep through the night
    d. Limit the baby's growth

28-3 A hospital policy that can interfere with breastfeeding progress and duration is:
    a. Distribution of formula samples
    b. Single-room maternity care
    c. Beginning breastfeeding during the first period of reactivity after birth
    d. Encouraging mothers to breastfeed newborns on demand based on feeding readiness cues

28-4 A pregnant woman wants to breastfeed her baby, but her husband is not convinced that there are any scientific reasons to do so. The nurse can give the couple printed information comparing breastfeeding and bottle feeding. Which of the following statements is true? Bottle feeding using commercially prepared infant formulas:
    a. Increases the risk that the infant will develop allergies
    b. Helps the infant sleep through the night
    c. Assures that the infant is getting iron in a form that is easily absorbed
    d. Requires that multivitamin supplements be given to the infant

28-5 A postpartum woman telephones about her 4-day-old baby. She is not scheduled for a weight check until the baby is 10 days old, and she is worried about whether or not breastfeeding is going well. Effective breastfeeding is indicated by the newborn who:
a. Sleeps for 6 hours at a time between feedings
b. Has at least three breast milk stools every 24 hours
c. Gains 1 to 2 ounces per week
d. Has at least four wet diapers per day

28-6 A primiparous woman is delighted with her newborn son and wants to begin breastfeeding as soon as possible. The nurse can facilitate the baby's correct latch-on by helping the woman hold the baby:
a. With his arms folded together over his chest
b. Curled up in a fetal position
c. With his head cupped in her hand
d. With his head and body in alignment

28-7 A breastfeeding woman develops engorged breasts at 3 days postpartum. Which of the following actions would help this woman achieve her goal of reducing the engorgement? The woman:
a. Skips feedings to let her sore breasts rest
b. Avoids using a breast pump
c. Breastfeeds her baby every 2 hours
d. Reduces her fluid intake for 24 hours

28-8 At a 2-month, well-baby examination, it was discovered that a breastfed infant had only gained 10 ounces in the last 4 weeks. The mother and the nurse agree that, in order to gain weight faster, the baby needs to:
a. Begin solid foods
b. Have a bottle of formula after every feeding
c. Add at least one extra breastfeeding session every 24 hours
d. Start iron supplements

28-9 Parents have been asked by the neonatologist to provide breast milk for their newborn son, who was born prematurely at 32 weeks' gestation. The nurse who instructs them about pumping, storing, and transporting the milk needs to assess their knowledge about lactation. Which of the following statements is valid?
a. A premature baby more easily digests breast milk than formula.
b. A glass of wine just before pumping will help reduce stress and anxiety.
c. The mother should only pump as much as the baby can drink.
d. The mother should pump every 2 to 3 hours, including during the night.

28-10 A new mother wants to be sure that she is meeting her daughter's needs while feeding her commercially prepared infant formula. The nurse should evaluate the mother's knowledge about appropriate infant care. The mother meets her child's needs when she:
a. Adds rice cereal to her formula at 2 weeks of age to ensure adequate nutrition
b. Warms the bottles using a microwave oven
c. Burps her infant during and after the feeding as needed
d. Refrigerates any leftover formula for the next feeding

# CHAPTER 29

## Assessment for Risk Factors

29-1  A woman arrives at the clinic seeking confirmation that she is pregnant. The following information is obtained: She is 24 years old. Her BMI is 17.5. She admits to having used cocaine "several times" during the past year and drinks alcohol occasionally. Her blood pressure is 108/70 mm Hg, her pulse is 72 beats per minute, and her respirations are 16 breaths per minute. Family history is positive for diabetes mellitus and cancer; her sister recently gave birth to a baby with a neural tube defect. Which characteristics place the woman in a high risk category?
   a. Blood pressure, age, BMI
   b. Drug/alcohol use, age, family history
   c. Family history, blood pressure, BMI
   d. Family history, BMI, drug/alcohol abuse

29-2  A 39-year-old primigravida thinks that she is about 8 weeks pregnant, although she has had irregular menstrual periods all of her life. She has a history of smoking approximately one pack of cigarettes a day but tells you that she is trying to cut down. Her laboratory data are within normal limits. Which of the following diagnostic techniques could be employed with this pregnant woman at this time?
   a. Ultrasound examination
   b. Maternal serum alpha-fetoprotein screening
   c. Amniocentesis
   d. Nonstress test

29-3  A 26-year-old pregnant woman, gravida 2, para 1 0 0 1, is 28 weeks pregnant when she experiences bright red painless vaginal bleeding. Upon her arrival at the hospital, what would be an expected diagnostic procedure?
   a. Amniocentesis for fetal lung maturity
   b. Ultrasound for placental location
   c. Contraction stress test
   d. Internal fetal monitoring

29-4  The nurse sees a woman for the first time when she is 30 weeks pregnant. The woman has smoked throughout the pregnancy, and now fundal height measurements are suggestive of growth restriction in the fetus. In addition to ultrasound to measure fetal size, what would be another tool useful in confirming the diagnosis?
   a. Doppler blood flow analysis
   b. Contraction stress test
   c. Amniocentesis
   d. Daily fetal movement counts

29-5 A 41-week pregnant multigravida presents in the labor and delivery unit after a nonstress test indicated that her fetus could be experiencing some difficulties in utero. Which diagnostic tool would yield more detailed information about the fetus?
   a. Ultrasound for fetal anomalies
   b. Biophysical profile
   c. Maternal serum alpha-fetoprotein screening
   d. Percutaneous umbilical blood sampling

29-6 At 35 weeks of pregnancy, a woman experiences preterm labor. Although tocolytics are administered and she is placed on bed rest, she continues to experience regular uterine contractions, and her cervix is beginning to dilate and efface. What would be an important test for fetal well-being at this time?
   a. Percutaneous umbilical blood sampling
   b. Ultrasound for fetal size
   c. Amniocentesis for fetal lung maturity
   d. Nonstress test

29-7 A 38-year-old woman is at 16 weeks' gestation. Because of the woman's age, which of the following diagnostic tests and procedures is the obstetrician most likely to perform at this time?
   a. Ultrasound
   b. Contraction stress test
   c. Chorionic villus sampling
   d. Triple marker test

29-8 A laboring woman's membranes rupture, and meconium is noted in the amniotic fluid. The baby's heart rate and variability are noted to be normal on the fetal monitor. How should care providers respond to this occurrence?
   a. Prepare the woman for an immediate cesarean birth.
   b. Assess the woman's vital signs more frequently.
   c. Perform a vaginal examination.
   d. Anticipate the need for early suctioning at the time of birth.

29-9 A 40-year-old pregnant woman is 10 weeks pregnant. Which diagnostic tool would be appropriate to suggest to her at this time?
   a. Biophysical profile
   b. Amniocentesis
   c. Maternal serum alpha-fetoprotein
   d. Chorionic villus sampling

29-10 A 30-year-old gravida 3, para 2 0 0 2 is at 18 weeks' gestation by dates. At this time, what screening test should be suggested to her?
   a. Biophysical profile
   b. Amniocentesis for genetic anomalies
   c. Maternal serum alpha-fetoprotein screening
   d. Screening for diabetes mellitus

29-11 A maternal serum alpha-fetoprotein test indicates an elevated level. It is repeated and again is reported as higher than normal. What would be the next step in the assessment sequence to determine the well-being of the fetus?
   a. Percutaneous umbilical blood sampling
   b. Ultrasound for fetal anomalies
   c. Biophysical profile for fetal well-being
   d. Amniocentesis for genetic anomalies

# CHAPTER 30

## Hypertensive Disorders in Pregnancy

30-1 A primigravida is being monitored in her prenatal clinic for pregnancy-induced hypertension (PIH). Which of the following should concern her nurse?
   a. Blood pressure increase to 138/86 mm Hg
   b. Weight gain of 0.5 kg during the past 2 weeks
   c. A dipstick value of 3+ for protein in her urine
   d. Pitting pedal edema at the end of the day

30-2 The labor of a pregnant woman with preeclampsia is going to be induced. Before initiating the Pitocin infusion, the nurse reviews the woman's latest laboratory test findings that reveal a platelet count of 90,000, an elevated AST level, and a falling hematocrit. The nurse notifies the physician because the lab results are indicative of:
   a. Eclampsia
   b. Disseminated intravascular coagulation
   c. HELLP syndrome
   d. Idiopathic thrombocytopenia

30-3 The nurse has educated a pregnant woman at 30 weeks' gestation regarding signs and symptoms of preeclampsia and warning signs of possible complications. The nurse determines that the woman needs more instruction when she states:
   a. "If I have changes in my vision, I will notify my physician."
   b. "I will weigh myself every morning before breakfast after voiding and call my doctor if I notice a weight gain of 0.5 kg or greater in 1 week."
   c. "I will count my baby's movements twice a day, in the morning and in the evening after I eat."
   d. "If I have a headache, I will take Tylenol."

30-4 A woman with preeclampsia has a seizure. The nurse's primary duty during the seizure is to:
   a. Insert an oral airway
   b. Suction the mouth to prevent aspiration
   c. Administer oxygen by mask
   d. Stay with the client and call for help

30-5 A pregnant woman has been receiving a magnesium sulfate infusion for treatment of severe preeclampsia. On assessment the nurse finds the following vital signs: T = 37.3° C, P = 88, R = 10, BP = 148/90, absent DTRs, and no ankle clonus. The client complains, "I'm so thirsty and warm." The nurse:

a. Calls for a stat magnesium sulfate level
b. Administers oxygen
c. Discontinues the magnesium sulfate infusion
d. Prepares to administer hydralazine

30-6 A woman with severe preeclampsia has been receiving magnesium sulfate by intravenous infusion for 8 hours for preeclampsia. The nurse assesses the woman and documents the following findings: T = 37.1° C, P = 96, R = 24, BP = 155/112, 3+ DTRs, and no ankle clonus. The nurse calls the physician, anticipating an order for:

a. Hydralazine
b. Magnesium sulfate bolus
c. Diazepam
d. Calcium gluconate

30-7 A woman at 39 weeks' gestation with a history of PIH is admitted to the labor and birth unit. She suddenly experiences increased contraction frequency of every 1 to 2 minutes, dark red vaginal bleeding, and a tense, painful abdomen. The nurse suspects the onset of:

a. Eclamptic seizure
b. Rupture of the uterus
c. Active labor stage
d. Abruptio placentae

30-8 A woman with worsening preeclampsia is admitted to the hospital's labor and birth unit. The physician explains the plan of care regarding severe preeclampsia, including the induction of labor, to the woman and her husband. The nurse determines that the couple needs further information when the woman's husband says:

a. "I will help my wife use the breathing techniques that we learned in our childbirth classes."
b. "I will give my wife clear liquids to drink during labor."
c. "Since we will be here for awhile, I will call my friend so that we can all watch the football game here in the room."
d. "I will stay with my wife during her labor just as we planned."

30-9 A woman with severe preeclampsia is receiving magnesium sulfate infusion. The nurse becomes concerned after assessment when the woman exhibits:

a. A sleepy, sedated affect
b. A respiratory rate of 10 breaths per minute
c. Deep tendon reflexes of 2+
d. Absent ankle clonus

# CHAPTER 31

## Antepartal Hemorrhagic Disorders

31-1 A woman presents to the emergency department complaining of bleeding and cramping. Initial nursing history is significant for a last menstrual period 6 weeks ago. On sterile speculum examination, the primary care provider finds that the cervix is closed. The anticipated plan of care for this woman would be based on a probable diagnosis of which type of spontaneous abortion?
   a. Incomplete
   b. Inevitable
   c. Threatened
   d. Septic

31-2 A pregnant woman is being discharged from the hospital after placement of cerclage because of a history of recurrent pregnancy loss secondary to an incompetent cervix. Discharge teaching should emphasize that:
   a. Any vaginal discharge should be reported immediately to her care provider
   b. The presence of any uterine cramping or low backache may indicate preterm labor and should be reported
   c. She will need to make arrangements for care at home because her activity level will be restricted
   d. She will be scheduled for a cesarean birth

31-3 The perinatal nurse is giving discharge instructions to a woman status post–suction curettage secondary to a hydatidiform mole. The woman asks why she must take oral contraceptives for the next 12 months. The best response for the nurse would be:
   a. "If you get pregnant within 1 year, the chances of a successful pregnancy are very small. Therefore, if you desire a future pregnancy, it would be better for you to use the most reliable method of contraception available."
   b. "The major risk to you after a molar pregnancy is a type of cancer that can only be diagnosed by measuring the same hormone that your body produces during pregnancy. If you were to get pregnant, it would make the diagnosis of this cancer more difficult."
   c. "If you can avoid a pregnancy for the next year, the chance of developing a second molar pregnancy is rare. Therefore, to improve your chance of a successful pregnancy, it is better not to get pregnant at this time."
   d. "Oral contraceptives are the only form of birth control that will prevent a recurrence of a molar pregnancy."

31-4 The clinical manifestation of a placenta previa that differs from a placental abruption is the absence of:
   a. Bleeding
   b. Intensifying abdominal pain
   c. Uterine activity
   d. Cramping

31-5 Which of the following laboratory markers is indicative of disseminated intravascular coagulation?
   a. Bleeding time of 10 minutes
   b. Presence of fibrin split products
   c. Thrombocytopenia
   d. Hyperfibrinogenemia

31-6 In caring for the woman with DIC, the nurse should anticipate which of the following orders?
   a. Administration of blood
   b. Preparation of client for invasive hemodynamic monitoring
   c. Restriction of intravascular fluids
   d. Administration of steroids

31-7 Methotrexate is recommended as part of the treatment plan for which of the following obstetric complications?
   a. Complete hydatidiform mole
   b. Missed abortion
   c. Unruptured ectopic pregnancy
   d. Abruptio placentae

# CHAPTER 32

## Endocrine and Metabolic Disorders

32-1 In assessing the knowledge of a pregestational woman with diabetes concerning changing insulin needs during pregnancy, the nurse recognizes that further teaching is warranted when the client states:
   a. "I will need to increase my insulin dosage during the first 3 months of pregnancy."
   b. "Insulin dosage will likely need to be increased during the second and third trimesters."
   c. "Episodes of hypoglycemia are more likely to occur during the first 3 months."
   d. "Insulin needs should return to normal within 7 to 10 days after birth if I am bottle feeding."

32-2 Preconception counseling is critical to the outcome of diabetic pregnancy because poor glycemic control before and during early pregnancy is associated with:
   a. Frequent episodes of maternal hypoglycemia
   b. Congenital anomalies in the fetus
   c. Polyhydramnios
   d. Hyperemesis gravidarum

32-3 In planning for the care of a 30-year-old woman with pregestational diabetes, the nurse recognizes that the most important factor affecting pregnancy outcome is the:
   a. Mother's age
   b. Number of years since diabetes was diagnosed
   c. Amount of insulin required prenatally
   d. Degree of glycemic control during pregnancy

32-4  During a prenatal visit, the nurse is explaining dietary management to a woman with pregestational diabetes. The nurse evaluates that teaching has been effective when the woman states:
a. "I will need to eat 600 more calories per day since I am pregnant."
b. "I can continue with the same diet as before pregnancy, as long as it is well-balanced."
c. "Diet and insulin needs change during pregnancy."
d. "I will plan my diet based on results of urine glucose testing."

32-5  In teaching the woman with pregestational diabetes about desired glucose levels, the nurse explains that a normal fasting glucose level, such as before breakfast, is in the range of:
a. 65 to 95 mg/dl
b. 90 to 120 mg/dl
c. 120 to 150 mg/dl
d. 150 to 180 mg/dl

32-6  The nurse is reviewing a pregnant woman's health history at her first prenatal visit at 10 weeks' gestation. Which of the following would indicate that the woman is at risk for developing gestational diabetes during this pregnancy?
a. She is 28 years old.
b. Her first baby was delivered by cesarean.
c. There is a family history of type I diabetes.
d. Her last baby weighed 4.5 kg (10 lb) at birth.

32-7  Screening at 24 weeks revealed that a pregnant woman has gestational diabetes mellitus (GDM). In planning her care, the nurse and the woman mutually agree that an expected outcome is to prevent injury to the fetus as a result of GDM. The nurse identifies that the fetus is at greatest risk for:
a. Macrosomia
b. Congenital anomalies of the central nervous system
c. Preterm birth
d. Low birth weight

32-8  A 26-year-old primigravida has come to the clinic for her regular prenatal visit at 12 weeks. She appears thin and somewhat nervous; she reports that she eats a well-balanced diet although her weight is 5 pounds less than her last visit. The results of laboratory studies confirm that she has a hyperthyroid condition. Based on the available data, the nurse formulates a plan of care. Which of the following nursing diagnoses is most appropriate for the woman at this time?
a. Fluid volume deficit
b. Altered nutrition: less than body requirements
c. Altered nutrition: more than body requirements
d. Sleep pattern disturbance

32-9  Maternal phenylketonuria is an important health concern during pregnancy because:
a. It is a recognized cause of preterm labor
b. The fetus may develop neurologic problems
c. A pregnant woman is more likely to die without dietary control
d. Women with phenylketonuria are usually retarded and should not reproduce

# CHAPTER 33

## Medical-Surgical Problems in Pregnancy

33-1  When caring for a pregnant woman with cardiac problems, the nurse must be alert for signs and symptoms of cardiac decompensation, which are:
   a. A regular heart rate and hypertension
   b. An increased urinary output, tachycardia, and dry cough
   c. Shortness of breath, bradycardia, and hypertension
   d. Dyspnea, crackles, and an irregular weak pulse

33-2  Prophylaxis of subacute bacterial endocarditis (SBE) is given before and after birth when a pregnant woman has:
   a. Valvular disease
   b. Congestive heart disease
   c. Arrhythmias
   d. Postmyocardial infarction

33-3  Postpartum care of the woman with cardiac disease:
   a. Is the same for any pregnant woman
   b. Includes rest, stool softeners, and monitoring the effect of activity
   c. Includes ambulating frequently, alternating with active ROM
   d. Includes limiting visits of the infant to once per day

33-4  A woman was anemic during her pregnancy. She had been taking iron for 3 months before the birth. She gave birth by cesarean 2 days ago and has been having problems with constipation. After assisting her back to bed from the bathroom, the nurse notes that the woman's stools are dark (greenish black). The nurse would:
   a. Perform a guaiac test and record the results
   b. Recognize the finding as abnormal and report it to the primary health care provider
   c. Recognize the finding as normal, as a result of iron therapy
   d. Check the woman's next stool to validate the observation

33-5  In assisting with labor and birth of a woman with pulmonary disease, which drug would not be used because it causes bronchospasm?
   a. Pitocin
   b. Aminophylline
   c. Morphine
   d. Fentanyl

33-6  In providing nutritional counseling for the pregnant woman experiencing cholecystitis, the nurse would:
   a. Assess the client's dietary history for adequate calories and proteins
   b. Instruct the client that the bulk of calories should come from proteins
   c. Instruct the client to eat a low-fat diet and to avoid fried food
   d. Instruct the client to eat a low-cholesterol, low-salt diet

33-7 In caring for a pregnant woman with sickle cell anemia with the increased blood viscosity, the nurse is concerned about the development of a thromboembolism. The nursing care would include:
   a. Monitoring the client for a negative Homan's sign
   b. Massaging calves when the woman complains of pain
   c. Applying antiembolic stockings
   d. Maintaining a restriction on fluid intake

33-8 Appendicitis is more difficult to diagnose during pregnancy because the appendix is:
   a. Covered by the uterus
   b. Displaced to the left
   c. Low and to the right
   d. High and to the right

33-9 Postoperative care of the pregnant woman who requires abdominal surgery for appendicitis includes which additional assessment?
   a. Intake and output, intravenous site
   b. Signs and symptoms of infection
   c. Vital signs and incision
   d. Fetal heart rate and uterine activity

# CHAPTER 34

## Obstetric Critical Care

34-1 The nurse caring for a pregnant woman at 32 weeks' gestation with the diagnosis of severe preeclampsia with pulmonary edema is assisting with the insertion of a pulmonary artery catheter. As the catheter enters the right ventricle, the main priority of nursing assessments is to:
   a. Assess fetal response to the procedure
   b. Monitor for premature ventricular contractions
   c. Monitor maternal vital signs, especially blood pressure changes
   d. Observe for complaint of sudden chest pain

34-2 A pregnant woman at 38 weeks' gestation has severe preeclampsia with refractory oliguria. A pulmonary artery catheter is inserted and the following hemodynamic profile is obtained: CVP, 2 mm Hg; PAP, 17/4 mm Hg; PCWP, 4 mm Hg; CO, 5.1 L/min. One hour after treatment, the hemodynamic profile changes to the following: CVP, 2 mm Hg; PAP, 25/7 mm Hg; PCWP, 7 mm Hg; CO, 6.4 L/min. The nurse evaluates the woman's condition as:
   a. Improving, as the hemodynamic profile is normal
   b. Improving; the cardiac output is greater but with hypervolemia
   c. No better, as right preload has not changed
   d. Worsening, as pulmonary edema is rapidly developing

34-3 The nurse caring for a critically ill pregnant woman at 36 weeks' gestation with a pulmonary artery catheter in place obtains the following hemodynamic profile: CVP, 3 mm Hg; PAP, 40/18 mm Hg; PCWP, 18 mm Hg; CO, 7 L/min. Which hemodynamic value(s) is (are) normal?
a. CVP only
b. CO and CVP
c. PAP and PCWP
d. PAP only

34-4 The nurse caring for a critically ill pregnant woman at 36 weeks' gestation with a pulmonary artery catheter in place obtains the following hemodynamic profile: CVP, 3 mm Hg; PAP, 40/18 mm Hg; PCWP, 18 mm Hg; CO, 7 L/min. The nurse interprets the hemodynamic profile as correlating with:
a. High left preload
b. High right preload
c. Low left preload
d. Normal right preload

34-5 The nurse caring for a critically ill pregnant woman at 36 weeks' gestation with a pulmonary artery catheter in place obtains the following hemodynamic profile: CVP, 3 mm Hg; PAP, 40/18 mm Hg; PCWP, 18 mm Hg; CO, 7 L/min. This hemodynamic profile correlates with the client having the most difficulty with maintaining adequate:
a. Blood pressure to perfuse tissues
b. Contractility of her myocardium
c. Delivery of blood to tissues
d. Oxygen exchange

34-6 The nurse caring for a critically ill pregnant woman at 36 weeks' gestation with a pulmonary artery catheter in place obtains the following hemodynamic profile: CVP, 3 mm Hg; PAP, 40/18 mm Hg; PCWP, 18 mm Hg; CO, 7 L/min. The nurse administers a diuretic drug as ordered for the client. From evaluation of the hemodynamic profile, the nurse recognizes that this drug was given to treat:
a. Cardiogenic pulmonary edema
b. Hypovolemia
c. Noncardiogenic pulmonary edema
d. Preeclampsia or eclampsia

34-7 The nurse assessing for internal hemorrhage after blunt abdominal trauma in the pregnant woman at 28 weeks' gestation will most closely observe for:
a. Alteration in maternal vital signs, especially blood pressure
b. Complaints of abdominal pain
c. Changes in FHR patterns
d. Vaginal bleeding

34-8 A pregnant woman at 33 weeks' gestation is brought to the birthing unit after a minor automobile accident. She has no pain and no vaginal bleeding, her vital signs are stable, and FHR is good. The nurse should plan to:
   a. Monitor the woman for a ruptured spleen
   b. Obtain a physician order to discharge her home
   c. Transfer her to the trauma unit
   d. Use continuous electronic fetal monitoring for 2 to 4 hours

34-9 A pregnant woman at term is transported to the emergency room after a severe vehicular accident. The obstetric nurse responds and rushes to the ER with a fetal monitor. A cardiopulmonary arrest occurs as the OB nurse arrives. The first thing for the ER and OB team to do is to:
   a. Obtain IV access and start aggressive fluid resuscitation
   b. Quickly apply the fetal monitor to determine if the fetus is alive
   c. Start cardiopulmonary resuscitation
   d. Transfer her to the operating room for an emergency cesarean birth in case the fetus is still alive

# CHAPTER 35

## Mental Health Disorders and Substance Abuse

35-1 Common symptoms of postpartum blues are:
   a. Anxiety, panic attacks, insomnia, and disinterest in the infant
   b. Delusions, hallucinations, disorganized speech, and catatonic behavior
   c. Flight of ideas, distractibility, psychomotor agitation, and a decreased need for sleep
   d. Mood swings, anxiety, tears, and fatigue

35-2 Immediate intervention for the pregnant woman with bipolar disorder is necessary when the following symptoms are present:
   a. Dehydration and lack of sleep
   b. Decreased appetite and flight of ideas
   c. Hyperactivity and distractibility
   d. Pressured speech and grandiosity

35-3 One of the main concerns when a woman is diagnosed with postpartum depression with psychotic features is that she may:
   a. Have outbursts of anger
   b. Neglect her hygiene
   c. Harm her infant
   d. Lose interest in her husband

35-4 An appropriate nursing diagnosis for a pregnant woman who is verbalizing suicidal thoughts is risk for:
   a. Injury to fetus related to potential maternal suicide
   b. Altered parenting related to suicidal threats
   c. Ineffective coping related to poor impulse control
   d. Self-care deficit related to preservation of suicidal thoughts

35-5 Psychotropic medications, such as antidepressants, may be given to the pregnant woman if she is:
a. Unable to care for herself
b. Followed by a case manager
c. In a psychiatric hospital
d. Threatening a suicide attempt

35-6 During inpatient psychiatric hospitalization, it is important for the new mother to have:
a. Contact with her significant other
b. Supervised and guided visits with her baby
c. No contact with anyone who irritates her
d. The baby with her at all times

35-7 Alcohol withdrawal may be manifested as:
a. Nausea and vomiting, agitation, restlessness, and tremors of the hands
b. Drinking binges, delusions, panic attacks, and tears
c. Overprotective responses, sleepiness, fatigue, and distractibility
d. Emotional highs, grandiosity, delusions, and calmness

35-8 What is an opiate that causes euphoria, relaxation, drowsiness, and detachment from reality?
a. Heroin
b. Alcohol
c. PCP
d. Cocaine

# CHAPTER 36

## Preterm Labor and Birth

36-1 Which of the following women is most likely to be at risk for preterm labor?
a. One who has a rupture of membranes at 30 weeks' gestation
b. One who is Native American and 30 years old
c. One whose mother has diabetes and hypertension
d. One who is Hispanic with a history of urinary tract infections

36-2 In planning for home care of a woman with preterm labor, which of the following concerns needs to be addressed?
a. Nursing assessments will be different than those done in the hospital setting.
b. Restricted activity and medications will be necessary to prevent recurrence of preterm labor.
c. Prolonged bed rest may cause negative physiologic effects.
d. Home health care providers will be necessary.

36-3 The nurse providing care for a woman with preterm labor on terbutaline would include which of the following interventions to identify side effects of the drug?
a. Assess deep tendon reflexes
b. Assess breath sounds
c. Assess for bradycardia
d. Assess for hypoglycemia

36-4 In evaluating the effectiveness of magnesium sulfate for treatment of preterm labor, which of the following findings would alert the nurse to possible side effects?
a. Urine output of 160 ml in 4 hours
b. Deep tendon reflexes 2+ and no clonus
c. Respiratory rate of 16 breaths per minute
d. Serum magnesium level of 10 mg/dl

36-5 A woman in preterm labor at 30 weeks' gestation receives two 12-mg doses of betamethasone intramuscularly. The purpose of this pharmacologic treatment is to:
a. Stimulate fetal surfactant production
b. Reduce maternal and fetal tachycardia associated with ritodrine administration
c. Suppress uterine contractions
d. Maintain adequate maternal respiratory effort and ventilation during magnesium sulfate therapy

36-6 A woman at 26 weeks' gestation is being assessed to determine if she is experiencing preterm labor. Which of the following findings indicates that preterm labor is occurring?
a. Estriol is found in maternal saliva.
b. Irregular mild uterine contractions are occurring every 12 to 15 minutes.
c. Fetal fibronectin is present in vaginal secretions.
d. The cervix is effacing and dilated to 2 cm.

# CHAPTER 37

## Labor and Birth Complications

37-1 A primigravida at 40 weeks' gestation is having uterine contractions every $1\frac{1}{2}$ to 2 minutes and says that they are very painful. Her cervix is dilated 2 cm and has not changed in 3 hours. The woman is crying and wants an epidural. What is the likely status of this woman's labor?
a. She is exhibiting a protracted active phase.
b. She is experiencing a normal latent stage.
c. She is exhibiting hypertonic uterine dysfunction.
d. She is experiencing pelvic dystocia.

37-2 Which of the following assessments is least likely to be associated with a breech presentation?
a. Meconium-stained amniotic fluid
b. Fetal heart tones heard at or above the maternal umbilicus
c. Preterm labor and birth
d. Postterm gestation

37-3 A woman is having her first baby. She has been in labor for 15 hours. Two hours ago her vaginal examination revealed the cervix to be dilated to 5 cm, 100% effaced, and the presenting part to be at station 0. Five minutes ago her vaginal examination result indicated that there had been no change. What abnormal labor pattern is associated with this description?
a. Prolonged latent phase
b. Protracted active phase
c. Arrest of active phase
d. Protracted descent

37-4 In evaluating the effectiveness of oxytocin induction, the nurse would expect:
  a. Contractions lasting 40 to 90 seconds, 2 to 3 minutes apart
  b. The intensity of contractions to be at least 110 to 130 mm Hg
  c. Labor to progress at least 2 cm/hr dilation
  d. That at least 30 mU/min of oxytocin will be needed to achieve cervical dilation

37-5 In planning for an expected cesarean birth for a woman who has given birth by cesarean previously and who has a fetus in the transverse presentation, the nurse would include which of the following information?
  a. "Since this is a repeat procedure, you are at the lowest risk for complications."
  b. "Even though this is your second cesarean birth, you may wish to review the preoperative and postoperative procedures."
  c. "Since this is your second cesarean birth, you will recover faster."
  d. "You will not need preoperative teaching since this is your second cesarean birth."

37-6 For a woman at 42 weeks' gestation, which of the following findings would be a concern to the nurse?
  a. Fetal heart rate of 116 bpm
  b. Cervix dilated 2 cm and 50% effaced
  c. Score of 8 on the biophysical profile
  d. One fetal movement noted in 1 hour of assessment by the mother

37-7 A pregnant woman's amniotic membranes rupture. Prolapsed cord is suspected. Which of the following interventions would be the top priority?
  a. Place the woman in the knee-chest position.
  b. Cover the cord in sterile gauze soaked in saline.
  c. Prepare the woman for a cesarean birth.
  d. Start oxygen by face mask.

37-8 Prepidil has been ordered for a pregnant woman at 43 weeks' gestation. The nurse recognizes that this medication will be administered to:
  a. Enhance uteroplacental perfusion in an aging placenta
  b. Increase amniotic fluid volume
  c. Ripen the cervix in preparation for labor induction
  d. Stimulate the amniotic membranes to rupture

# CHAPTER 38

## Postpartum Complications

38-1 The perinatal nurse is caring for a woman in the immediate postbirth period. Assessment reveals that the woman is experiencing profuse bleeding, The most likely etiology for the bleeding is:
  a. Uterine atony
  b. Uterine inversion
  c. Vaginal hematoma
  d. Vaginal laceration

38-2 A primary nursing responsibility when caring for a woman experiencing an obstetric hemorrhage is to:
a. Establish venous access
b. Monitor maternal vital signs
c. Prepare the woman for surgical intervention
d. Start an infusion of Methergine

38-3 Late postpartum hemorrhage is most likely caused by:
a. Subinvolution of the placental site
b. Defective vascularity of the decidua
c. Cervical lacerations
d. Coagulation disorders

38-4 The most common cause of postpartum hemorrhage is:
a. Uterine atony
b. DIC
c. Lacerations
d. Retained placenta

38-5 Which of the following women is at greatest risk for early postpartum hemorrhage?
a. A primiparous woman (G 2 P-1-0-0-1) being prepared for an emergency cesarean birth for fetal distress
b. A woman with severe preeclampsia on magnesium sulfate whose labor is being induced
c. A multiparous woman (G 3 P-2-0-0-2) with an 8-hour labor
d. A primigravida in spontaneous labor with preterm twins

38-6 The first and most important nursing intervention when a nurse observes profuse postpartum bleeding is to:
a. Call the woman's primary health care provider
b. Administer the standing order for an oxytocic
c. Palpate the uterus and massage it if boggy
d. Assess maternal blood pressure and pulse for signs for hypovolemic shock

38-7 When caring for a postpartum woman experiencing hemorrhagic shock, the nurse recognizes that the most objective and least invasive assessment of adequate organ perfusion and oxygenation is:
a. Absence of cyanosis in the buccal mucosa
b. Cool, dry skin
c. Diminished restlessness
d. Urinary output of at least 30 ml/hour

38-8 The most effective and least expensive treatment of puerperal infection is prevention. Which of the following is important in this strategy?
a. Large doses of vitamin C during pregnancy
b. Prophylactic antibiotics
c. Strict aseptic technique, including handwashing, by all health care personnel
d. Limited protein and fat intake

38-9 One of the first symptoms of puerperal infection to assess for in the postpartum woman is:
   a. Fatigue
   b. Pain
   c. Profuse vaginal bleeding
   d. Temperature of 38° C (100.4° F) or higher on two successive days starting 24 hours after birth

38-10 Acute mastitis can be avoided by:
   a. Washing nipples and breasts with mild soap and water once a day
   b. Using proper breastfeeding techniques
   c. Wearing a nipple shield for the first few days of breastfeeding
   d. Wearing a supportive bra 24 hours a day

# CHAPTER 39

## Acquired Problems of the Newborn

39-1 A macrosomic infant is born after a difficult, forceps-assisted delivery. After stabilization, the infant is weighed, and the birth weight is 4550 grams (9 pounds, 6 ounces). The nurse's most appropriate action is to:
   a. Leave the infant in the room with the mother
   b. Take the infant immediately to the nursery
   c. Perform a gestational age assessment to determine if the infant is large for gestational age
   d. Monitor blood glucose levels frequently and observe closely for signs of hypoglycemia

39-2 A 3.8-kg infant was delivered vaginally at 39 weeks after a 30-minute second stage. There was a nuchal cord. After birth, the infant is noted to have petechiae over the face and upper back. Information given to this infant's parents should be based on the knowledge that petechiae:
   a. Are benign if they disappear within 48 hours of birth
   b. Result from increased blood volume
   c. Should always be further investigated
   d. Usually occur with forceps delivery

39-3 When planning care for an infant with a fractured clavicle, the nurse should recognize that in addition to gentle handling:
   a. Prone positioning will facilitate bone alignment
   b. No special treatment is necessary
   c. Parents should be taught range-of-motion exercises
   d. The shoulder should be immobilized with a splint

39-4 Infants of mothers with diabetes are at higher risk for developing:
   a. Anemia
   b. Hyponatremia
   c. Macrosomia
   d. Sepsis

39-5 A baby was born 2 hours ago at 37 weeks' gestation, weighing 4.1 kg. The baby appears chubby with a flushed complexion and is very tremulous. The tremors are most likely the result of:
a. Birth injury
b. Hypocalcemia
c. Hypoglycemia
d. Seizures

39-6 A pregnant woman at 37 weeks' gestation has had ruptured membranes for 26 hours. A cesarean section is performed for failure to progress. Fetal heart rate before birth is 180 with limited variability. At birth, the newborn had Apgar scores of 6 and 7 at 1 and 5 minutes and is noted to be pale and tachypneic. Based on the maternal history, the cause of this newborn's distress is most likely to be:
a. Hypoglycemia
b. Phrenic nerve injury
c. Respiratory distress syndrome
d. Sepsis

39-7 The most important nursing action in preventing neonatal infection is:
a. Good handwashing
b. Isolation of infected infants
c. Separate gown technique
d. Standard Precautions

39-8 A pregnant woman presents in labor at term, having had no prenatal care. After birth, her infant is noted to be small for gestational age with small eyes, a thin upper lip, and microcephaly. Based on her infant's physical findings, this woman should be questioned regarding her use of which substance during pregnancy?
a. Alcohol
b. Cocaine
c. Heroin
d. Marijuana

39-9 A plan of care for an infant experiencing symptoms of drug withdrawal should include:
a. Administering chloral hydrate for sedation
b. Feeding q 4-6 h to allow extra rest
c. Swaddling the infant snugly and holding tightly
d. Playing soft music during feeding

# CHAPTER 40

## Hemolytic Disorders and Congenital Anomalies

40-1 Kernicterus occurs if:
a. The kidney excretes bilirubin
b. Bilirubin collects in the liver
c. Bilirubin deposits are concentrated in the cardiac muscle
d. Bilirubin deposits are in the brain

40-2 Which of the following supports the diagnosis of pathologic jaundice?
   a. Serum bilirubin concentrations greater than 2 mg/dl in cord blood
   b. Serum bilirubin levels increasing more than 1 mg/dl in 24 hours
   c. Serum bilirubin levels greater than 10 mg/dl in a full-term newborn
   d. Clinical jaundice evident within 24 hours of birth

40-3 The most common cause of pathologic hyperbilirubinemia is:
   a. Hepatic disease
   b. Hemolytic disorders in the newborn
   c. Postmaturity
   d. Congenital heart defect

40-4 Which of the following infants would be more likely to have Rh incompatibility?
   a. Infant of an Rh-negative mother and a father who is Rh positive and homozygous for the Rh factor
   b. Infant who is Rh negative and mother is Rh negative
   c. Infant of an Rh-negative mother and a father who is Rh positive and heterozygous for the Rh factor
   d. Infant who is Rh positive and mother who is Rh positive

40-5 A major nursing intervention for an infant born with myelomeningocele is to:
   a. Protect the sac from injury
   b. Prepare the parents for the child's paralysis from the waist down
   c. Prepare the parents for the closure of the sac at around 2 years old
   d. Assess for cyanosis

40-6 The priority nursing diagnosis for a newborn diagnosed with a diaphragmatic hernia would be:
   a. Risk for altered parent-infant attachment
   b. Altered nutrition: less than body requirements
   c. Risk for infection
   d. Impaired gas exchange

40-7 An infant diagnosed with erythroblastosis fetalis would characteristically exhibit:
   a. Edema
   b. Immature red blood cells
   c. Enlargement of the heart
   d. Ascites

# CHAPTER 41

## Nursing Care of the High Risk Newborn

41-1 A 36-week gestation infant has increasing respirations (80 to 100 breaths per minute with marked substernal retractions). The infant is given oxygen by nasal CPAP. Which of the following arterial oxygen levels would indicate hypoxia?
   a. $PaO_2$ of 67
   b. $PaO_2$ of 89
   c. $PaO_2$ of 45
   d. $PaO_2$ of 73

41-2 A premature infant who requires an incubator and gavage feedings will be transferred closer to home. What physiologic parameter would indicate that the infant was stable for transfer?
a. Oxygen saturation greater than 92% when crying
b. Respiratory rate greater than 60 breaths per minute when sleeping
c. Three apnea spells in the past 24 hours
d. Oxygen saturation 85% to 90% when sleeping

41-3 On day 3 of life, a newborn continues to require 100% oxygen by nasal cannula. The parents ask if they can hold their baby during his next gavage feeding. Given that this newborn is physiologically stable, what response would the nurse give?
a. "Parents are not allowed to hold their infants who are dependent on oxygen."
b. "You may only hold your baby's hand during the feeding."
c. "Feedings cause more stress, so the baby must be closely monitored."
d. "You may hold your baby during the feeding."

41-4 A premature infant with respiratory distress syndrome receives artificial surfactant. How would the nurse explain surfactant therapy to the parents?
a. Surfactant improves the ability of your baby's lungs to exchange oxygen and carbon dioxide.
b. The drug keeps your baby from requiring too much sedation.
c. Surfactant is used to reduce episodes of periodic breathing.
d. Your baby needs this medication to fight a possible respiratory tract infection.

41-5 A 1550 g infant is to be weaned from the incubator to an open crib. Which of the following should the nurse prepare ahead of the weaning process?
a. A crib with prewarmed blankets
b. A shirt and a cap
c. An incubator servo control probe
d. A digital rectal thermometer

41-6 When providing an infant with a gavage feeding, which of the following should be documented each time?
a. The infant's abdominal circumference after the feeding
b. The infant's heart rate and respirations
c. The infant's suck and swallow coordination
d. The infant's response to the feeding

41-7 An infant is to receive gastrostomy feedings. What intervention should the nurse institute to prevent bloating, gastrointestinal reflux into the esophagus, vomiting, and respiratory compromise?
a. Rapid bolusing of the entire amount in 15 minutes
b. Warm cloths to the abdomen for the first 10 minutes
c. Slow, small, warm bolus feedings over 30 minutes
d. Cold, medium bolus feedings over 20 minutes

41-8 A premature infant never seems to sleep longer than an hour at a time. Each time a light is turned on, an incubator closes, or people talk near her crib, she wakes up and cries inconsolably until held. The correct nursing diagnosis is ineffective coping related to:
a. Severe immaturity
b. Environmental stress
c. Physiologic distress
d. Interpersonal interactions

41-9 Which of the following combinations of expressing pain could be demonstrated in a neonate?
a. Low-pitched crying, tachycardia, eyelids open wide
b. Cry face, flaccid limbs, closed mouth
c. High-pitched cry, withdrawal, change in heart rate
d. Cry face, eye squeeze, no change in blood pressure

41-10 A 26-week gestation infant arrives from the delivery room intubated. The nurse weighs the infant, places him under the radiant warmer, and attaches him to the ventilator at the prescribed settings. A pulse oximeter and cardiorespiratory monitor are placed. The pulse oximeter is recording oxygen saturations of 80%. The prescribed saturations are 92%. The nurse's most appropriate action would be to:
a. Listen to breath sounds and ensure patency of the endotracheal tube, increase oxygen, and notify physician
b. Continue to observe and make no changes until the saturations are 75%
c. Continue with the admission process to ensure that a thorough assessment is completed
d. Notify the parents that their infant is not doing well

41-11 A newborn was admitted to the NICU after being delivered at 29 weeks' gestation to a 28-year-old multiparous, married, Caucasian female whose pregnancy was uncomplicated until premature rupture of membranes and preterm birth. The newborn's parents arrive for their first visit after the birth. The parents walk toward the bedside but remain approximately 5 feet away from the bed. The nurse's most appropriate action would be to:
a. Wait quietly at the newborn's bedside until the parents come closer
b. Go to the parents, introduce himself or herself, and gently encourage them to come meet their infant; explain the equipment first and then focus on the newborn
c. Leave the parents at the bedside while they are visiting so that they can have some privacy
d. Tell the parents only about the newborn's physical condition and caution them to avoid touching their baby

41-12 Necrotizing enterocolitis (NEC) is an inflammatory disease of the gastrointestinal mucosa. The signs of NEC are nonspecific. Some generalized signs include:
a. Hypertonia, tachycardia, and metabolic alkalosis
b. Abdominal distention, temperature instability, and grossly bloody stools
c. Hypertension, absence of apnea, and ruddy skin color
d. Scaphoid abdomen, no residual with feedings, and increased urinary output

41-13 An infant was being discharged from the NICU after 70 days of hospitalization. This infant was born at 30 weeks' gestation with several conditions associated with prematurity, including respiratory distress syndrome, mild bronchopulmonary dysplasia, and retinopathy of prematurity requiring surgical treatment. The infant's mother asks the nurse during discharge teaching if her baby will meet developmental milestones on time as her son did who was born at term. The nurse's most appropriate response would be:
a. "Your baby will develop exactly like your first child did."
b. "Your baby does not appear to have any problems at the present time."
c. "Your baby will need to be corrected for prematurity. Your baby is currently 40 weeks' post-conceptional age and can be expected to be doing what a 40-week infant would be doing."
d. "Your baby will never be normal."

41-14 A pregnant woman was admitted for induction of labor at 43 weeks' gestation with sure dates. A nonstress test in the obstetrician's office revealed a nonreactive tracing. Upon artificial rupture of membranes, thick meconium-stained fluid was noted. The nurse caring for the baby after birth should anticipate which of the following?
a. Meconium aspiration, hypoglycemia, and dry cracked skin
b. Excessive vernix caseosa covering the skin, closed sleepy eyes, and respiratory distress syndrome
c. Golden yellow to green stained skin and nails, absence of scalp hair, and increased amount of subcutaneous fat
d. Hyperglycemia, hyperthermia, and an alert wide-eyed appearance

# CHAPTER 42

## Loss and Grief

42-1 A family is visiting the surviving two triplets. The third triplet died 2 days ago. Which of the following would indicate that the family had begun to grieve for the dead infant?
a. Referring to the two live infants as twins
b. Asking about the dead triplet's current status
c. Bringing in play clothes for all three infants
d. Referring to the dead infant in the past tense

42-2 A newborn in the NICU is dying as a result of massive infection. The parents speak to the neonatologist and know their son's prognosis. When the father sees his son, he says, "He looks just fine to me. I can't understand what all this is about." The nurse's initial assessment is:
a. The father is in denial
b. The physician did not give the parents a complete picture of their son's prognosis
c. The father is in the shock and numbness dimension of mourning
d. The father is avoiding facing the reality of his son's death

42-3 A newborn in the NICU is dying as a result of massive infection. The parents speak to the neonatologist and know their son's prognosis. When the father sees his son, he says, "He looks just fine to me. I can't understand what all this is about." An appropriate response by the nurse at this time might be:
a. "Didn't the doctor tell you about your son's problems?"
b. "This must be a difficult time for you. Tell me how you feel."
c. To ignore the statement
d. "You'll have to face up to the fact that he is going to die sooner or later."

42-4 A woman is diagnosed with having a stillborn. At first she appears stunned by the news, cries a little, and then she asks you to call her mother. The phase of bereavement that the woman is experiencing is called:
a. No phase of bereavement; it hasn't "hit" her yet
b. Shock and numbness
c. Searching and yearning
d. Disorganization

42-5 Which is the most appropriate phrase that can be said to bereaved parents?
a. "You have an angel in heaven."
b. "I understand how you must feel."
c. "You're young and can have other children."
d. "I'm sorry."

42-6 After giving birth to a stillborn baby, the woman turns to the nurse and says, "I just finished painting the baby's room. Do you think that caused my baby to die?" The nurse's best response to this woman is:
a. "That's an old wives' tale; lots of women are around paint during pregnancy, and this doesn't happen to them."
b. "Maybe."
c. Silence
d. "I can understand your need to find an answer to what caused this. What else are you thinking about?"

42-7 When should the nurse offer a tissue to a crying mother who has just given birth to a stillborn baby?
a. When she asks for one
b. As soon as she starts crying
c. When she starts to look for a tissue
d. A nurse should never offer a tissue to a crying client

42-8 How many times should a family be offered the options for their memories of saying good-bye?
a. Only once
b. Twice
c. Three times
d. If they say no, they should not be asked again

42-9 What options for saying good-bye would the nurse want to discuss with a woman who is diagnosed with having a stillborn girl?
a. The nurse shouldn't discuss any options at this time; there is plenty of time after the baby is born.
b. "Would you like a picture taken of your baby after birth?"
c. "When your baby is born, would you like to see and hold her?"
d. "What funeral home do you want notified after the baby is born?"

42-10 A woman experienced a miscarriage at 10 weeks' gestation and had a dilation and curettage (D&C). She states that she is just fine and wants to go home as soon as possible. When assessing her responses to her loss, she tells you that she had purchased some baby things and had picked out a name. Based on your assessment of her responses, what nursing intervention would you do for her first?
a. Ready her for discharge.
b. Notify pastoral care to offer her a blessing.
c. Ask her if she would like to see what was obtained from her D&C.
d. Ask her what name she had picked out for her baby.

# Test Bank Answer Key

## CHAPTER 1

1-1. a
1-2. b
1-3. c
1-4. a
1-5. d
1-6. c
1-7. b
1-8. d
1-9. c
1-10. c
1-11. d

## CHAPTER 2

2-1. a
2-2. d
2-3. c
2-4. b
2-5. b
2-6. a
2-7. c
2-8. d
2-9. c
2-10. b

## CHAPTER 3

3-1. d
3-2. b
3-3. a
3-4. b
3-5. c
3-6. c
3-7. a
3-8. d
3-9. b
3-10. d
3-11. c

## CHAPTER 4

4-1. c
4-2. b
4-3. d
4-4. c
4-5. b

## CHAPTER 5

5-1. a
5-2. d
5-3. c
5-4. b
5-5. c
5-6. b
5-7. d

## CHAPTER 6

6-1. d
6-2. a
6-3. c
6-4. d
6-5. a
6-6. c
6-7. a
6-8. c
6-9. b
6-10. b
6-11. d
6-12. c
6-13. b
6-14. d
6-15. a
6-16. b
6-17. c
6-18. b

## CHAPTER 7

7-1. a
7-2. d
7-3. a
7-4. a
7-5. d
7-6. b
7-7. a
7-8. c
7-9. c
7-10. b
7-11. d
7-12. b

## CHAPTER 8

8-1. d
8-2. a
8-3. c
8-4. a
8-5. b
8-6. a
8-7. c
8-8. d
8-9. c
8-10. b
8-11. a
8-12. d

# CHAPTER 9

9-1. a
9-2. d
9-3. b
9-4. c
9-5. b
9-6. b
9-7. c
9-8. c
9-9. d
9-10. a
9-11. a
9-12. b
9-13. d
9-14. d
9-15. a

# CHAPTER 10

10-1. b
10-2. a
10-3. d
10-4. b
10-5. c
10-6. b
10-7. c

# CHAPTER 11

11-1. a
11-2. c
11-3. b
11-4. a
11-5. d
11-6. b
11-7. c
11-8. b
11-9. a
11-10. d

# CHAPTER 12

12-1. c
12-2. d
12-3. c
12-4. d
12-5. b
12-6. d
12-7. a
12-8. b

# CHAPTER 13

13-1. b
13-2. a
13-3. d
13-4. b
13-5. b
13-6. a
13-7. c
13-8. a
13-9. d

# CHAPTER 14

14-1. c
14-2. b
14-3. c
14-4. a
14-5. b
14-6. c
14-7. a
14-8. a
14-9. b
14-10. c

# CHAPTER 15

15-1. b
15-2. c
15-3. d
15-4. a
15-5. b
15-6. b
15-7. a
15-8. b
15-9. d
15-10. b

# CHAPTER 16

16-1. d
16-2. c
16-3. a
16-4. d
16-5. b
16-6. a
16-7. b
16-8. d
16-9. c
16-10. d

# CHAPTER 17

17-1. b
17-2. c
17-3. b
17-4. a
17-5. d
17-6. c
17-7. b
17-8. b
17-9. a
17-10. b
17-11. b
17-12. d
17-13. b
17-14. d
17-15. a
17-16. b
17-17. d
17-18. c
17-19. b
17-20. a
17-21. b
17-22. d

# CHAPTER 18

18-1. a
18-2. b
18-3. c
18-4. d
18-5. a
18-6. c

18-7. c
18-8. a

# CHAPTER 19

19-1. d
19-2. c
19-3. c
19-4. b
19-5. a
19-6. c
19-7. d
19-8. a
19-9. d
19-10. a

# CHAPTER 20

20-1. d
20-2. d
20-3. a
20-4. a
20-5. a
20-6. c
20-7. c
20-8. b
20-9. b
20-10. d
20-11. a

# CHAPTER 21

21-1. a
21-2. c
21-3. d
21-4. a
21-5. a
21-6. b
21-7. c
21-8. a
21-9. c
21-10. a
21-11. d

# CHAPTER 22

22-1. c
22-2. c
22-3. d
22-4. b
22-5. a
22-6. c
22-7. c
22-8. a
22-9. d
22-10. d
22-11. a
22-12. b
22-13. c
22-14. b
22-15. a
22-16. d
22-17. a
22-18. a
22-19. b
22-20. a
22-21. b

# CHAPTER 23

23-1. a
23-2. d
23-3. b
23-4. d
23-5. c
23-6. c
23-7. b
23-8. c
23-9. d
23-10. a

# CHAPTER 24

24-1. c
24-2. d
24-3. d
24-4. a
24-5. b
24-6. d
24-7. d

24-8. a
24-9. a
24-10. d
24-11. c
24-12. a

# CHAPTER 25

25-1. d
25-2. d
25-3. b
25-4. b
25-5. c
25-6. a
25-7. b
25-8. c
25-9. a
25-10. d
25-11. a

# CHAPTER 26

26-1. b
26-2. a
26-3. c
26-4. c
26-5. b
26-6. d
26-7. c
26-8. a
26-9. d
26-10. b
26-11. b
26-12. d
26-13. c

# CHAPTER 27

27-1. c
27-2. b
27-3. c
27-4. c
27-5. a
27-6. a
27-7. c

27-8. d
27-9. c
27-10. d
27-11. a

## CHAPTER 28

28-1. b
28-2. b
28-3. a
28-4. a
28-5. b
28-6. d
28-7. c
28-8. c
28-9. a
28-10. c

## CHAPTER 29

29-1. d
29-2. a
29-3. b
29-4. a
29-5. b
29-6. c
29-7. d
29-8. d
29-9. d
29-10. c
29-11. b

## CHAPTER 30

30-1. c
30-2. c
30-3. d
30-4. d
30-5. c
30-6. a
30-7. d
30-8. c
30-9. b

## CHAPTER 31

31-1. c
31-2. b
31-3. b
31-4. b
31-5. b
31-6. a
31-7. c

## CHAPTER 32

32-1. a
32-2. b
32-3. d
32-4. c
32-5. a
32-6. d
32-7. a
32-8. b
32-9. b

## CHAPTER 33

33-1. d
33-2. a
33-3. b
33-4. c
33-5. c
33-6. c
33-7. c
33-8. d
33-9. d

## CHAPTER 34

34-1. b
34-2. a
34-3. b
34-4. a
34-5. d
34-6. a
34-7. c
34-8. d
34-9. c

## CHAPTER 35

35-1. d
35-2. a
35-3. c
35-4. a
35-5. d
35-6. b
35-7. a
35-8. a

## CHAPTER 36

36-1. a
36-2. c
36-3. b
36-4. d
36-5. a
36-6. d

## CHAPTER 37

37-1. c
37-2. d
37-3. c
37-4. a
37-5. b
37-6. d
37-7. a
37-8. c

## CHAPTER 38

38-1. a
38-2. b
38-3. a
38-4. a
38-5. b
38-6. c
38-7. d
38-8. c
38-9. d
38-10. b

# CHAPTER 39

39-1. d
39-2. a
39-3. b
39-4. c
39-5. c
39-6. d
39-7. a
39-8. a
39-9. c

# CHAPTER 40

40-1. d
40-2. d
40-3. b
40-4. a
40-5. a
40-6. d
40-7. b

# CHAPTER 41

41-1. c
41-2. a
41-3. d
41-4. a
41-5. b
41-6. d
41-7. c
41-8. b
41-9. d
41-10. a
41-11. b
41-12. b
41-13. c
41-14. a

# CHAPTER 42

42-1. d
42-2. a
42-3. b
42-4. b
42-5. d
42-6. d
42-7. c
42-8. c
42-9. c
42-10. d